Emerging Technologies in Renal Stone Management

Editors

OJAS SHAH
BRIAN R. MATLAGA

UROLOGIC CLINICS
OF NORTH AMERICA

www.urologic.theclinics.com

Consulting Editor
SAMIR S. TANEJA

May 2019 • Volume 46 • Number 2

ELSEVIER

1600 John F. Kennedy Boulevard • Suite 1800 • Philadelphia, Pennsylvania, 19103-2899

http://www.theclinics.com

UROLOGIC CLINICS OF NORTH AMERICA Volume 46, Number 2
May 2019 ISSN 0094-0143, ISBN-13: 978-0-323-67864-3

Editor: Kerry Holland
Developmental Editor: Laura Kavanaugh

Urologic Clinics of North America (ISSN 0094-0143) is published quarterly by Elsevier Inc., 360 Park Avenue South, New York, NY 10010-1710. Months of issue are February, May, August, and November. Business and Editorial Offices: 1600 John F. Kennedy Blvd., Suite 1800, Philadelphia, PA 19103-2899. Periodicals postage paid at New York, NY and additional mailing offices. Subscription prices are $387.00 per year (US individuals), $757.00 per year (US institutions), $100.00 per year (US students and residents), $450.00 per year (Canadian individuals), $946.00 per year (Canadian institutions), $520.00 per year (foreign individuals), $946.00 per year (foreign institutions), and $240.00 per year (Canadian and foreign students/residents). Foreign air speed delivery is included in all *Clinics* subscription prices. All prices are subject to change without notice. **POSTMASTER:** Send address changes to *Urologic Clinics of North America*, Elsevier Health Sciences Division, Subscription Customer Service, 3251 Riverport Lane, Maryland Heights, MO 63043. **Customer Service: 1-800-654-2452 (US). From outside the United States, call 1-314-447-8871. Fax: 1-314-447-8029. E-mail: JournalsCustomerServiceusa@elsevier.com (for print support)** and **JournalsOnlineSupport-usa@elsevier.com (for online support)**.

Reprints. For copies of 100 or more, of articles in this publication, please contact the Commercial Reprints Department, Elsevier Inc., 360 Park Avenue South, New York, New York 10010-1710. Tel.: 212-633-3874; Fax: 212-633-3820; E-mail: reprints@elsevier.com.

Urologic Clinics of North America is covered in MEDLINE/PubMed (*Index Medicus*), *Excerpta Medica, Current Contents/Clinical Medicine, Science Citation Index,* and *ISI/BIOMED*.

Contributors

CONSULTING EDITOR

SAMIR S. TANEJA, MD
The James M. Neissa and Janet Riha Neissa
Professor of Urologic Oncology, Professor of
Urology and Radiology, Director, Division of
Urologic Oncology, Vice Chair, Department of
Urology, NYU Langone Medical Center, New
York, New York, USA

EDITORS

OJAS SHAH, MD
George F. Cahill Professor of Urology, Director,
Division of Endourology and Stone Disease,
Professor and Director of Endourology,
Department of Urology, Columbia University
Irving Medical Center, New York Presbyterian
Hospital, New York, New York, USA

BRIAN R. MATLAGA, MD, MPH
The Stephens Professor of Urology, Director,
The Stephens Center for Stone Disease,
James Buchanan Brady Urological Institute,
Department of Urology, Johns Hopkins
University School of Medicine, Baltimore,
Maryland, USA

AUTHORS

ALI H. ALDOUKHI, MBBS, MS
Research Fellow, Department of Urology,
University of Michigan, Medical Sciences
Unit I, Ann Arbor, Michigan, USA

MICHAEL R. BAILEY, PhD, MS
Adjunct Associate Professor, Department of
Urology, University of Washington School of
Medicine; Senior Principal Engineer, Center
for Industrial and Medical Ultrasound, Applied
Physics Laboratory; Associate Professor,
Department of Mechanical Engineering,
University of Washington, Seattle,
Washington, USA

D. DUANE BALDWIN, MD
Department of Urology, Loma Linda University
Health, Loma Linda University Medical
Center, Loma Linda, California, USA

DAVID B. BAYNE, MD, MPH
Fellow in Endourology, Urology,
University of California San Francisco,
San Francisco, California, USA

KRISTIAN M. BLACK, BS
MD Student, Department of Urology,
University of Michigan, Medical
Sciences Unit I, Ann Arbor, Michigan,
USA

MICHAEL S. BOROFSKY, MD
Department of Urology, University of
Minnesota, Minneapolis, Minnesota,
USA

BEN H. CHEW, MD, MSC
Department of Urologic Sciences,
Vancouver, British Columbia, Canada

THOMAS L. CHI, MD
Associate Professor, Urology, University
of California San Francisco, San Francisco,
California, USA

JESSICA C. DAI, MD
Resident, Department of Urology, University of
Washington School of Medicine, University of
Washington, Seattle, Washington, USA

VINCENT DE CONINCK, MD, FEBU
Service d'Urologie, Sorbonne Université, Assistance-Publique Hôpitaux de Paris, Hôpital Tenon, GRC no. 20, Groupe de Recherche Clinique sur la Lithiase Urinaire, Paris, France; Department of Urology, AZ Klina, Brasschaat, Belgium

BRIAN H. EISNER, MD
Department of Urology, Massachusetts General Hospital, Boston, Massachusetts, USA

CONNOR FORBES, MD
Department of Urologic Sciences, Vancouver, British Columbia, Canada

KHURSHID R. GHANI, MBChB, MS, FRCS
Associate Professor, Department of Urology, University of Michigan, Ann Arbor, Michigan, USA

GUIDO GIUSTI, MD
Department of Urology, IRCCS San Raffaele Hospital, Ville Turro Division, Milan, Italy

MOHAMMAD HAJIHA, MD
Department of Urology, Loma Linda University Health, Loma Linda University Medical Center, Loma Linda, California, USA

JONATHAN D. HARPER, MD
Associate Professor, Chief of Endourology and Minimally Invasive Surgery, Department of Urology, University of Washington School of Medicine, University of Washington, Seattle, Washington, USA

KELLY A. HEALY, MD, FACS
Assistant Professor, Department of Urology, Columbia University Medical Center, New York Presbyterian Hospital, New York, New York, USA

ETIENNE XAVIER KELLER, MD, FEBU
Service d'Urologie, Sorbonne Université, Assistance-Publique Hôpitaux de Paris, Hôpital Tenon, GRC no. 20, Groupe de Recherche Clinique sur la Lithiase Urinaire, Paris, France; Department of Urology, University Hospital Zurich, University of Zurich, Zurich, Switzerland

SARI S. KHALEEL, MD, MS
Department of Urology, University of Minnesota, Minneapolis, Minnesota, USA

BODO E. KNUDSEN, MD, FRCSC
Henry A. Wise II Endowed Chair in Urology, Department of Urology; Director, OSU Comprehensive Kidney Stone Program; Associate Professor, The Ohio State University Wexner Medical Center, Columbus, Ohio, USA

KEVIN KOO, MD, MPH, MPhil
Department of Urology, Johns Hopkins University School of Medicine, Baltimore, Maryland, USA

AMY E. KRAMBECK, MD
Michael O. Koch Professor, Department of Urology, Indiana University, Methodist Hospital, Indianapolis, Indiana, USA

DIRK LANGE, PhD
Department of Urologic Sciences, Vancouver, British Columbia, Canada

TIM LARGE, MD
Endourology Fellow, Department of Urology, Indiana University, Methodist Hospital, Indianapolis, Indiana, USA

MICHAEL E. LIPKIN, MD, MBA
Division of Urologic Surgery, Duke University Medical Center, Durham, North Carolina, USA

BRIAN R. MATLAGA, MD, MPH
The Stephens Professor of Urology, Director, The Stephens Center for Stone Disease, James Buchanan Brady Urological Institute, Department of Urology, Johns Hopkins University School of Medicine, Baltimore, Maryland, USA

BROOKE MOORE, BA
Department of Urology, Massachusetts General Hospital, Boston, Massachusetts, USA

SILVIA PROIETTI, MD
Department of Urology, IRCCS San Raffaele Hospital, Ville Turro Division, Milan, Italy

KYMORA B. SCOTLAND, MD, PhD
Department of Urologic Sciences, Vancouver, British Columbia, Canada

MICHELLE JO SEMINS, MD
Assistant Professor, Department of Urology,
University of Pittsburgh Medical Center,
Pittsburgh, Pennsylvania, USA

OJAS SHAH, MD
George F. Cahill Professor of Urology, Director,
Division of Endourology and Stone Disease,
Professor and Director of Endourology,
Department of Urology, Columbia University
Irving Medical Center, New York Presbyterian
Hospital, New York, New York, USA

ALEXANDER C. SMALL, MD
Urology Resident, Department of Urology,
Columbia University Medical Center, New York
Presbyterian Hospital, New York, New York,
USA

MATHEW D. SORENSEN, MD, MS, FACS
Associate Professor, Residency Director,
Department of Urology, University of
Washington School of Medicine, University of
Washington, Puget Sound Veterans Affairs
Hospital, Seattle, Washington, USA

SAMANTHA L. THOROGOOD, BA
Medical Student, Department of Urology,
Columbia University Medical Center, New York
Presbyterian Hospital, New York, New York,
USA

OLIVIER TRAXER, MD
Service d'Urologie, Sorbonne Université,
Assistance-Publique Hôpitaux de Paris,
Hôpital Tenon, GRC no. 20, Groupe de
Recherche Clinique sur la Lithiase Urinaire,
Paris, France

DANIEL A. WOLLIN, MD
Division of Urologic Surgery, Duke University
Medical Center, Durham, North Carolina, USA;
Division of Urologic Surgery, VA Boston
Healthcare System, West Roxbury,
Massachusetts, USA

TODD SAMUEL YECIES, MD
Resident Physician, Department of Urology,
University of Pittsburgh Medical Center,
Pittsburgh, Pennsylvania, USA

Contents

resistance to fracture with bending, and tip configuration are all important factors that contribute to a fiber's overall performance. Understanding these characteristics assists the end user with proper fiber selection for procedures.

Next-generation holmium laser systems provide the user with a range of parameters that can help optimize fragmentation efficiency. Ureteroscopic strategies broadly consist of fragmentation with active retrieval, or dusting, which uses low pulse energy settings to break stones into fine fragments for spontaneous passage. Techniques for dusting include dancing, chipping, and popcorning. The Moses technology is a multipulse mode that may help reduce retropulsion and increase fragmentation. The thulium fiber laser is an emerging laser technology that provides an extensive parameter range for dusting. Future studies are needed to define the role of these technologies and techniques for laser lithotripsy.

Percutaneous nephrolithotomy is the treatment of choice for large renal stones. Larger, straight access tracts allow for use of rigid pneumatic and ultrasonic lithotripsy devices. Through advanced technologies, more efficient fragmentation has become possible, allowing for a variety of treatment options depending on stone location, size, and composition. As novel methods of lithotripsy enter the clinical sphere, it is a requirement that the operating urologist understand the available surgical options and the associated mechanisms used to best treat their patients. This article discusses the mechanisms of basic pneumatic and ultrasonic devices, and examines the data regarding current and novel combination lithotrites.

This comprehensive review updates the advances in extracorporeal lithotripsy, including improvements in external shockwave lithotripsy and innovations in ultrasound based lithotripsy, such as burst wave lithotripsy, ultrasonic propulsion, and histotripsy. Advances in endoscopic technology and training have changed the surgical approach to nephrolithiasis; however, improvements and innovations in extracorporeal lithotripsy maintain its status as an excellent option in appropriately selected patients.

 Video content accompanies this article at http://www.urologic.theclinics.com.

Although advances in percutaneous nephrolithotomy have occurred, the initial renal access remains a challenging and high-risk step. This risk and technical difficulty have resulted in a minority of urologists obtaining their own access. Therefore, continued innovation in access techniques that simplify the procedure, lower risk, and reduce radiation exposure is needed. This article provides a high-level overview of recent advances in percutaneous renal access. The techniques are organized based on approach (antegrade or retrograde) and the imaging modality used, such as fluoroscopy, ultrasonography, computed tomography, and other novel techniques (laser, electromagnetic, and robotics).

phantom, animal, and human studies are reviewed herein. New developments in these rapidly growing areas of ultrasound research are also highlighted.

Nephrolithiasis is an increasingly common condition worldwide and mobile technology is revolutionizing how patients with kidney stone are being diagnosed and managed. Emerging platforms include software applications to increase adherence to stone prevention, mobile compatible hardware, online social media communities, and telemedicine. Applications and hardware specifically relevant to increasing hydration, diet modification, medication adherence, and rapid diagnosis (ie, mobile ultrasound and endoscopy) have the greatest potential to reduce stone recurrence and expedite treatment. Social media and online communities have also been rapidly adopted by patients and providers to promote education and support.

Diagnosis, treatment, and follow-up are all influential in determining the overall cost to the health care system for kidney stones. New innovations in the field of nephrolithiasis have been abundant, including disposable ureteroscopes, ultrasound-guided approaches to percutaneous nephrolithotomy, and advanced laser lithotripters. Identifying cost-effective treatment strategies encourages practitioners to be thoughtful about providing value-based high-quality care and remains on important principle in the treatment of urinary stone disease.

UROLOGIC CLINICS OF NORTH AMERICA

Foreword

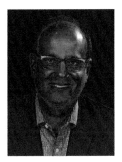

Samir S. Taneja, MD
Consulting Editor

Stone disease is truly the "bread and butter" of global Urology. Not only does it serve as an essential component of the history of our specialty but also one could consider it the very nidus that lamellated into the expansive field in which we now practice. Prior to being physicians, urologists evolved from barbers who would travel the countryside offering haircuts and bladder stone removals. We have, fortunately, moved on from the time that stones were blindly extracted by traveling barbers, through the urethra or a perineal stab incision, resulting in mortality in more than half the patients due to bleeding or sepsis. Stone management now employs, arguably, the most sophisticated technological tools and innovative strategies in all of Urology.

The management of urinary stone disease has become a perfect fusion of science, technology, and surgical expertise. The understanding of the biological basis of stone formation, the advances in medical management of stone prevention, the development of elegant tools to address every problem incurred, and the specialized expertise of the stone surgeon have elevated the level of care from simple stone extraction to an elegant individualized management strategy. Unlike other areas of urologic specialization, regardless of the degree of expertise and artistry achieved by the specialized endourologist, stone surgery remains a staple of daily practice for most American urologists, creating a demand that they continue to elevate their skill set as well.

In this issue of the *Urologic Clinics*, the editors have focused the articles on describing what the future of this highly evolved field may hold. In doing so, they provide not only a comprehensive review of the current "state-of-the-art" but also a glimpse into what the practicing urologist should anticipate down the road. In this regard, I would expect this issue would be of great value to every practicing urologist and urology trainees. I am indebted the guest editors and all the authors for providing us with such a valuable resource.

Samir S. Taneja, MD
Department of Urology
NYU Langone Health
222 East 41st Street, 12th Floor
New York, NY 10017, USA

E-mail address:
samir.taneja@nyumc.org

Urol Clin N Am 46 (2019) xiii
https://doi.org/10.1016/j.ucl.2019.03.002
0094-0143/19/© 2019 Published by Elsevier Inc.

Preface
A Vision of the Future of Stone Management

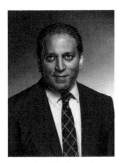
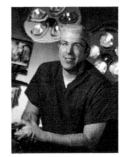

Ojas Shah, MD   Brian R. Matlaga, MD, MPH
Editors

In recent years, we have seen tremendous advances in the management of patients suffering from urinary stone disease. For example, ureteroscopy has moved from a procedure that had limited efficacy for complex stone burdens to the most commonly performed procedure for stones at any location in the collecting system. Similarly, percutaneous nephrolithotomy has evolved from a morbid intervention associated with high complication rates and prolonged hospitalization to an efficient stone removal approach that can claim excellent clinical outcomes. Certainly, there was an evolution of surgical technique that was a driver of these advances in stone management. However, at the same time, the surgical technology integral to those procedures was also advancing at a great rate. These synergistic advances in surgical technique and technology have combined to provide a meaningful improvement in the care our patients receive.

In this issue of the *Urologic Clinics of North America*, we endeavor to provide you with a vision of what the future of stone management may hold. In particular, our goal is to give a broad exposure to emerging technologies that will impact how we treat our patients in the coming years. To that end, many of our contributing authors focus on advances in the field of surgical stone management. These articles address advances in endoscope platforms, lithotripsy approaches, and stone manipulation, as well as factors fundamental to surgical approaches, such as percutaneous access and ureteral stent drainage.

However, we also wish to provide a view of where the field of stone management is moving outside of the operating room as well. From a diagnostic standpoint, advances in imaging technologies, such as computed tomography and ultrasonography, as well as maneuvers to mitigate radiation exposure, will affect how we evaluate our patients. As the world we live in is becoming ever more interconnected with mobile technologies, these, too, will have a role to play in our approach to patient management. And, finally, given the increasing economic pressures that are being applied to the health care system, an understanding of what the future of cost-effectiveness in stone management will look like is particularly important.

Taken all together, we hope that this issue of the *Urologic Clinics* will provide you with an interesting and enjoyable education on the future technologies of stone management.

Ojas Shah, MD
Division of Endourology and Stone Disease
Department of Urology
Columbia University Irving Medical Center
161 Fort Washington Avenue, 11th Floor
New York, NY 10032, USA

Brian R. Matlaga, MD, MPH
The Stephens Center for Stone Disease
James Buchanan Brady Urological Institute
Johns Hopkins Medicine
600 North Wolfe Street
Baltimore, MD 21287, USA

E-mail addresses:
os2302@cumc.columbia.edu (O. Shah)
bmatlaga@jhmi.edu (B.R. Matlaga)

Urol Clin N Am 46 (2019) xv
https://doi.org/10.1016/j.ucl.2019.03.001
0094-0143/19/© 2019 Published by Elsevier Inc.

urologic.theclinics.com

Next-Generation Fiberoptic and Digital Ureteroscopes

Etienne Xavier Keller, MD, FEBU[a,b,1],
Vincent De Coninck, MD, FEBU[a,c,1], Olivier Traxer, MD[a,*]

KEYWORDS

- Ureteroscopy • Irrigation • Pressure • Temperature • Deflection • Robotics • Ergonomics
- Single use

KEY POINTS

- Major technological innovations in ureteroscopy include, but are not limited to, bundled optical fibers for flexible image transmission, rod lens design for enhanced image quality, active tip deflection, and integration of miniaturized digital image sensors.
- Efficacy of ureteroscopy may be improved by warranting constant clear vision. Visibility is intimately related to irrigation flow, which in turn is affected by the size of instruments and working channels.
- Robot-assisted multiple-axis tip defection may present as a solution for full range of motion of ureteroscopes in order to warrant unhindered access to all renal cavities.
- Safety of ureteroscopy might be improved by the integration of pressure and temperature control.
- Single-use instruments might vanish concerns about sterility and availability of reusable ureteroscopes.

INTRODUCTION

Ureteroscopy is a widely adopted operation technique for upper urinary tract disorders. Its current efficacy and safety profile originate from a history of tremendous, continuous, and rapid technological innovations. This article presents an overview of emerging technologies and current innovations that may define next-generation ureteroscopes. Understanding the principles that define current ureteroscopy is key to establishing the directions of future developments. Therefore, each topic is introduced by a brief summary of current achievements and limitations, before proposing potential solutions.

FROM PAST TO PRESENT

A chronologic summary of the most important past achievements and innovations relating to ureteroscopes is presented in **Table 1**.[1–15] Awareness about these developments is essential to defining next-generation ureteroscopes.

Disclosure: Dr O. Traxer is a consultant for Coloplast, Rocamed, Olympus, EMS, Boston Scientific, and IPG.
Funding support: Dr E.X. Keller is supported by a travel grant from the University Hospital Switzerland and by a grant from the Kurt and Senta Herrmann Foundation, Liechtenstein. Dr V. De Coninck is supported by a European Urological Scholarship Programme scholarship from the European Association of Urology and by a grant from the Belgische Vereniging voor Urologie (BVU).
[a] Service d'Urologie, Sorbonne Université, Assistance-Publique Hôpitaux de Paris, Hôpital Tenon, GRC n°20, Groupe de Recherche Clinique sur la Lithiase Urinaire, 4 rue de la Chine, Paris 75020, France; [b] Department of Urology, University Hospital Zurich, Zurich, Switzerland; [c] Department of Urology, AZ Klina, Brasschaat, Belgium
[1] These authors contributed equally.
* Corresponding author. Sorbonne Université, Service d'Urologie, Assistance-Publique Hôpitaux de Paris, Hôpital Tenon, 4 rue de la Chine, Paris 75020, France.
E-mail address: olivier.traxer@aphp.fr

Urol Clin N Am 46 (2019) 147–163
https://doi.org/10.1016/j.ucl.2018.12.001

Table 1
Past achievements and innovations relating to ureteroscopes

Authors, Year	Origin	Achievement or Innovation	Details on Material	Details on Technique
Young et al,[1] 1912 (reported 1929)	United States	First ureteroscopy	9.5-Fr pediatric cystoscope	Inadvertent visualization of the ureter and renal pelvis
Hopkins,[2] 1954	United Kingdom	Bundled optical fibers	A bundle of glass fibers transmits optical images along a flexible axis	Birth of flexible endoscopy
Hopkins,[3] 1959	United Kingdom	Rod lens design	Air lenses are interposed between a series of cylindrical (rod) glass lenses	Substantially enhanced image quality and 4× higher light transmission
Marshall,[4] 1960	United States	First flexible ureteroscopy	9-Fr fiberoptic ureteroscope, passive deflection, no working channel	Only diagnostic, not therapeutic
Storz,[3] 1960	Germany	Cold light source	An external light source transmits very bright light through a fiberoptic cable	Solved the previous problem of fragile and heat-generating electric bulbs at the tips of endoscopes
Hopkins,[3] 1961	United Kingdom	Antireflective coating of glass lenses	Coating supporting light to exit lenses instead of being reflected back in the lens	80× higher light transmission
Storz,[3] 1967	Germany	Commercialization of rod lens cystoscopes	Fully operational cystoscope including a cold light source	—
Takagi et al,[5] 1968	Japan	First flexible ureteroscopy with active deflection	No working channel	Only diagnostic, not therapeutic
Goodman,[6] 1977; Lyon et al,[7] 1978	United States	First therapeutic ureteroscopy (fulguration of ureteral tumors)	12–16-Fr dilators, 11-Fr pediatric cystoscope, and 14-Fr resectoscope	Limited to the lower ureter

Teichmann[8] 1979	Germany	First intraureteral lithotripsy	Electrohydraulic and ultrasonic lithotripters	Limited to the lower ureter
Lyon et al,[9] 1979	United States	First ureteroscopic extraction of urinary stones	10–16-Fr dilators, 13-Fr pediatric cystoscope, 14.5-Fr resectoscope, and stone baskets	Limited to the lower ureter
Perez-Castro and Martinez-Pineiro,[10,11] 1980–82	Spain	First therapeutic ureteroscopy including the renal pelvis	12-Fr rigid ureteroscope, 50-cm length, 4-Fr working channel, 0° and 70° rod lens optics	Therapeutic ureteroscopy of the whole upper urinary tract, except for lower pole calyces
Bagley,[12] 1987; Preminger,[13] 1987; Aso et al,[14] 1987	United States and Japan	First therapeutic, flexible ureteroscopy	6.5-Fr up to 13.5-Fr flexible scopes, passive or active deflection, 1.2-Fr up to 6-Fr working channel	Therapeutic flexible ureteroscopy with stone retrieval (basket or forceps)
Humphreys et al,[15] 2008	United States	First report of the clinical use of a digital ureteroscope	8.7-Fr flexible ureteroscope, digital image sensor at the tip, 3.6-Fr working channel, light-emitting diode illumination	—

FUTURE DIRECTIONS
Size Reduction

Anatomic considerations

Retrograde access to the kidney inherently implies the passing of instruments within the confinements of the ureter.[16] Although this path allows clinicians to guide instruments with ease toward the kidney, the ureter also represents a natural bottleneck that dictates the sizing of instruments used in ureteroscopy. Development of the endourologic armamentarium has therefore always integrated the necessity of miniaturizing components, with a particular dedication to the design of the tip of ureteroscopes.

Distal tip design

Several companies provide their ureteroscopes with a tapered tip, allowing a size reduction at the distal tip (**Table 2**) (**Fig. 1**A). Most ureteroscopes are round in cross section, although some companies have integrated the notion that the ureter is not merely a cylindrical tube but is a flaccid cavity that may accept any shape of instrument. This observation forms the rationale for providing oval instruments (**Fig. 1**B). This design may be advantageous for an optimal and compact orchestration of components within the scope and may also allow an improved accommodation of the ureteroscope to the angulations of the ureter.

Scope size

The distal tip of most flexible ureteroscopes is less than or equal to 9 Fr (see **Table 2**), which remarkably corresponds with the findings of a study based on CT-scan measurements, where the native ureteral diameter was less than or equal to 9 Fr in 96% of all patients.[17] Nevertheless, based on experience from daily practice, most of the currently available flexible ureteroscopes are too large to warrant primary access to the kidney in all patients. Further reducing the size of ureteroscopes would therefore lower the rate of ureteroscopic insertion failure, leading to higher single-session success rates.

Impact of scope size on irrigation flow

Size reduction of ureteroscopes is also key to improving a fundamental determinant for successful ureteroscopy: irrigation flow. To understand this counterintuitive assertion, the following should be recalled: an increase in irrigation inflow can be easily achieved (eg, irrigation hand pumps) but must be compensated for by an equal increase in irrigation outflow (**Fig. 2**A) to avoid hazardous increases in intrarenal pressure (**Fig. 2**B, E).[18–20] Most importantly, irrigation outflow is dictated by the free space left between the outer contours of the ureteroscope and the inner wall of the ureter. The use of a ureteral access sheath achieves an optimal patency of this free space and therefore achieves a significant improvement in irrigation outflow.[21–23] At a constant irrigation inflow, this decreases intrarenal pressure (**Fig. 2**D).[24] It is not safe to increase the size of ureteral access sheaths as a way to improve irrigation outflow, because large ureteral access sheaths entail the risk of serious ureteral wall damage.[25] Henceforth, the ureter must be considered as a fixed anatomic constraint where improved irrigation outflow (and therefore overall irrigation fluid turnover in the kidney) goes along with a size reduction of ureteroscopes (see **Fig. 2**C, F).

The necessity of an instrument size reduction as a way of improving irrigation flow becomes particularly valid considering the increasing enthusiasm for high-frequency stone lasering.[26,27] When large amounts of stone dust are produced, irrigation is key to maintaining uninterrupted clear visibility. This concept is also valid for conservative management of upper urinary tract tumors, where bleeding from laser vaporization may rapidly preclude visibility if irrigation flow is not sufficient.

Working channel size

With a few exceptions, the working channel size of currently available flexible ureteroscopes is 3.6 Fr (see **Table 2**). Arguably, reducing the working channel size represents a straightforward solution to allow an overall size reduction of ureteroscopes. Ureteroscopes with a smaller working channel should achieve equally good performance as conventional 3.6-Fr working channel ureteroscopes for stone and tumor treatment, since ancillary devices such as laser fibers or baskets are expected to become smaller in the years to come. The resulting cross-sectional size reduction of instruments occupying the working channel would therefore not impact on irrigation flow through the ureteroscope. The thulium fiber laser is currently being explored as an alternative to holmium:yttrium-aluminum-garnet (YAG) for lithotripsy.[28] This new laser offers the possibility of laser energy delivery through fibers as small as 50 μm, which is substantially smaller than the inferior size limit of fibers for holmium:YAG (≥200 μm).[29]

Pressure Control

Risks of high pressure

A growing body of evidence suggests high intrarenal pressure as a serious threat for patients undergoing ureteroscopy.[30–33] The underlying physiopathology is not fully understood, but high intrarenal pressure has been shown to lead to pyelovenous backflow, forniceal rupture, as well as

Table 2

Characteristics of currently available flexible ureteroscopes

Brand	Model	Type Fiberoptic	Type Digital	Tip Flat	Tip Tapered	Cross Section Round	Cross Section Oval	Scope Size (Fr) Tip	Scope Size (Fr) Shaft	Scope Size[a] (Fr)	Working Channel Position[a] 3 o'clock	Working Channel Position[a] 9 o'clock	Working Channel Position Additional Working Channel	Deflection Angulation[a] Upward/Downward (°)
Olympus	URF-P5	Yes	—	—	Yes	Yes	—	5.3	8.4	3.6	—	Yes	—	180/275
	URF-P6	Yes	—	—	Yes	Yes	—	4.9	7.95	3.6	—	Yes	—	275/275
	URF-P7	Yes	—	—	Yes	Yes	—	4.9	7.95	3.6	—	—	—	275/275
	URF-V	—	Yes	—	Yes	Yes	—	8.5	9.9	3.6	—	Yes	—	180/275
	URF-V2	—	Yes	—	Yes	Yes	—	8.5	8.4	3.6	—	Yes	—	275/275
	URF-V3	—	Yes	—	Yes	Yes	—	8.5	8.4	3.6	—	Yes	—	275/275
Storz	Flex X2/X2s	Yes	—	Yes	—	—	Yes	7.5	7.5	3.6	—	Yes	—	270/270
	Flex Xc	—	Yes	Yes	—	—	Yes	8.5	8.4	3.6	Yes	—	—	270/270
Wolf	Viper	Yes	—	—	Yes	Yes	—	6.0	8.8	3.6	Yes	—	—	270/270
	Boa vision	—	Yes	—	Yes	Yes	—	6.6	8.7	3.6	—	Yes	—	270/270
	Cobra	Yes	—	—	Yes	Yes	—	6.0	9.9	Twice 3.3	Yes	—	12 o'clock	270/270
	Cobra vision	—	Yes	—	Yes	Yes	—	5.2	9.9	2.4 and 3.3	—	Yes	6 o'clock	270/270
Boston Scientific	Lithovue	—	Yes	—	Yes	Yes	—	7.7	9.5	3.6	Yes	—	—	270/270
Pusen	Uscope	—	Yes	—	Yes	Yes	—	9.0	9.5	3.6	Yes	—	—	270/270
PolyScope	—	Yes	—	Yes	—	Yes	—	8	8	3.8	Yes	—	—	>250

[a] As given by manufacturer.

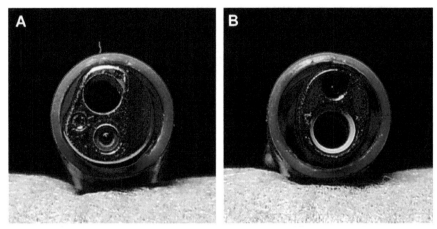

Fig. 1. Comparison of the shape of the distal tip. (*A*) Round and tapered tip (Olympus URF-V2). (*B*) Oval and flat tip. Both ureteroscopes were placed in a 10/12 ureteral access sheath (Coloplast Retrace) for demonstration purposes.

tubular and interstitial intrarenal backflow.[18] Normal intrarenal pressure usually ranges between approximately 0 and 10 cm H_2O.[34] Gross pyelovenous backflow becomes evident at more than 40 cm H_2O,[35] and forniceal rupture may occur at more than 80 cm H_2O, although this has not been verified in humans.[36] Ultimately, high intrarenal pressure has been associated with systemic

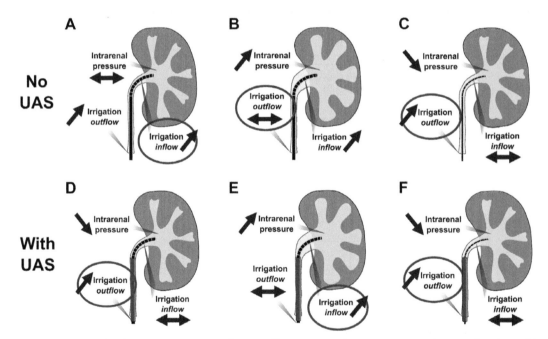

Fig. 2. The relationship between irrigation inflow, outflow, intrarenal pressure, ureteral access sheath, and instrument size. (*A*) Any inflow increase must be compensated by an equal outflow increase to maintain a stable intrarenal pressure. (*B*) If inflow is further increased (eg, to improve visibility) and outflow reaches its maximal transport capacity, then intrarenal pressure will increase. (*C*) At a constant inflow, a decrease in intrarenal pressure may be achieved by the use of a miniaturized ureteroscope, because this results in an increased outflow transport capacity. (*D*) Alternatively, at a constant irrigation inflow, a decrease in intrarenal pressure may be achieved by the use of a ureteral access sheath. (*E*) If inflow is further increased (eg, to improve visibility) and outflow reaches its maximal transport capacity, then intrarenal pressure will increase despite the use of a ureteral access sheath. (*F*) Again, at a constant inflow, a decrease in intrarenal pressure may be achieved by the use of a miniaturized ureteroscope, analogous to the scenario in (*C*). UAS, ureteral access sheath.

inflammatory response, septic shock, and even death.[37,38] The proposed mechanism is dissemination of pathogens by irrigation backflow.

Pressure control and irrigation flow

In order to prevent such complications, it seems necessary to integrate pressure control into ureteroscopy. To ensure low intrarenal pressure, clinicians may simply limit irrigation inflow pressure, which can easily be achieved by hanging irrigation bags such that the superior limit of saline solution is less than 40 cm H_2O higher than the level of the kidney. The drawback of this rudimental pressure control is that irrigation flow rate is substantially reduced whenever the working channel is occupied by auxiliary devices, as a direct consequence of pressure loss along the ureteroscope.[39] This reduction explains why irrigation pressure should be modulated in order to maintain sufficient irrigation flow.

Pressure sensor

A proposed solution for intrarenal pressure control is to place a pressure sensor within renal cavities during ureteroscopy. Such feedback control would permit continuous modulation of irrigation pressure or irrigation inflow rate (so-called pressure-controlled irrigation) (**Fig. 3**A). This concept has already been integrated in a sensor-equipped ureteral access sheath that additionally can control active irrigation suction, as a way of increasing irrigation outflow.[40] It seems straightforward that next-generation ureteroscopes will be equipped with similar pressure control sensors and will allow pressure-controlled irrigation. The benefit of such devices on operative time and complication rates remains to be established.

Pressure control as a limitation

In the short run, pressure-controlled irrigation may be seen as a future limitation to ureteroscopy, because it will result in an overall reduction of irrigation flow compared with contemporary (possibly excessive) habits of irrigation. This limitation is where size reduction of ureteroscopes will present all its advantages, as discussed earlier, and as has been shown in a study in which size reduction of semirigid ureteroscopes achieved an effective reduction of intrarenal pressure.[41]

The hazards of pressure-controlled irrigation systems

A serious hazard of pressure-controlled irrigation systems occurs whenever the urinary tract patency is disrupted (eg, forniceal rupture or ureteral wall perforation; **Fig. 3**B). In such cases, irrigation fluid may escape from intrarenal cavities toward the retroperitoneum, leading to a falsely negative feedback signal from the intrarenal pressure sensor, which may in turn result in hazardous excesses of irrigation inflow. This situation may result in unrecognized extravasation of a substantial amount of irrigation fluid (**Fig. 3**C).

Temperature Control

Heat generated by lasers

With increasing power range of newly marketed laser generators, concerns have arisen about the risks entailed by temperature dissipation during laser lithotripsy. In several in vitro studies, irrigation fluid temperature increase occurred within seconds after laser activation and reached plateau phases that mostly depended on irrigation flow rate and irrigation fluid temperature.[42–45] Damage to tissues (cell death) not only depends on maximal temperature increase but also depends on time of exposure to high temperature levels.[46] One in vitro study took into account this thermal-dose effect on tissue and found continuous laser activation for 60 seconds with low power settings (10 W) to be safe, even when no irrigation flow

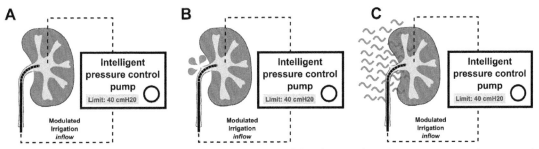

Fig. 3. The hazards of pressure-controlled irrigation systems. (*A*) As long as the urinary tract patency is conserved, the pump can reliably modulate irrigation inflow according to measured intrarenal pressure. (*B*) In case of disruption of urinary tract patency, irrigation fluid escapes to the retroperitoneum. The pump would then eventually try to compensate a falsely negative feedback signal from the intrarenal pressure sensor by hazardous increase in irrigation inflow. (*C*) This situation may result in unrecognized extravasation of a substantial amount of irrigation fluid.

was present.[43] At 20 W, a minimum irrigation flow of 7 to 8 mL/min (irrigation fluid at 23°C) was necessary to stay within a safe thermal-dose range. At 40 W, tissue theoretically has been put at risk of thermal damage, even if irrigation flow was increased to 14 to 15 mL/min.

Temperature sensor to control what?

To date, no reports of thermal tissue damage have been made in conjunction with temperature increase of irrigation fluid during laser lithotripsy in humans, unless laser was purposely fired in close proximity with tissue. This raises a question: should temperature control be recommended for ureteroscopy? Arguably, next-generation ureteroscopes integrating a temperature sensor at the tip of the instrument should be concievable. If so, which parameter would the measured intrarenal temperature affect and to what extent? Should a feedback control allow for deactivating the laser generator at a given temperature cutoff? Should this control irrigation flow as a way to cool down intrarenal cavities? Should this adapt the temperature of inflowing irrigation fluid? An element of response comes from the thermal dose effect theory, which should allow the calculation of a safe laser power range that could be used in conjunction with a given inflowing irrigation fluid temperature and flow rate. Future studies are warranted to verify the necessity and utility of intrarenal fluid temperature control during ureteroscopy.

Active Suction of Stone Dust

What is stone dust?

In recent years, there has been growing enthusiasm for dusting laser lithotripsy techniques among endourologists following the observation that stone dust is capable of spontaneously evacuating, which therefore removes the necessity of time-consuming stone fragment retrieval.[47] Nevertheless, no study available to date has precisely defined what should be considered to be stone dust. A consequence of this is that clinically significant residual fragments might be left in place after dusting lithotripsy.

Stone-free dusting

To ensure full clearance of all stone fragments after dusting lithotripsy, it would be desirable to develop a device or a technique capable of active suction of stone dust. The opening diameter of such an aspiration device should be in close relation with the size that would define stone dust. At the end of the procedure, active suction of stone dust would allow the identification of any remaining residual fragments that would be too large

and therefore be at risk of not evacuating spontaneously (**Fig. 4**). The authors propose this concept as a way of increasing stone-free rates after dusting lithotripsy. Nevertheless, active suction of stone dust through currently available ureteroscopes is not recommended, because clogging of stone dust within the working channel may occur and may cause instrument failure with the necessity of instrument repair. Next-generation ureteroscopes might overcome this limitation and allow safe active suction of stone dust.

Multiple-Axis Tip Deflection

One-plane deflection

Flexible ureteroscopes have been developed such that deflection is only be possible in 1 plane. The rationale for this design comes from the observation that rotation of the instrument's handle permits clinicians to orientate the tip of the scope in any other plane. Consequently, for a right-handed operator, posteriorly and anteriorly situated calyces in a right kidney can be visualized by a light supination (**Fig. 5**A) and extensive supination (**Fig. 5**B) of the ureteroscope, respectively. The opposite is true for the left kidney.

The complexity of renal cavities

The pyelocaliceal system is not to be thought of as a system with radiations (calyces) centered on a fixed point (pelvis). It must instead be understood as a central cavity (pelvis) with multiple sinusoidal radiations (infundibulum) ending on surfaces (calyces) that may adopt various orientations. This complexity explains why certain renal cavities are not amendable to some ureteroscopes. This finding has become particularly valid for digital scopes, which have been shown to have a decreased end-tip deflection compared with fiberoptic scopes,[48] which is caused by the bulky and rigid configuration of the digital camera unit at the tip of digital ureteroscopes. Nonetheless, it seems evident from daily practice that, in certain cases, some additional degree of deflection in another plane would have been key for treatment success. The ability of multiple-axis tip deflection therefore seems to be one of the greatest achievements that should be incorporated in next-generation flexible ureteroscopes.

Variable Working Channel Positions

Anatomic considerations

In line with the consideration outlined earlier, the success of a given ureteroscopic treatment is dictated by the interrelation between anatomy and proprieties of ureteroscopes. The invariable

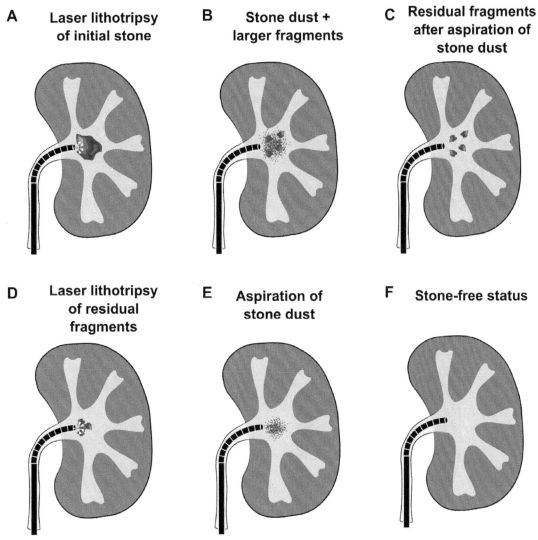

Fig. 4. Aspiration of stone dust. (*A*) Laser lithotripsy of the initial stone mass. (*B*) After a period of lithotripsy, a mixture of stone dust and larger fragments may be found. (*C*) After aspiration of stone dust, larger residual fragments become apparent. (*D*) These larger residual fragments can now selectively be addressed by laser lithotripsy. (*E*) Residual fragments are now rendered to stone dust. (*F*) Stone-free status can now be achieved by aspiration of stone dust.

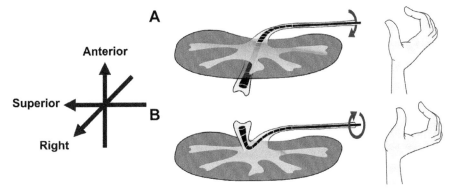

Fig. 5. Orienting the deflected scope in another plane. While the deflected scope is within a right-sided kidney, a light supination movement at the scope's handle gives access to posteriorly situated calyces (*A*), whereas an extensive supination gives access to anteriorly situated calyces (*B*).

configuration of the working channel at the tip of the scope remains a problem to be resolved in next-generation ureteroscopes. For treatment in a right-sided kidney, gravity typically displaces stones or stone fragments in a 3-o'clock position (**Fig. 6**A). This location is ideally accessible for accessory instruments inserted in scope with a working channel at about 3 o'clock (see **Table 2**). The opposite is true for a left-sided kidney, where scopes with a working channel at about 9 o'clock offer a better access (**Fig. 6**B). Implementation of the ability to vary the position of the working channel at the tip of the scope would therefore be a major future improvement.

Memory of the deflection axis
The earlier depicted concept of multiple-axis tip deflection may represent a viable solution for variable working channel positions; if next-generation ureteroscopes are able to memorize and maintain a given position, then a simple rotation of the scope's shaft would make the working channel rotate in the field of view without any change of the position of the deflectable tip within the kidney. This concept is reminiscent of robotic arms used in laparoscopy, where the needle driver can be rotated such that the position of the arm remains unchanged within the pneumoperitoneum (referred to as EndoWrist technology by Intuitive Surgical).

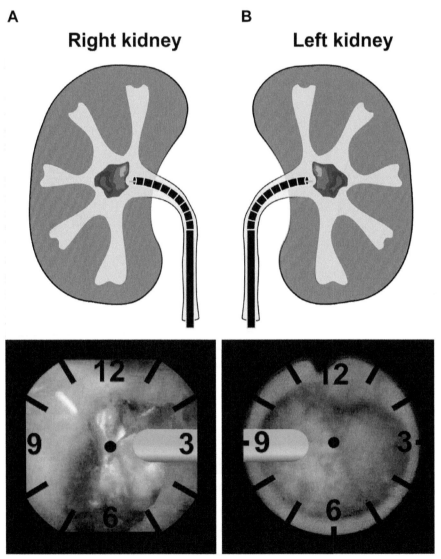

Fig. 6. The importance of the working channel position. Gravity typically displaces stones or stone fragments to a 3-o'clock position in a right-sided kidney (*A*). Stones are in a 9 o'clock position in a left-sided kidney (*B*). The respective position of the working channel for a given ureteroscope makes these stones most amenable to laser lithotripsy (blue laser fiber) in either one side or the other.

Robotics

Definition of a robot

A robot can be understood either as a device capable of autonomous or automated operability based on the interpretation of information captured by sensors or as a device that can mimic, assist, or augment the human hand's range of motion and skills. For ureteroscopy, the former can be rudimentarily exemplified by an irrigation device capable of intelligent control of intrarenal pressure.[40] The second definition of a robot corresponds with a device capable of influencing the motion and function of a ureteroscope based on tactile, visual, or auditive inputs emanating from a human being.

Limitations of current platforms

Two platforms have been developed for robot-assisted ureteroscopy: the Sensei-Magellan (Hansen Medical Inc, CA) and the Roboflex Avicenna (ELMED, Ankara, Turkey). The former was initially designed for angiographic purposes. The first report about its adaptation for robot-assisted ureteroscopy in humans was in 2008, but any further development of this platform has been discontinued.[49] The Roboflex Avicenna has been CE (Conformité Européene)-marketed in 2013, after having proved the feasibility and safety of robot-assisted ureteroscopy.[50–52] The operator sits at a console and steers 2 joysticks or a central wheel that enable deflection, rotation, insertion, and retraction of a ureteroscope. A touch screen and foot pedals additionally allow speed of movements to be changed and a laser fiber to be advanced, retracted, and activated. Improved operator comfort and reduced radiation exposition have been named as possible advantages compared with conventional ureteroscopy.[50] However, both Sensei-Magellan and Roboflex Avicenna platforms failed to offer any serious advantage in terms of maneuverability, because these platforms robotically steer the same ureteroscopes that can be manipulated manually. In expert hands, these robotic platforms may therefore even represent a disadvantage, because the tactile feedback of the scope is missing. Other limitations are the acquisition and maintenance costs, as well as the space requirements within operating facilities. These limitations may explain why robotic platforms for ureteroscopy have not yet been widely adopted by endourologists.

The robotic ureteroscope

Robotic next-generation ureteroscopes should offer greater advantages than conventional ureteroscopes. Most importantly, these should include an augmented range of motion of the deflectable tip. A scope capable of multiple-axis tip deflection, as proposed earlier, would perfectly exemplify robot-assisted ureteroscopy: the operator would navigate along the upper urinary tract by means of a handheld control that could be freely moved in space, then the positioning information would be transmitted to software that would transmit the calculated range of movement to the robotic ureteroscope. The robotic ureteroscope would then position itself in the intended position, as long as the range of motion of the multiple-axis tip deflection allows it. Such handheld controls should also ideally integrate haptics (force feedback) to prevent any hazards such as organ perforation or ureteral avulsion. Alternative or additional controls would be visual or auditive signals. A simple example of an auditive control would be to modulate irrigation flow by vocal orders to the robotic platform. A simple example of a visual control would be to activate narrow-band imaging (NBI) on a short period of rapid blink of the operator's eyes.

Enhanced Ergonomics

Looking in the eyepiece

The handle of a flexible ureteroscope is conventionally held by the dominant hand at the level of the thorax, with the operating shaft exiting on its lower part. The deflection mechanism is conventionally found at the upper part of the handle and is steered by the thumb.[53] This design originates from the historical necessity of the operator to visualize the image brought by optic fibers through the eyepiece at the top of the instrument's handle. Nowadays, the necessity to look directly into the eyepiece has been removed, because the image can be caught either by a camera fixed at the eyepiece of fiberoptic scopes or by an image sensor at the distal tip of digital scopes.[54] It thus seems surprising that the design of the handle of ureteroscopes has remained unchanged in recent decades, with one exception being the Poly-Scope, which is held like a syringe.[55]

Weight of ureteroscopes

Despite their similar construct design, the weight of currently available ureteroscopes varies greatly: 309 to 352 g (mean, 335 g) for fiberoptic ureteroscopes and 278 to 943 g (mean, 700 g) for digital ureteroscopes.[56] Another 266 to 798 g (mean, 447 g) is added to fiberoptic scopes when a camera head is attached to the eyepiece. These weight differences have been associated with decreased muscle activity in favor of lighter ureteroscopes.[57] Ultimately, reduced muscle strain may prevent fatigue of the operator and increase surgical productivity, as has been found in a study on ergonomic stance during laryngoscopy.[58] Although this ergonomics-related productivity advantage remains to be established for ureteroscopy, weight differences between scopes might represent part of the explanation of why digital ureteroscopes led to significantly shorter operative times in several clinical studies.[59–61]

In summary, the design and ergonomics of next-generation ureteroscopes could be completely rethought, particularly if robot-assisted ureteroscopy, as explained earlier, becomes available.

Image Quality

Optical image transmission

Apart from maneuverability characteristics, image quality is a key factor affecting the efficacy, safety, and versatility of ureteroscopy. The first major advance opening the path to flexible endoscopy was bundling of optical fibers between the distal tip and the proximal eyepiece.[2] This pivotal innovation, along with the rod lens construct found in rigid ureteroscopes, was introduced by Harold H. Hopkins.[3] Thin, flexible glass fibers were covered by a cladding with low refraction index, allowing light transmission over a long distance with minimal losses. For illumination purposes, light is transmitted noncoherently through fiber optics. For image capture, the bundle of glass fibers must be orchestrated coherently in order to produce an identical matrix of glass fibers at both ends of the instrument.

Electronic image sensors

The next pivotal innovation was electronic image sensors such as charge-coupled device (CCD) or complementary metal-oxide semiconductor (CMOS) sensors.[54] These sensors transform light (photons) into electron charges that create voltage-dependent signals captured by semiconductors. Each sensor is composed of an array of single photo units (pixels) capturing primary colors: red, green, and blue (RGB). After software processing, these pixels eventually produce a digital image. One of the greatest advantages of these image sensors is the possibility to transport images for distant projection (eg, on a liquid crystal display [LCD]). Miniaturization of image sensors has eventually allowed their integration at the tip of ureteroscopes, thus palliating any image quality losses conveyed by optical fibers. A parallel development was the replacement of optical fibers by light-emitting diodes (LEDs) for illumination purposes.

From fiberoptic to digital technology

The replacement of optical fibers by a few electronic cables within the shaft of digital ureteroscopes theoretically represents a space saving that could allow a size reduction of ureteroscopes. Nevertheless, the smallest currently available ureteroscope is based on fiberoptic technology (see **Table 2**). This apparent paradox is explained by the currently bulky design of the image sensor unit at the tip of currently available digital ureteroscopes, which has also been shown to cause significant loss of end deflection.[48]

Digital ureteroscopes achieve better image quality than fiberoptic ones.[62] This superiority may represent part of the reason why digital ureteroscopes achieved a significantly shorter operative time in several clinical studies.[59–61] As for detection of upper tract urothelial carcinoma, most investigators agree that digital ureteroscopes seem to achieve better tumor detection, although the potential benefits in terms of tumor recurrence rate and survival remain to be established.[63]

Next-generation ureteroscopes are likely to integrate ultraminiaturized digital image sensors with increasing image resolution, catching up with current display resolution standards such as full high definition (1920 × 1080 pixels) or 4k (4096 × 2160 pixels). The 1:1 ratio of images captured by current digital ureteroscopes might be changed to another format. Ultimately, whether fiberoptic ureteroscopes will present any residual advantages in future remains a question.

Enhanced Imaging Technology

Because upper tract urothelial carcinoma is amendable to ureteroscopic management, real-time image enhancement technologies have been integrated to ureteroscopes in pursuit of better tumor detection. These technologies include NBI, photodynamic diagnosis (PDD), and Image 1-S technology (formerly Storz Professional Image Enhancement System (SPIES)).

Narrow-band imaging

NBI was first conceived in 1999.[64] To understand its mode of operation, 3 basic principles have to be understood. First, the light source (usually a xenon lamp) is color filtered to illuminate tissues with only 2 bandwidths: 415 nm (blue-violet) and 540 nm (green). These 2 bandwidths correspond with 2 distinct absorption peaks of hemoglobin,[65] such that poorly vascularized tissues reflect a substantially higher proportion of the emitted narrow-band light compared with highly vascular tissue (**Fig. 7**A). Second, the reflected light is selectively recorded by a camera as follows: 415-nm bandwidth signals (blue-violet light) are assigned to the blue and green color channel; 540-nm bandwidth signals (green light) are assigned to the red color channel.[64] Consequently, the final image on an LCD display has a different color scheme than the light that is reflected by tissues. Third, the depth of light propagation in tissues is associated

A

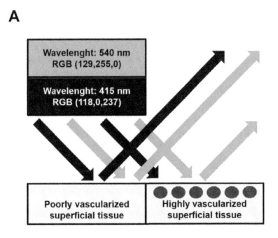

B

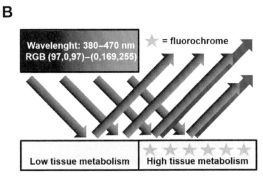

Fig. 7. NBI and PDD: illumination by color-filtered light sources. (*A*) For NBI, 2 light bandwidths are emitted: 415 nm (blue-violet) and 540 nm (green). These 2 bandwidths correspond with 2 distinct absorption peaks of hemoglobin, such that highly vascularized tissues reflect a substantially lower proportion of light compared with poorly vascular tissue, especially for blue-violet light, which is more subject to scattering in superficial tissues than green light. (*B*) For PDD, light with a spectral range from 380 to 470 nm is emitted and exits a fluorochrome that accumulates in tissue with high metabolic activity. On relaxation of the fluorochrome, a photon with a wavelength corresponding with red-pink is emitted. Highly metabolic tumor tissue can therefore be revealed by its red-pink fluorescence.

with its wavelength: the longer the wavelength, the deeper the propagation and the less scattering in superficial tissue. Therefore, the 415-nm light is mainly scattered within and reflected by superficial tissues, thus accounting for the fluorescentlike blue-green shine of the mucosae in the processed image on LCD. In highly vascularized tissues, the 415-nm light is mostly absorbed by hemoglobin after scattering, whereas the 540 nm-light propagates deeper through tissues, thus revealing highly vascularized tumors in red in the processed image on LCD. This difference in tissue penetration also explains the brownish appearance of superficial

capillary networks (eg, carcinoma in situ) and the cyan appearance of thicker blood vessels in deeper connective tissues. The net result of these 3 principles is a contrast enhancement that may help in the recognition of highly vascularized tumors.[66]

Photodynamic diagnosis
The PDD also relies on contrasting tumor tissue with normal tissue. For this, a fluorochrome (typically porphyrin-related fluorochrome 5-aminoaevulinic acid and its derivate hexaminolevulinate) is accumulated in cells with high metabolism that are going to be revealed by endoscopic illumination with a blue-violet color spectrum (380–470 nm). This blue-violet light excites the fluorochrome, which later emits a photon when relaxation of the fluorochrome occurs. This photon is characterized by a longer wavelength, thus producing a different color (red-pink) (**Fig. 7**B). Consequently, highly metabolic tumor tissue is revealed by its red-pink fluorescence.

Spectral light modulation
It should be noted that both NBI and PDD are not amenable to ureteroscopes that rely on illumination by LEDs, because the spectral range of LEDs cannot be modulated. It remains of interest to note the 3 colors emitted by an RGB LED: peaks are typically found at 625 nm (range, 620–630 nm) for red, 525 nm (520–230 nm) for green, and 425 nm (420–430 nm) for blue.[67] It therefore seems conceivable that specific LEDs could be manufactured to allow tissue enhancement in next-generation ureteroscopes.

Image 1-S technology
The Image 1-S technology is based on the reprocessing of the image captured by the digital sensor in order to enhance contrast domains that affect the human eye's interpretation of the rendered image. It does not necessitate a modification of the white light spectrum and therefore any light source can be used for illumination. Of the 5 available reprocessing modalities, the so-called Clara + Chroma mode has been shown to reach a significantly better subjective image quality score in vitro.[68]

Multimodal image enhancement
Compelling evidence for superiority in terms of tumor recurrence rate and survival is currently not available for any of the image enhancement technologies presented earlier.[69] Nevertheless, enhanced imaging will be further explored for next-generation ureteroscopes and will extend their field of application to urinary stone disease (eg, stone composition analysis). Multimodal

approaches integrating differing imaging modalities may provide a solution for better characterization of tissues.[70] Physical integration of auxiliary devices into ureteroscopes might be amenable. In particular, optical coherence tomography (OCT) and confocal laser endomicroscopy (CLE) for tumor detection may become readily available technologies if integrated in ureteroscopes.

Three-Dimensional Visualization

Three-dimensional (3D) visualization has not yet been integrated into any ureteroscope. It is not clear whether this is a consequence of physical constraints rendering the development of such scopes difficult, or whether it is explainable by a lack of interest by end users. Should 3D visualization be part of next-generation ureteroscopes, it would be of great interest to assess whether this might offer any advantage in terms of therapeutic efficacy and safety. One domain that could take advantage of 3D vision would be the detection of papillary upper urinary tract tumors. Of interest, a recent meta-analysis on studies comparing 3D with two-dimensional laparoscopic and thoracoscopic surgeries found significantly shorter operating time, less blood loss, and shorter hospital stay in favor of 3D imaging systems.[71]

From Reusable to Single Use

Current advantages of single-use ureteroscopes

Single-use flexible ureteroscopes represent a decisive milestone for ureteroscopy in the current decade.[72] Rather than a technological innovation, single-use ureteroscopes have led to a complete rethinking of operative room logistics.[73] They offer the advantages of being readily available, always sterile, and without traces of instrument wear. These advantages may prevent postponement of interventions, eliminate the risk of nosocomial infection caused by instrument contamination, and guarantee full operational (deflection) range of instruments for each operation. Also, single-use ureteroscopes do not require a dedicated sterilization process, which may be associated with unrecognized supplementary costs and inadvertent breakage of scopes. In addition, their implementation for treating locations that involve forcing maneuvers may cap the risks entailed by eventual instrument damage and repair costs of reusable scopes. In terms of quality, some of the currently available single-use ureteroscopes have visibility and maneuvering proprieties comparable with contemporary digital reusable flexible ureteroscopes.[74]

Further potential advantages

Further potential advantages of next-generation single-use ureteroscopes should be explored: for instance, a given manufacturer could provide a scope in a declination of various working channel positions (eg, scopes with a 3-o'clock working channel for interventions on the right kidney and scopes with a 9-o'clock working channel for interventions on the left kidney, respectively; discussed earlier, and see **Fig. 6**), therefore considerably enhancing versatility for the end-user at no additional price.

A single-use future

It is therefore conceivable that next-generation ureteroscopes are to become single use only, thereby entirely replacing reusable scopes. Awareness of sterility issues of reusable scopes and pricing policy will presumably be the pivotal variables determining the time point of this shift.

The hazards of single-use ureteroscopes

The downside of single-use devices is the risk of the appearance on the market of low-cost devices with low built quality. Technical weaknesses of such low-cost devices may become apparent only after repeated use or when facing a challenging case. This situation might expose the operator to the risk of unexpected instrument deficiencies such as spontaneous loss of vision or deflection mechanism failure. Also, because of low instrument replacement costs, surgeons may be tempted to force maneuvering and risk instrument breakage when facing difficult access to a urinary cavity. Instrument failures may lead to disastrous complications, eventually leading to open surgical extraction of a retained ureteroscope. Therefore, it is of utmost importance to handle single-use ureteroscopes with the same great care as for reusable ureteroscopes. Forcing instruments should only be done in expert hands.

SUMMARY

Major achievements and technological innovations from recent decades have shaped what has become modern ureteroscopy: a versatile, efficient, and safe operation technique for upper urinary tract disease. Necessity of further development of instruments and techniques arises from several domains relating to ureteroscopy: anatomic constraints, intrarenal pressure and temperature, maneuverability and ergonomics of ureteroscopes, image quality, image processing, and sterility of instruments. Any addition or improvement to these domains must be ascertained to fulfill the intended advantages with full consideration of possible secondary hazards. Emerging technologies are, therefore, now shaping what ureteroscopy will be in the future.

REFERENCES

1. Young HH, McKay RW. Congenital valvular obstruction of the prostatic urethra. Surg Gynecol Obstet 1929;(48):509.
2. Hopkins HH. A flexible fibrescope, using static scanning. Nature 1954;173(4392):39–41.
3. Goddard JC. A series of fortunate events: Harold Hopkins. J Clin Ultrasound 2018;11(1_suppl):4–8.
4. Marshall VF. Fiber optics in urology. J Urol 1964;91:110–4.
5. Takagi T, Go T, Takayasu H, et al. Small-caliber fiberscope for visualization of the urinary tract, biliary tract, and spinal canal. Surgery 1968;64(6):1033–8.
6. Goodman TM. Ureteroscopy with pediatric cystoscope in adults. Urology 1977;9(4):394.
7. Lyon ES, Kyker JS, Schoenberg HW. Transurethral ureteroscopy in women: a ready addition to the urological armamentarium. J Urol 1978;119(1):35–6.
8. Teichmann HH. [Intraureteral Lithotripsy]. Urologe A 1979;19:231–3.
9. Lyon ES, Banno JJ, Schoenberg HW. Transurethral ureteroscopy in men using juvenile cystoscopy equipment. J Urol 1979;122(2):152–3.
10. Perez-Castro Ellendt E, Martinez-Pineiro JA. [Transurethral ureteroscopy. A current urological procedure]. Arch Esp Urol 1980;33(5):445–60.
11. Perez-Castro Ellendt E, Martinez-Pineiro JA. Ureteral and renal endoscopy. A new-approach. Eur Urol 1982;8(2):117–20.
12. Bagley DH. Active versus passive deflection in flexible ureteroscopy. J Endourol 1987;1(1):15–8.
13. Preminger GM. Ureteral stone extraction utilizing nondeflectable flexible fiberoptic ureteroscopes. J Endourol 1987;1(1):31–5.
14. Aso Y, Ohtawara Y, Fukuta K, et al. Operative fiberoptic nephroureteroscopy: removal of upper ureteral and renal calculi. J Urol 1987;137(4):629–32.
15. Humphreys MR, Miller NL, Williams JC Jr, et al. A new world revealed: early experience with digital ureteroscopy. J Urol 2008;179(3):970–5.
16. Giusti G, Proietti S, Villa L, et al. Current standard technique for modern flexible ureteroscopy: tips and tricks. Eur Urol 2016;70(1):188–94.
17. Zelenko N, Coll D, Rosenfeld AT, et al. Normal ureter size on unenhanced helical CT. AJR Am J Roentgenol 2004;182(4):1039–41.
18. Tokas T, Herrmann TRW, Skolarikos A, et al. Pressure matters: intrarenal pressures during normal and pathological conditions, and impact of increased values to renal physiology. World J Urol 2018. [Epub ahead of print].
19. Tokas T, Skolarikos A, Herrmann TRW, et al. Pressure matters 2: intrarenal pressure ranges during upper-tract endourological procedures. World J Urol 2018. [Epub ahead of print].
20. Proietti S, Dragos L, Somani BK, et al. In vitro comparison of maximum pressure developed by irrigation systems in a kidney model. J Endourol 2017. [Epub ahead of print].
21. Sener TE, Cloutier J, Villa L, et al. Can we provide low intrarenal pressures with good irrigation flow by decreasing the size of ureteral access sheaths? J Endourol 2016;30(1):49–55.
22. Ng YH, Somani BK, Dennison A, et al. Irrigant flow and intrarenal pressure during flexible ureteroscopy: the effect of different access sheaths, working channel instruments, and hydrostatic pressure. J Endourol 2010;24(12):1915–20.
23. De Coninck V, Keller EX, Rodriguez-Monsalve M, et al. Systematic review on ureteral access sheaths: facts and myths. BJU Int 2018;122(6):959–69.
24. Rehman J, Monga M, Landman J, et al. Characterization of intrapelvic pressure during ureteropyeloscopy with ureteral access sheaths. Urology 2003;61(4):713–8.
25. Traxer O, Thomas A. Prospective evaluation and classification of ureteral wall injuries resulting from insertion of a ureteral access sheath during retrograde intrarenal surgery. J Urol 2013;189(2):580–4.
26. Aldoukhi AH, Roberts WW, Hall TL, et al. Holmium laser lithotripsy in the new stone age: dust or bust? Front Surg 2017;4:57.
27. Doizi S, Keller EX, De Coninck V, et al. Dusting technique for lithotripsy: what does it mean? Nat Rev Urol 2018;15(11):653–4.
28. Traxer O, Keller EX. Thulium fiber laser: the new player for kidney stone treatment? A comparison with Holmium:YAG laser. World J Urol 2019. [Epub ahead of print].
29. Wilson C, Kennedy JD, Irby P, et al. Miniature ureteroscope distal tip designs for potential use in thulium fiber laser lithotripsy. J Biomed Opt 2018;23(7):1–9.
30. Rao PN. Fluid absorption during urological endoscopy. Br J Urol 1987;60(2):93–9.
31. Schwalb DM, Eshghi M, Davidian M, et al. Morphological and physiological changes in the urinary tract associated with ureteral dilation and ureteropyeloscopy: an experimental study. J Urol 1993;149(6):1576–85.
32. Cybulski P, Honey RJ, Pace K. Fluid absorption during ureterorenoscopy. J Endourol 2004;18(8):739–42.
33. Jung HU, Frimodt-Moller PC, Osther PJ, et al. Pharmacological effect on pyeloureteric dynamics with a

clinical perspective: a review of the literature. Urol Res 2006;34(6):341–50.

34. Kiil F. Pressure recordings in the upper urinary tract. Scand J Clin Laboratory Invest 1953;5(4):383–4.

35. Boccafoschi C, Lugnani F. Intra-renal reflux. Urol Res 1985;13(5):253–8.

36. Thomsen HS, Dorph S, Olsen S. Pyelorenal backflow in normal and ischemic rabbit kidneys. Invest Radiol 1981;16(3):206–14.

37. Zhong W, Leto G, Wang L, et al. Systemic inflammatory response syndrome after flexible ureteroscopic lithotripsy: a study of risk factors. J Endourol 2015; 29(1):25–8.

38. Omar M, Noble M, Sivalingam S, et al. Systemic inflammatory response syndrome after percutaneous nephrolithotomy: a randomized single-blind clinical trial evaluating the impact of irrigation pressure. J Urol 2016;196(1):109–14.

39. Pasqui F, Dubosq F, Tchala K, et al. Impact on active scope deflection and irrigation flow of all endoscopic working tools during flexible ureteroscopy. Eur Urol 2004;45(1):58–64.

40. Huang J, Xie D, Xiong R, et al. The application of suctioning flexible ureteroscopy with intelligent pressure control in treating upper urinary tract calculi on patients with a solitary kidney. Urology 2018;111:44–7.

41. Caballero-Romeu JP, Galan-Llopis JA, Soria F, et al. Micro-ureteroscopy vs. ureteroscopy: effects of miniaturization on renal vascularization and intrapelvic pressure. World J Urol 2018;36(5):811–7.

42. Buttice S, Sener TE, Proietti S, et al. Temperature changes inside the kidney: what happens during holmium:yttrium-aluminium-garnet laser usage? J Endourol 2016;30(5):574–9.

43. Aldoukhi AH, Ghani KR, Hall TL, et al. Thermal response to high-power holmium laser lithotripsy. J Endourol 2017;31(12):1308–12.

44. Wollin DA, Carlos EC, Tom WR, et al. Effect of laser settings and irrigation rates on ureteral temperature during holmium laser lithotripsy, an in vitro model. J Endourol 2018;32(1):59–63.

45. Molina WR, Silva IN, Donalisio da Silva R, et al. Influence of saline on temperature profile of laser lithotripsy activation. J Endourol 2015;29(2):235–9.

46. Sapareto SA, Dewey WC. Thermal dose determination in cancer therapy. Int J Radiat Oncol Biol Phys 1984;10(6):787–800.

47. Dauw CA, Simeon L, Alruwaily AF, et al. Contemporary practice patterns of flexible ureteroscopy for treating renal stones: results of a worldwide survey. J Endourol 2015;29(11):1221–30.

48. Dragos LB, Somani BK, Sener ET, et al. Which flexible ureteroscopes (digital vs. fiber-optic) can easily reach the difficult lower pole calices and have better end-tip deflection: in vitro study on K-Box. A PETRA evaluation. J Endourol 2017;31(7):630–7.

49. Desai MM, Grover R, Aron M, et al. Robotic flexible ureteroscopy for renal calculi: initial clinical experience. J Urol 2011;186(2):563–8.

50. Saglam R, Muslumanoglu AY, Tokatli Z, et al. A new robot for flexible ureteroscopy: development and early clinical results (IDEAL stage 1-2b). Eur Urol 2014;66(6):1092–100.

51. Proietti S, Dragos L, Emiliani E, et al. Ureteroscopic skills with and without Roboflex Avicenna in the K-box® simulator. Cent European J Urol 2017;70(1):76–80.

52. Geavlete P, Saglam R, Georgescu D, et al. Robotic flexible ureteroscopy versus classic flexible ureteroscopy in renal stones: the initial Romanian experience. Chirurgia 2016;111(4):326–9.

53. Doizi S, Traxer O. Flexible ureteroscopy: technique, tips and tricks. Urolithiasis 2018;46(1):47–58.

54. Tan YH, Preminger GM. Advances in video and imaging in ureteroscopy. Urol Clin North Am 2004; 31(1):33–42.

55. Bader MJ, Gratzke C, Walther S, et al. The PolyScope: a modular design, semidisposable flexible ureterorenoscope system. J Endourol 2010;24(7):1061–6.

56. Proietti S, Somani B, Sofer M, et al. The "Body Mass Index" of flexible ureteroscopes. J Endourol 2017; 31(10):1090–5.

57. Ludwig WW, Lee G, Ziemba JB, et al. Evaluating the ergonomics of flexible ureteroscopy. J Endourol 2017;31(10):1062–6.

58. Smith LJ, Trout JM, Sridharan SS, et al. Comparison of microsuspension laryngoscopy positions: a randomized, prospective study. Laryngoscope 2015; 125(3):649–54.

59. Somani BK, Al-Qahtani SM, de Medina SD, et al. Outcomes of flexible ureterorenoscopy and laser fragmentation for renal stones: comparison between digital and conventional ureteroscope. Urology 2013;82(5):1017–9.

60. Binbay M, Yuruk E, Akman T, et al. Is there a difference in outcomes between digital and fiberoptic flexible ureterorenoscopy procedures? J Endourol 2010;24(12):1929–34.

61. Usawachintachit M, Isaacson DS, Taguchi K, et al. A prospective case-control study comparing Litho-Vue, a single-use, flexible disposable ureteroscope, with flexible, reusable fiber-optic ureteroscopes. J Endourol 2017;31(5):468–75.

62. Talso M, Proietti S, Emiliani E, et al. Comparison of flexible ureterorenoscope quality of vision: an in vitro study. J Endourol 2018;32(6):523–8.

63. Mandalapu RS, Remzi M, de Reijke TM, et al. Update of the ICUD-SIU consultation on upper tract urothelial carcinoma 2016: treatment of low-risk upper tract urothelial carcinoma. World J Urol 2017;35(3): 355–65.

64. Gono K. Narrow band imaging: technology basis and research and development history. Clin Endosc 2015;48(6):476–80.

65. Faber DJ, Mik EG, Aalders MC, et al. Light absorption of (oxy-)hemoglobin assessed by spectroscopic optical coherence tomography. Opt Lett 2003; 28(16):1436–8.

66. Traxer O, Geavlete B, de Medina SG, et al. Narrow-band imaging digital flexible ureteroscopy in detection of upper urinary tract transitional-cell carcinoma: initial experience. J Endourol 2011;25(1):19–23.

67. Kim S, Kim J, Lim W, et al. In vitro bactericidal effects of 625, 525, and 425 nm wavelength (red, green, and blue) light-emitting diode irradiation. Photomed Laser Surg 2013;31(11):554–62.

68. Emiliani E, Talso M, Baghdadi M, et al. Evaluation of the Spies™ modalities image quality. Int Braz J Urol 2017;43(3):476–80.

69. Bus MT, de Bruin DM, Faber DJ, et al. Optical diagnostics for upper urinary tract urothelial cancer: technology, thresholds, and clinical applications. J Endourol 2015;29(2):113–23.

70. Pradere B, Poulon F, Comperat E, et al. Two-photon optical imaging, spectral and fluorescence lifetime analysis to discriminate urothelial carcinoma grades. J Biophotonics 2018;11(11):e201800065.

71. Liang H, Liang W, Lei Z, et al. Three-dimensional versus two-dimensional video-assisted endoscopic surgery: a meta-analysis of clinical data. World J Surg 2018;42(11):3658–68.

72. Emiliani E, Traxer O. Single use and disposable flexible ureteroscopes. Curr Opin Urol 2017;27(2): 176–81.

73. Doizi S, Traxer O. Re: evaluation of a novel single-use flexible ureteroscope. Eur Urol 2017;72(1): 152–3.

74. Proietti S, Dragos L, Molina W, et al. Comparison of new single-use digital flexible ureteroscope versus nondisposable fiber optic and digital ureteroscope in a cadaveric model. J Endourol 2016;30(6): 655–9.

Single-Use Ureteroscopes

Brooke Moore, BA[a], Silvia Proietti, MD[b], Guido Giusti, MD[b],
Brian H. Eisner, MD[a],*

KEYWORDS

- Single-use • Reusable • Ureteroscopy • Kidney stones

KEY POINTS

- Ureteroscopy is frequently used for the treatment and management of stone disease and other endourologic conditions.
- Conflicting evidence exists on the performance characteristics of reusable ureteroscopes relative to single-use ureteroscopes.
- Theoretical advantages of single-use ureteroscopes include eliminating the need for sterilization and improving operating room efficiency and throughput. However, this must be balanced against the cost of purchasing a single-use instrument for each flexible ureteroscopy.

INTRODUCTION

Since its initial description by Young in 1912, the ureteroscope has facilitated the diagnosis and treatment of various urologic diseases.[1] Marshall's design of the fiber-optic ureteroscope in 1964 marked the beginning of many significant instrumental improvements, particularly in regard to image quality, durability, and performance.[2] Such advancements have promoted its widespread use for the management of various conditions including stone disease, hematuria, and upper tract urothelial carcinoma (UTUC).

With time the indications for flexible ureteroscopy have expanded, and recent reports have noted that ureteroscopy has surpassed shockwave lithotripsy for the treatment of stone disease in some countries.[3] With this increased use of ureteroscopy has come the realization that repair costs for reusable ureteroscopes may be very costly, depending on the frequency of ureteroscope breakage.[4,5] Compounding initial and repair costs, as well as sterilization and reprocessing expenditures, are raising awareness about the long-term economic viability of reusable ureteroscopes. In fact, the high cost and limited durability of the currently available, nondisposable, flexible ureteroscopes are significant variables that limit the establishment of flexible ureteroscopy programs in some countries.[6]

To address these cost-related concerns, manufacturers recently developed digital single-use ureteroscopes. However, single-use flexible ureteroscopes are relatively new to the market; therefore, comparisons between single-use and reusable ureteroscopes are correspondingly few to date. Herein we review the available evidence for the single-use ureteroscope as an alternative tool for the management of kidney stones, including recent data regarding image quality, performance, ergonomics, cost, efficiency, infection control, environmental impact, and reported experiences.

IMAGE QUALITY

Precise visualization of calculi is essential for the successful management of kidney stones. Optical performance of single-use and conventional ureteroscopes has been assessed by image resolution, color reproducibility, contrast, field of view, and distortion in ex vivo, in vitro, and in vivo

Disclosure Statement: Dr. Giusti - Consultant for Boston Scientific, Coloplast, Cook, Lumenis, Olympus, Rocamed; Dr. Eisner - consultant for Boston Scientific, Olympus, Kalera Medical, Sonomotion

[a] Department of Urology, Massachusetts General Hospital, 55 Fruit Street, GRB 1102, Boston, MA 02114, USA;
[b] Department of Urology, IRCCS San Raffaele Hospital, Ville Turro Division, Milan, Italy
* Corresponding author.
E-mail address: beisner@mgh.harvard.edu

Urol Clin N Am 46 (2019) 165–174
https://doi.org/10.1016/j.ucl.2018.12.002

models.[7–11] In a blinded review of ex vivo renal images from a porcine model, 13 fellowship-trained endourologists determined that the image quality of the single-use ureteroscope, LithoVue (Boston Scientific, Quincy, MA, USA), was significantly better than that of reusable, fiber-optic scopes (P5, Olympus, Tokyo, Japan; P6, Olympus; Flex X2, Storz, Tuttlingen, Germany; Cobra, Richard Wolf, Knittlingen, Germany).[11] The same reviewers also described comparable image quality between LithoVue and digital, reusable ureteroscopes (Flex-XC, Storz; V2, Olympus; Boa, Richard Wolf) and concluded that LithoVue produced a clinically acceptable image ex vivo.[11]

Subsequent in vitro assessments of image quality have led to similar findings. Dale and colleagues[9] used a standardized 1951 USAF Test Pattern Card at varying distances to demonstrate that LithoVue resolution was comparable with Flex-XC and superior to Cobra (**Fig. 1**). Using a multifrequency grid distortion target, studies further concluded that LithoVue produced less image distortion than its reusable counterparts.[9] An expansion of this study found that an alternative single-use ureteroscope, NeoFlex (Neoscope, San Jose, CA, USA), produced sharper resolution than LithoVue, Flex-XC, and Cobra. However, no significant difference in color reproducibility was noted between any of the studied instruments.[10]

Similarly, Talso and colleagues[8] used standardized grids, as well as stones of varying composition, to assess the image resolution and contrast of seven different fiber-optic and digital flexible ureteroscopes (fURS). The resulting data revealed that the optical performance of LithoVue was better than that of the fiber-optic ureteroscopes P6, Flex X2, and Cobra, as well as the digital ureteroscope, V2 (Olympus).[8] However, investigators also noted that LithoVue received significantly lower visual performance scores than reusable digital ureteroscopes Storz Flex-XC and Olympus URF-V ($P<.0001$).[8] This data variability indicates a need for further comparative assessments of image quality in an in vivo model.

In vivo data on image quality is scarce. In a study designed by Wiseman and colleagues,[7] six endourologists performed flexible ureteroscopy on three anesthetized pigs using LithoVue and P5 ureteroscopes. Although both instruments allowed for the successful visualization and treatment of stones, operators gave LithoVue a mean score of 6.86, indicating superior image quality and performance when compared with a reusable fiber-optic flexible ureteroscope (Olympus P5).[7] Field of view and depth of view, as well as access and navigational ability, all contributed to the instruments' scores.

In summary, published studies have noted that single-use ureteroscopes, such as LithoVue, demonstrate superior optical characteristics when compared with reusable fiber-optic flexible ureteroscopes and comparable visual quality to reusable digital flexible ureteroscopes.[7–9,11] It is noteworthy, however, that to date no publications have corroborated these results in live human patients.

PERFORMANCE

Given the complex renal anatomy, access to all parts of the renal collecting system, especially lower-pole calyces, can be challenging.

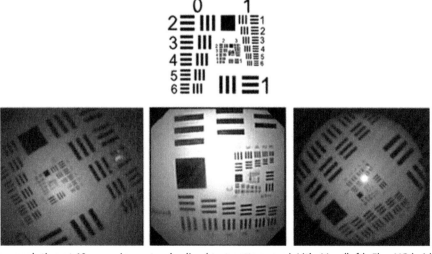

Fig. 1. Image resolution at 10 mm using a standardized test pattern card. LithoVue (left); Flex-XC (middle); Cobra (right). (*From* Dale J, Kaplan AG, Radvak D, et al. Evaluation of a novel single-use flexible ureteroscope. J Endourol 2017. https://doi.org/10.1089/end.2016.0237; with permission.)

Comparative data on ureteroscope deflection, maneuverability, flow rate, and stone clearance has been collected to assess the performance of single-use flexible ureteroscopes.[6,9,10,12–14] In addition to examining image quality, Dale and colleagues[9] assessed the deflection of LithoVue, Storz Flex-XC, and Wolf Cobra with and without instruments inside the working channel. LithoVue exhibited the greatest degree of deflection with an empty working channel, as well as with a laser inside the working channel, although it demonstrated inferior deflection to Storz Flex-XC with nitinol based in the working channel (**Table 1**).[9] Other studies have demonstrated that LithoVue deflection is superior to that of both Olympus P5 and URF-V in a cadaveric model.[6] When navigating four renal units of recently deceased female cadavers, surgeons noted no statistical difference in angle between all ureteroscopes ($P > .05$), and preferred LithoVue for maneuverability in more trials than Olympus P5 and URF-V.[6] This preferential performance emphasizes the potential of LithoVue for the treatment of challenging kidney stones.

In a recently published case report, Leveillee and Kelly[12] described similar maneuverability when LithoVue was used to treat a large lower-pole renal stone with a 365-μm laser fiber in a 35-year-old woman. They noted no loss in deflection or subsequent procedural complications, as well as a stone-free rate of 100% 1 week after the procedure[12] (**Fig. 2**).

Irrigation rates influence visibility as well as wound healing and hydration, and therefore affect the success of single-use ureteroscopes in managing kidney stones. Dale and colleagues[9] reported that LithoVue flow rates were superior to those of both Storz Flex-XC and Wolf Cobra; these values were confirmed by both an empty channel and a 200 μm laser fiber in the working channel ($P = .003$, $P<.001$). Additional findings noted that the fiber-optic, single-use ureteroscope, YC-FR-A (YouCare Tech, Wuhan, China), produced a

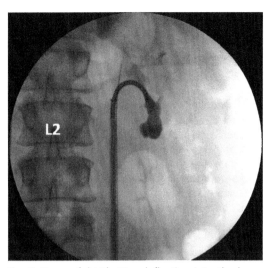

Fig. 2. Successful LithoVue deflection into the lower renal pole of a 35-year-old woman. (*From* Leveillee RJ, Kelly EF. Impressive performance: new disposable digital ureteroscope allows for extreme lower-pole access and use of 365 μm holmium laser fiber. J Endourol Case Rep 2016;2(1):116; with permission.)

flow rate of 59 mL/min, which was superior to that of LithoVue, Flex-XC, NeoFlex, and Cobra.[10,13] Despite this initially high flow rate with an empty working channel, investigators described significant decreases once instruments were added to the working channel (28.7 and 16.7 mL/min, respectively).[13]

COST ANALYSIS

Because of concerns about the high cost and limited lifespan of reusable flexible ureteroscopes, the cost-benefit of these instruments remains a significant variable that limits further dissemination of flexible ureteroscopy.[6] Many factors, including sterilization technique, procedure type, surgeon experience, and prior ureteroscope refurbishment, contribute to the reduced durability and subsequent repair cost of reusable ureteroscopes.[5,6,15,16] Comparative cost assessments of single-use and reusable ureteroscopes are crucial in assessing the suitability of these instruments for kidney stone treatment.

Ureteroscope reprocessing requires a balance between adequate sterilization and prevention of costly damage.[15,17] Abraham and colleagues[17] investigated the effects of two reprocessing methods, SSP1 (Steris, Mentor, OH, USA) and Cidex OPA (ASP, Irvine, CA, USA), on the optical quality, physical structure, and deflection of identical Storz flexible ureteroscopes. During this study period, investigators described notable physical destruction and a significant decline in the optical

Table 1 Ureteroscope deflection angles with and without instruments in the working channel			
	LithoVue	Flex-XC	Cobra
Empty	276	263	253
200 μm laser fiber	−2	−9	−2
1.9F nitinol basket	−5	0	−5
2.0F NPL probe	−2	−5	−3
2.4F NPL probe	−3	−27	−19

From Dale J, Kaplan AG, Radvak D, et al. Evaluation of a novel single-use flexible ureteroscope. J Endourol 2017. https://doi.org/10.1089/end.2016.0237; with permission.

quality of the fURS sanitized with SSP1.[17] Conversely, no physical damage to the fURS sterilized with Cidex OPA was noted.[17] These findings suggest that, despite its widespread use, SSP1 reprocessing may contribute to the elevated repair costs associated with reusable ureteroscopes.

In addition to decreased durability and increased repair expenditures, reprocessing also includes time-related costs. Isaacson and colleagues[15] used time-driven activity-based costing to isolate the most expensive steps in ureteroscope reprocessing. Investigators incorporated variables such as time, salary, protective equipment, and in-house repair labor to calculate a

monetary value for each step[15] (**Fig. 3**). Using this method, each reprocessing event was estimated to cost US$96.13.[15] It should be noted that the estimated reprocessing cost did not consider direct repair cost, which was calculated to be approximately $9420 per repair.[15] Nevertheless, these costs are avoided by the use of single-use ureteroscopes.

The type of procedure and location of the target stone can also influence ureteroscope durability.[6,16] Subsequent investigations by Hennessey and colleagues[16] noted that lower-pole and staghorn stones were the most significant risk factors for flexible ureteroscope damage. In fact,

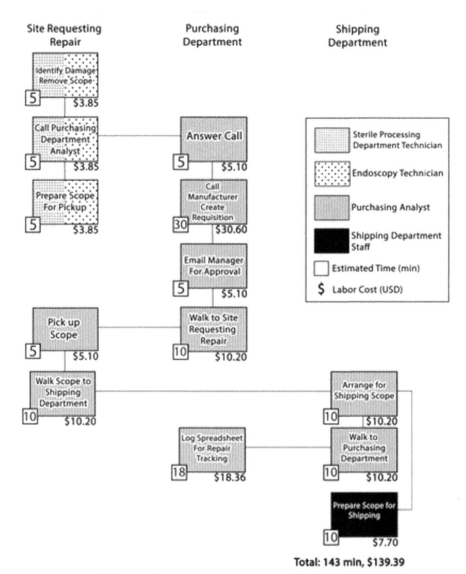

Total: 143 min, $139.39

Fig. 3. Repair process map following the identification and removal of a damaged reusable ureteroscope. Estimated labor costs and time required for each step are indicated. (*From* Isaacson D, Zetumer S, Sherer B, et al. Defining the costs of reusable flexible ureteroscope reprocessing using time-driven activity-based costing. J Endourol 2017;31(10):1029; with permission.)

ureteroscope damage was reported in 8% of cases involving lower-pole calculi; conversely, no ureteroscope damage resulted from the management of middle calyx or upper pole stones.[16] Therefore, the employment of single-use ureteroscopes for particularly challenging cases may help to reduce procedure-induced repair costs.[16]

The depreciating durability of reusable flexible ureteroscopy following refurbishment or repair is an additional concern for institutions.[4–6] In a prospective study conducted by Carey and colleagues,[5] which examined data from 501 ureteroscope cases, investigators described an average of 6.9 uses for each newly refurbished, fiber-optic ureteroscope before additional repairs were needed. This longevity is significantly shorter than the 40- to 50-case lifespan of a new flexible ureteroscope.[4,5] Similar reports describe an average of 11 procedures for each ureteroscope following an initial repair, and between 4.75 and 7.7 uses for older models.[4] Furthermore, repair costs per flexible ureteroscope vary between approximately $4000 and $7500, prompting significant expenditures for care centers with ureteroscope programs.[4,5,18] In addition to initial purchase price, the repair and maintenance costs associated with depreciating ureteroscope lifespan must also be considered.

Prior investigations incorporated these variables into their comparative cost analyses to address the financial burdens of both reusable and single-use ureteroscopes.[16,18–20] Hennessey and colleagues[16] evaluated LithoVue as an alternative to the conventional digital reusable ureteroscope, Olympus URF-V, in terms of its durability and economic benefit. Investigators collected data on initial ureteroscope cost, as well as on repairs and reprocessing expenditures; ultimately, they concluded that the total repair cost of the seven flexible ureteroscopes during the 30-month study period was $121,490, with an average cost of approximately $519/case.[16] Minor repair costs, as well as the salaries and benefits of reprocessing staff, were not included in their calculations. Further comparative analyses revealed that the economic benefit of LithoVue depends highly on case volume, as well as the starting price, of this single-use ureteroscope.[16,19] Consequently, if used 28 times, LithoVue may provide an economic benefit at an initial price of $896; however, that benefit may be lost if the original cost increases to $1867 (**Fig. 4**).[16]

Similarly, Martin and colleagues[19] developed an algorithm to effectively examine the cost-benefit of single-use ureteroscopes. Using data from 348 flexible ureteroscope cases, investigators calculated the economic burden of Flex-XC compared

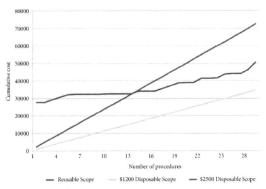

Fig. 4. Cumulative cost of LithoVue at an initial price of US$896 (1200 AUD) and $1867 (2500 AUD) compared with the cumulative cost of the reusable fURS, Olympus V. (*From* Hennessey DB, Fojecki GL, Papa NP, et al. Single-use disposable digital flexible ureteroscopes: an ex vivo assessment and cost analysis. BJU Int 2018;121 Suppl 3:59; with permission.)

with that of LithoVue.[19] Many factors, such as initial costs, repair costs, average number of cases before ureteroscope failure, reprocessing costs, and estimated benefits, were considered.[19] Excluding the initial price, investigators determined that the cost of each reusable fURS case was $848.10.[19] The initial LithoVue cost was $1500, resulting in a break-even point of 99 ureteroscopic procedures; however, after this break-even point reusable ureteroscopes were favored.[19] Although investigators determined that Flex-XC was more economic than LithoVue, this study also used four new flexible ureteroscopes instead of refurbished or repaired models.[19] As a result, these conclusions may not be applicable for care centers with older ureteroscopes, lower case volume, or infrequent lower-pole cases.

By contrast, Taguchi and colleagues[20] used a microcosting analysis to demonstrate the economic comparability of LithoVue and the reusable fiber-optic ureteroscope, Olympus P6. The study used a bottom-up approach that enabled investigators to directly measure the activity duration of all relevant steps and attribute a price per unit to each stage.[20] Calculations included the cost of the initial acquisition, instrument disposal, reprocessing, repairs, operating room, and labor/benefits.[20] Ultimately, investigators found no significant difference between the total cost of LithoVue per case and the total cost of Olympus P6 per case ($2852 and $2799, respectively).[20] The great variability of these cost-benefit analyses is common across studies, and suggests a significant need for further research in this area.[4,5,16,18,20–22]

EFFICIENCY

Delays and unexpected complications are common occurrences in operating rooms worldwide. These obstacles are often attributed to reprocessing events, postoperative complications, or the surprising discovery of unsuitable instruments.[15,23,24] Such occurrences have direct implications on patient satisfaction, operating cost, and procedural efficiency. To better quantify the effects of single-use ureteroscopes on care center efficiency, Usawachintachit and colleagues[23] assessed postoperative complications and procedural times of patients undergoing urologic treatments. The studied cases used both LithoVue and the reusable fiber-optic ureteroscope, Olympus P6.[23] Investigators reported that LithoVue produced a significantly lower postoperative complication rate than Olympus P6 ($P<.05$).[23] Moreover, mean procedural time was significantly shorter for LithoVue cases compared with Olympus P6 (54.1 min and 64.5 min, respectively; $P<.05$).[23] The described 10% to 20% reduction in procedural time may improve patient satisfaction and provide economic benefits arising from reduced operating room usage.[20,23] Furthermore, a shortened procedural time has the potential to increase daily case load and subsequently improve access for patients needing ureteroscopy.[23] Omission of reprocessing events, as well as a lighter design that enables faster performance, may explain the observed reduction in LithoVue procedural time.[15,23]

In addition to reprocessing and postoperative complications, unexpected instrument damage also contributes to decreased care center efficiency. In a prospective endourology study, examiners followed 103 consecutive urologic cases that required 119 unwrapped ureteroscopes.[24] In 10% of cases, at least two ureteroscopes were unwrapped before a suitable instrument was identified.[24] In one exceptionally challenging episode, the procedure was rescheduled after four unacceptable instruments were opened.[24] Investigators described various problems that made the reusable ureteroscopes unsuitable for use, including crushed shafts, camera dislodgments, and digital image failures.[24] The ensuing delays have detrimental effects on institutional expenditures as well as patient comfort and satisfaction.[23,24]

INFECTIOUS COMPLICATIONS

Invasive procedures require direct contact between a surgical device and a patient's tissues. To limit the transmission of infectious agents, practices must effectually disinfect surgical equipment after each procedure. Despite great sterilization efforts, communicable outbreaks are still described globally.[25–27] In fact, recent studies noted persistent contamination on gastroscopes and colonoscopes in spite of strict reprocessing guidelines.[28] These findings have incited additional investigations into the sterility of many other types of surgical equipment, including ureteroscopes, and may support the use of disposable instruments.

In the last decade, associations have been described between various multidrug-resistant *Enterobacter cloacae* and *Pseudomonas aeruginosa* outbreaks and the poor sterilization of reusable ureteroscopes.[29,30] A more recent ex vivo chemical analysis of ureteroscopes at two large multispecialty academic centers in the midwestern United States detected microbial growth on 13% of sterilized instruments and protein on 100% of devices.[31] Investigators attributed these findings to structural irregularities, discoloration, and damage to the ureteroscope working channel.[31] However, contamination of these instruments occurred despite manual cleaning and hydrogen peroxide sterilization, suggesting that improvements to reprocessing techniques may be necessary.

These findings suggest that extensive visual inspections, as well as routine biochemical tests, are needed to better assess the patient readiness of surgical instruments.[28,31,32] The notable contamination revealed by these investigations underscores the importance of adhering to manufacturer sterilization guidelines; failure to do so may also contribute to endoscopy-related outbreaks.[33] The described challenges of adequate ureteroscope sanitation emphasize the potential value that single-use ureteroscopes may have in preventing infectious transmission. Future studies are important to determine whether the stated findings associated with reusable ureteroscopes are clinically significant, and whether single-use ureteroscopes may reduce the risk of infectious transmission from one patient to another.

ERGONOMICS

Ergonomics is the science of workplace, tools, and equipment designed to reduce worker discomfort, strain, and fatigue, and to prevent work-related injuries. Recently there has been increased focus on surgeons' occupational health and the ergonomics of flexible ureteroscopy has also been increasingly studied, with an ever-growing number of reports on hand problems among endourologists.[34,35] With this concern in mind, Ludwig and colleagues[36] evaluated biomechanical stress by using surface electromyography on urologists performing flexible ureteroscopy in a training model.

They found that both single-use flexible uretero-scopes and reusable digital flexible ureteroscopes have better ergonomic parameters than fiber-optic flexible ureteroscopes because they require significantly less muscle activation and fatigue.[36] The investigators noted that the etiology underlying this finding is not understood, but speculate that it is related to both LithoVue and reusable digital flexible ureteroscopes being lighter and easier to deflect than reusable fiber-optic ureteroscopes, in which fiber-optic bundles might generate a certain bending resistance.[36]

Another potential impact on ergonomics is the weight of the individual ureteroscope, which seems to be one of the most important factors in determining muscle fatigue. In a recent study by Proietti and colleagues,[37] LithoVue was significantly lighter (277.5 g) whereas the mean weights of fiber-optic and digital ureteroscopes were 335.2 g and 699.6 g, respectively ($P<.05$). Moreover, it should also be highlighted that one limitation of the study by Ludwig and colleagues[36] was that the procedures were relatively short in duration. Real-world flexible ureteroscopy procedures can be longer and, especially in high-volume centers, preformed sequentially in a single day; this inevitably results in an accumulation of muscular fatigue. In this scenario, the single-use ureteroscopes have the potential to decrease surgeon fatigue, improve performance, and potentially improve stone-free rates.[38]

ENVIRONMENTAL IMPACT

Despite increasing concerns regarding environmental health, little attention has been given to the comparative environmental impact of urologic instruments. Davis and colleagues[39] recently published the first study exploring this topic. In their comparative analysis, the investigators examined the carbon footprint of LithoVue and Olympus URV-F.[39] Data on the carbon cost of ureteroscope manufacturing, sterilization, repairs, replacements, and disposal were collected for each instrument.[39] Ultimately this study revealed that LithoVue had a slightly lower carbon footprint than Olympus URV-F (4.43 and 4.47, respectively) (**Table 2**).[39]

Given the narrow scope of this study, as well as the limited pool of prior data, further research is needed to fully understand the environmental impact of these devices. However, the broad significance of human-induced climate change suggests that the carbon footprint of endourologic instruments is an important variable to consider when assessing the appropriateness of both devices.

Table 2
The associated carbon footprint values of each processing step for LithoVue and Olympus URV-F

Process	Carbon Footprint (kg of CO_2 per Case)
Boston Scientific LithoVue single-use digital ureteroscope	
Manufacturing cost (weight of scope 0.3 kg)	3.83
Solid waste = 0.3 kg	0.3
Sterilization (6)	0.3
Total per case	4.43
URV-F*	
Manufacturing cost (weight of scope 1 kg)	0.06
Washing/sterilization** (165 L)	3.95
Repackaging with theater wrap (3)	<0.005
Repair cost (estimated 5 kg CO_2/repair)	0.45
Solid waste of flexible ureteroscope = 1 kg	0.005
Total per case	4.47

*, Life cycle of 180 uses and 11 repairs (i.e., 180/16).
**, Sterilization machine used—Olympus ETD4. Olympus ETD4 uses 9.2 kW per cycle = each cycle takes 70 minutes and sterilizes 2 scopes = 7.9 kW/hour = 7.9 kg CO2 7. URV-F = Olympus Flexible Video Ureteroscope.
From Davis NF, McGrath S, Quinlan M, et al. Carbon footprint in flexible ureteroscopy: a comparative study on the environmental impact of reusable and single-use ureteroscopes. J Endourol 2018;32(3):214–7.

REPORTED SERIES

Currently, most of the available evidence for single-use ureteroscopes focuses on specific attributes of the instrument or was gathered from an in vitro or ex vivo model. As a result, there are limitations to the described findings. To determine whether this novel device is a viable alternative for the treatment of kidney stones, physicians must consider the overall performance of single-use ureteroscopes during their unique procedures.

Multiple investigators have described clinical successes while using single-use ureteroscopes in nonrandomized studies. A recent multicenter, retrospective study conducted by Chi and colleagues[40] incorporated LithoVue data from 159 cases across 14 care centers to assess the clinical efficacy of this instrument. Investigators reported a 96.8% first-treatment success rate in terms of ability to access stone, structure, and UTUC lesion, leading them to conclude that LithoVue performed comparably with their historical reusable flexible ureteroscope experience in terms of reaching and treating the target of the procedure. Notably, however, this study lacks short-term and long-term follow-up data.

In a smaller pilot study, Salvadó and colleagues[41] noted similar successes using the Pusen single-use ureteroscope (Zhuhai Carelife Medical, Zhuhai, China). Specifically, investigators described a 100% stone-free rate in eight cases and an 80% stone-free rate in the remaining three.[41] Both studies suggested that single-use ureteroscopes may be a reasonable, cost-efficient alternative for the management of kidney stones and that further studies are necessary to corroborate these preliminary data.[41]

FUTURE DIRECTIONS

Ureteroscopy is frequently used for the treatment of kidney stones as well as for the management of other urologic diseases. Concerns surrounding the cost-benefit of reusable ureteroscopes has limited their widespread use and perpetuated the development of single-use ureteroscopes. The available evidence suggests that these new devices may serve as a suitable option for the treatment of stones as well as for other disorders.

Prior investigators consistently concluded that single-use ureteroscopes were superior to conventional fiber-optic devices in regard to image quality and performance.[7,9,11] However, discrepancies between studies were noted when the same characteristics were compared with digital flexible ureteroscopes.[6,8–10] This variability suggests that further research must be carried out to concretely determine the comparability of single-use ureteroscope image quality and performance. Moreover, the design of the described studies limits the applicability of these conclusions in an in vivo human model.[7–11,13,14]

Inconsistencies about the potential economic benefits of single-use ureteroscopes have also been revealed. Past research demonstrates significant variability in regard to the cost of reusable ureteroscopes per case, as well as variations in the average lifespan of reusable ureteroscopes following an initial repair.[4,5,19,20] There is also little agreement about an economic break-even point for the two instruments; in fact, the financial benefit of single-use ureteroscopes seems to depend highly on institution-specific initial costs and care center case load. Therefore, care centers may profit from conducting their own cost-benefit analyses to account for their specific initial costs and average procedure volumes.

The environmental impact of single-use ureteroscopes is another variable that mandates greater attention. Few data exist about the carbon footprint of any endourologic instrument; subsequently, it is challenging to predict the potential environmental implications of single-use ureteroscope manufacture and disposal. Given the extensive implications of climate change, considerable attention must be paid to the impact of these surgical devices on environmental health.

SUMMARY

The indications for single-use ureteroscopes may be vast. These devices could serve as a reasonable alternative for immunocompromised patients in whom infection risk must be considered, as well as for hospitals with high ureteroscope breakage rates. Single-use ureteroscopes may also be appropriate for procedures that carry an increased risk of instrument damage, such as challenging lower-pole stones. Furthermore, as the demand for single-use ureteroscopes increases, the cost of these new devices may be reduced. This is a considerable variable to note when assessing the economic benefits of this alternative. However, owing to the novelty of the single-use ureteroscope, insufficient data currently exist. As a result, it is difficult to adequately assess the comparability of these two instruments as well as the full range of benefits that the single-use ureteroscope may provide.

REFERENCES

1. Fuchs GJ. Milestones in endoscope design for minimally invasive urologic surgery: the sentinel role of a pioneer. Surg Endosc 2006;20(Suppl 2):S493–9.
2. Marshall VF. Fiber optics in urology. J Urol 1964; 91(1):110–4.
3. Ordon M, Urbach D, Mamdani M, et al. The surgical management of kidney stone disease: a population based time series analysis. J Urol 2014;192(5): 1450–6.
4. Carey RI, Gomez CS, Maurici G, et al. Frequency of ureteroscope damage seen at a tertiary care center. J Urol 2006;176(2):607–10.
5. Carey RI, Martin CJ, Knego JR. Prospective evaluation of refurbished flexible ureteroscope durability seen in a large public tertiary care center with multiple surgeons. Urology 2014;84(1):42–5.
6. Proietti S, Dragos L, Molina W, et al. Comparison of new single-use digital flexible ureteroscope versus nondisposable fiber optic and digital ureteroscope in a cadaveric model. J Endourol 2016;30(6):655–9.
7. Wiseman O, et al. MP51-03. Comparison of a new single-use digital flexible ureteroscope (LithoVue™)

to a non-disposable fibre-optic flexible ureteroscope in a live porcine model. J Urol 2016;195(4):e682.

8. Talso M, Proietti S, Emiliani E, et al. Comparison of flexible ureterorenoscope quality of vision: an in vitro study. J Endourol 2018;32(6):523–8.

9. Dale J, Kaplan AG, Radvak D, et al. Evaluation of a novel single-use flexible ureteroscope. J Endourol 2017. https://doi.org/10.1089/end.2016.0237.

10. Tom WR, Wollin DA, Jiang R, et al. Next-generation single-use ureteroscopes: an in vitro comparison. J Endourol 2017;31(12):1301–6.

11. Molina W, et al. Evaluating the image quality of a novel single-use digital flexible ureteroscope. J Endourol 2016;30(7):11.

12. Leveillee RJ, Kelly EF. Impressive performance: new disposable digital ureteroscope allows for extreme lower pole access and use of 365 μm holmium laser fiber. J Endourol Case Rep 2016;2(1): 114–6.

13. Wollin D, et al. PD35-09. Comparison of a novel single-use flexible ureteroscope to currently existing reusable and single-use flexible ureteroscopes. J Urol 2017;197(4):e666.

14. Schlager D, Hein S, Obaid MA, et al. Performance of single-use Flexorvue vs reusable Boavision ureteroscope for visualization of calices and stone extraction in an artificial kidney model. J Endourol 2017; 31(11):1139–44.

15. Isaacson D, Ahmad T, Metzler I, et al. Defining the costs of reusable flexible ureteroscope reprocessing using time-driven activity-based costing. J Endourol 2017;31(10):1026–31.

16. Hennessey DB, Fojecki GL, Papa NP, et al. Single-use disposable digital flexible ureteroscopes: an ex vivo assessment and cost analysis. BJU Int 2018;121(Suppl 3):55–61.

17. Abraham JB, Abdelshehid CS, Lee HJ, et al. Rapid communication: effects of Steris 1 sterilization and Cidex ortho-phthalaldehyde high-level disinfection on durability of new-generation flexible ureteroscopes. J Endourol 2007;21(9):985–92.

18. Kramolowsky E, McDowell Z, Moore B, et al. Cost analysis of flexible ureteroscope repairs: evaluation of 655 procedures in a community-based practice. J Endourol 2016;30(3):254–6.

19. Martin CJ, McAdams SB, Abdul-Muhsin H, et al. The economic implications of a reusable flexible digital ureteroscope: a cost-benefit analysis. J Urol 2017; 197(3 Pt 1):730–5.

20. Taguchi K, Usawachintachit M, Tzou DT, et al. Micro-costing analysis demonstrates comparable costs for LithoVue compared to reusable flexible fiberoptic ureteroscopes. J Endourol 2018;32(4): 267–73.

21. Gurbuz C, Atış G, Arikan O, et al. The cost analysis of flexible ureteroscopic lithotripsy in 302 cases. Urolithiasis 2014;42(2):155–8.

22. Tosoian JJ, Ludwig W, Sopko N, et al. The effect of repair costs on the profitability of a ureteroscopy program. J Endourol 2015;29(4):406–9.

23. Usawachintachit M, Isaacson DS, Taguchi K, et al. A prospective case-control study comparing Litho-Vue, a single-use, flexible disposable ureteroscope, with flexible, reusable fiber-optic ureteroscopes. J Endourol 2017;31(5):468–75.

24. Hubosky S, Healy K, Bagley D. MP3-10 defining the rate of encountering unacceptable reusable flexible ureteroscopes for immediate clinical use: 'Bad out of the Box'. J Endourol 2017;31(S2).

25. Rutala WA, Weber DJ. Disinfection and sterilization in health care facilities: an overview and current issues. Infect Dis Clin North Am 2016;30(3): 609–37.

26. Wendorf KA, Kay M, Baliga C, et al. Endoscopic retrograde cholangiopancreatography-associated AmpC Escherichia coli outbreak. Infect Control Hosp Epidemiol 2015;36(6):634–42.

27. Epstein L, Hunter JC, Arwady MA, et al. New Delhi metallo-beta-lactamase-producing carbapenem-resistant Escherichia coli associated with exposure to duodenoscopes. JAMA 2014;312(14): 1447–55.

28. Ofstead CL, Wetzler HP, Doyle EM, et al. Persistent contamination on colonoscopes and gastroscopes detected by biologic cultures and rapid indicators despite reprocessing performed in accordance with guidelines. Am J Infect Control 2015;43(8): 794–801.

29. Chang CL, Su LH, Lu CM, et al. Outbreak of ertapenem-resistant Enterobacter cloacae urinary tract infections due to a contaminated ureteroscope. J Hosp Infect 2013;85(2):118–24.

30. DasGupta R, French G, Glass J. Multi-resistant Pseudomonas aeruginosa outbreak in an endourology unit. Eur Urol Suppl 2008;7(3):323.

31. Ofstead CL, Heymann OL, Quick MR, et al. The effectiveness of sterilization for flexible ureteroscopes: a real-world study. Am J Infect Control 2017;45(8):888–95.

32. Ofstead CL, Wetzler HP, Heymann OL, et al. Longitudinal assessment of reprocessing effectiveness for colonoscopes and gastroscopes: results of visual inspections, biochemical markers, and microbial cultures. Am J Infect Control 2017;45(2):e26–33.

33. Wendelboe AM, Baumbach J, Blossom DB, et al. Outbreak of cystoscopy related infections with Pseudomonas aeruginosa: new Mexico, 2007. J Urol 2008;180(2):588–92 [discussion: 592].

34. Memon AG, Naeem Z, Zaman A, et al. Occupational health related concerns among surgeons. Int J Health Sci (Qassim) 2016;10(2):279–91.

35. Healy KA, Pak RW, Cleary RC, et al. Hand problems among endourologists. J Endourol 2011;25(12): 1915–20.

36. Ludwig WW, Lee G, Ziemba JB, et al. Evaluating the ergonomics of flexible ureteroscopy. J Endourol 2017;31(10):1062–6.

37. Proietti S, Somani B, Sofer M, et al. The "Body Mass Index" of flexible ureteroscopes. J Endourol 2017; 31(10):1090–5.

38. Seklehner S, Heißler O, Engelhardt PF, et al. Impact of hours worked by a urologist prior to performing ureteroscopy on its safety and efficacy. Scand J Urol 2016;50(1):56–60.

39. Davis NF, McGrath S, Quinlan M, et al. Carbon footprint in flexible ureteroscopy: a comparative study on the environmental impact of reusable and single-use ureteroscopes. J Endourol 2018;32(3):214–7.

40. Chi T, Stoller M, Abrahams H, et al. MP50-16 Initial Clinical Experience With a Single-Use Digital Flexible Ureteroscope. J Urol, 197(4S), p. e690.

41. Salvadó JA, et al. PD35-11. New digital single-use flexible ureteroscope (Pusen™): first clinical experience. J Urol 2017;197(4):e667.

Innovations in Disposable Technologies for Stone Management

Sari S. Khaleel, MD, MS, Michael S. Borofsky, MD*

KEYWORDS

- Nephrolithiasis • Stone • Kidney • Ureteroscopy • Technology • Sheath • Basket • Device

KEY POINTS

- Emerging technologies in disposable retrieval devices for stone management are aimed at making safer and more efficient stone removal.
- Efforts are being made to incorporate pressure control and suction capabilities through ureteral access sheaths to optimize irrigation and allow for suction of stone debris.
- Newer generation stone baskets are smaller, less traumatic, and more efficacious at removing and grasping stones. Future efforts are being made to incorporate stone measuring and allow single operator control.
- Application of bioadhesives are being explored and developed to improve efficiency of basket retrieval of small fragments and stone debris.

INTRODUCTION

Over the past decade, ureteroscopy has surpassed shock wave lithotripsy as the most commonly performed surgery for upper urinary tract stones in the United States.[1] This transition has primarily been enabled by improvements in scope size, design, and optics. However, another critical component that has facilitated the rise of ureteroscopy is the wide array of disposable devices that have improved the ability to treat stones with ever-increasing efficiency and precision. There have been several innovative new disposable technologies developed for percutaneous stone removal as well. The current armamentarium of disposable retrieval devices available to help manage renal and ureteral stones is vast and continues to improve and evolve at a rapid rate. Herein, an overview of the most recent and future disposable devices applicable to stone retrieval are reviewed.

Emerging Concepts in Ureteral Access Sheaths

Ureteral access sheaths (UASs) are one of the foundational disposable devices that allow stone retrieval by establishing secure passage for the scope from outside the body all the way to the upper urinary tract. The first UAS was developed in 1974 by Hisao Takayasu and Yoshio Aso as a "guide tube" to facilitate the insertion of the ureteroscope (URS) into the ureter. This initial model was made of polytetrafluoroethylene and had a diameter of 3 mm and a length of 38 cm, through which a flexible URS was advanced.[2] Since its initial introduction, the UAS has undergone significant technological modifications so as to minimize buckling, kinking, and potential for ureteral injury.

Current models are typically comprised of 2 disposable pieces: a tapered inner obturator that is passed over a working wire and an outer sheath that is meant to traverse the ureter and exit the body at the level of the urethral meatus. UASs

Disclosure Statement: M.S. Borofsky, Boston Scientific, Consultant; Auris Health, Consultant. S.S. Khaleel, none.
Department of Urology, University of Minnesota, 420 Delaware Street SE, MMC 394 Mayo, Minneapolis, MN 55455, USA
* Corresponding author.
E-mail address: mborofsk@umn.edu

Urol Clin N Am 46 (2019) 175–184
https://doi.org/10.1016/j.ucl.2018.12.003

come in a variety of sizes. Inner obturator diameters typically range from 9 to 14F, and outer sheath diameters commonly range from 11 to 16F.[3] In general, use of a UAS offers several advantages during ureteroscopic procedures including enabling repeated passes of the instrument to the kidney as well as easing movement and handling of the scope itself. It can also change the flow dynamics of irrigation allowing for better visibility at lower pressure within the kidney. Lower pressures in turn can decrease the risk of pyelovenous backflow and collecting system rupture, which have been associated with systemic inflammatory response and sepsis through dissemination of toxins and bacteria.[4,5] Use of a UAS has also been associated with reduced operative time and prolonged scope longevity.[4]

Despite these advantages, routine UAS use during ureteroscopy remains controversial.[6–8] Contrary arguments against routine use are mainly centered around potential for ureteral injury and perforation during placement. Recent and future UAS research is primarily focused on better understanding the benefits and harms associated with their use as well as innovation in design to enable better performance, particularly as it relates to stone removal.

UAS with suction capability
Basket extraction through a UAS is well recognized to be challenging, time consuming, and tedious. Stone dusting, whereby the stone is fragmented into miniscule (sub-mm) particles has been advocated as one way to avoid this process; yet, whether or not this stone debris ultimately will pass remains controversial.[9] An emerging idea to address this limitation is application of suction to the end of a UAS.

Zeng and colleagues[10] described a modified UAS with an evacuation side port designed to be used with a negative pressure vent attached to continuous negative suction to clear small stone fragments during and immediately post-ureteroscopic lithotripsy (**Fig. 1**). The authors used negative pressure settings of 150 to 200 mm Hg. During laser lithotripsy much of the stone debris would be aspirated through the side port. When stone fragments were too large to pass this way, they could be evacuated by withdrawing the scope to the bifurcation of the connection side port at the proximal end of the sheath thus allowing a pathway for stone evacuation through the side port. Among 74 patients with ureteral stones in whom the modified UAS was used, the immediate stone-free rate (SFR) was 97%, with a mean operative time of 27 minutes and no cases of retropulsion.[10] This sheath has since been brought to market as the

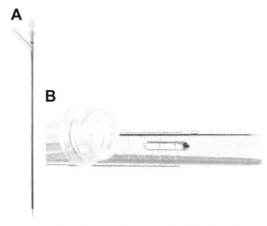

Fig. 1. Modified ureteral access sheath (A) and pressure vent (B) that improves stone retropulsion, a common issue encountered during URS with a traditional UAS. (*Adapted from* Zeng G, Wang D, Zhang T, et al. Modified access sheath for continuous flow ureteroscopic lithotripsy: a preliminary report of a novel concept and technique. J Endourol 2016;30(9):993; with permission.)

ClearPetra System (Well Lead Medical, China), The current commercially available devices feature models for ureteroscopy, percutaneous nephrolithotomy (PCNL), and cystoscopy.[11]

A separate UAS with suction capabilities was also described recently by Zhu and colleagues.[12] This sheath features 2 separate channels on its proximal end: 1 for suction and 1 to act as a pressure vent. The sheath has an inner 12F obturator and an outer sheath 14F in size. The authors used a matched-pair analysis to compare outcomes using the suctioning UAS to those using a standard UAS among 165 patients undergoing ureteroscopy. They found that the suction UAS cohort had a shorter mean operative time (50 vs 57 min) with a higher immediate SFR on postoperative day 1 (83% vs 72%). Stone-free rates at 1 month were comparable between the 2 groups. There was also a lower complication rate in the suction UAS cohort (12% vs 25%) with fewer infectious post-operative complications.

UAS with pressure control
The introduction of suction at the end of the sheath has also been part of a wider effort to use sheaths as a method of controlling renal pelvic pressure (RPP). A key benefit of ureteroscopy with a UAS compared with unsheathed ureteroscopy is the ability to insulate the kidney from high irrigation and intrapelvic pressures via increased irrigation outflow through the sheath. This is critical as higher RPP risks ureteral and parenchymal injury, as well as pyelovenous backflow, and the potential for systemic inflammatory response (8.1%) or

sepsis (0%–4.5%).[4,5,7,13] Physiologic RPP has been estimated at 4 to 7 mm Hg, with a recommended RPP safety threshold of 30 to 40 mm Hg to minimize the risk of pyelovenous backflow.[7] Prior studies have found that it is quite feasible to exceed these thresholds without a sheath with 1 study measuring an RPP of 59 cm H_2O under irrigation pressures of 200 cm H_2O,[14] and another identifying a peak RPP of 446 cm H_2O with forced irrigation for the purpose of improving vision.[15] In contrast, URS with a UAS can generally maintain an RPP below this threshold in most cases, even when the inflow pressures through the scope are high.[7] Nonetheless, the pressure dynamics during ureteroscopy remain somewhat ill-defined with the potential to vary depending on sheath size, ureteroscope shaft size (fiberoptic vs digital), location, and irrigation settings.

There are several ongoing efforts to develop a reliable and easy use of the device to monitor RPP during URS. Deng and colleagues,[13] developed a novel pressure sensing UAS with a platform that allows for automated or semiautomated real-time inflow pressure control by regulating irrigation flow and suctioning pressures. This UAS features a pressure transducer at its distal tip, along with 2 channels at its proximal end that are connected to a suction vacuum device and a pressure-monitoring feedback device, respectively (**Fig. 2**). This sheath has an outer diameter of 15F and an 11.5F working channel. It also comes in variable lengths.

One of the unique aspects of the sheath and suction platform is the ability to provide real-time RPP readings and automatically regulate pressure. The system is capable of providing a pressure warning value (default 20 mm Hg) and a pressure limit value (30 mm Hg). It also allows for a semiautomatic mode as well as pure perfusion and pure suction modes, the latter of which could theoretically facilitate stone removal through the sheath itself via suction. They tested the clinical feasibility of this system in a series of 93 patients. The authors claimed excellent SFRs (96% at 30 days) with reported clear visual fields in all cases with intelligent pressure monitoring that kept the RPP less than 20 mm Hg.[14] They have also reported favorable clinical data pertaining to use of this UAS/pressure-monitoring system among 40 patients with solitary kidneys.[16]

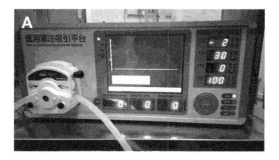
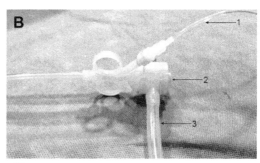
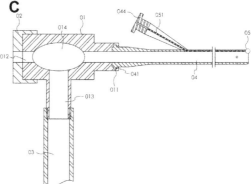

Fig. 2. Automated irrigation and suctioning platform developed by Deng and colleagues.[13] (*A*) Irrigation and suctioning platform. (*B*) Real picture of the UAS used by the system, which contains a channel for pressure monitoring and feedback (1), along with a working channel for the flexible ureteroscope (2), and a channel for vacuum suctioning (3). (*C*) Device design: 01, main body of suction joint; 02, seal cap; 03, suction pipe; 04, sheath pipe; 05, pressure transducer; 011, screw groove; 012, working cavity; 013, suction cavity; 014, curved cavity; 041, thread pipe; 044, conical interface; 051, signal line. UAS, ureteral access sheath. (*Adapted from* Deng X, Song L, Xie D, et al. A novel flexible ureteroscopy with intelligent control of renal pelvic pressure: an initial experience of 93 cases. J Endourol 2016;30(10):1068; with permission.)

Emerging Concepts in Stone Extraction

Baskets

Stone baskets are the main device used to move and retrieve stones from the upper urinary tract. Once made preferentially of reusable stainless steel, modern-day baskets have evolved significantly and are now generally smaller, less traumatic, single-use devices made of nitinol (nickel titanium). Modern baskets come in a variety of shapes and forms with slightly different mechanisms of action and intents for each (**Table 1**).

Table 1
Overview of currently available nitinol baskets and their unique features

Basket Shape	Manufacturer	Basket Name	Special Basket Features
Tipless (4-wire round)	Bard[a]	Skylite (1.9/2.4/3.0)	
	Boston Scientific	Zero Tip (1.9/2.4/3.0)	
	Cogentix Medical/ Laborie[b]	Unnamed Tipless (1.3/1.9/2.2)	
	Coloplast	Dormia No-Tip (1.5/2.2)	
	Cook	NCircle (1.5/2.2/3.0/4.5)	Also comes as delta (sturdier) version and helical (intertwined) configuration
	Olympus[c]	Ultra-Catch (1.8/2.2/3.0)	Twisted wires to maintain shape, rotation control handle
	Sacred Heart	Halo (1.5)	Rotation control handle
		Vantage (2.4)	Rotation control handle
Tipless (end engaging)	Boston Scientific	Dakota (1.9)	OpenSure handle capable of secondary opening to ensure release
	Cook	NGage (1.7/2.2)	
Tipless (unique)	Coloplast	Dormia No-Tip (3.0)	Twisted wire with flower design
	Olympus	X-Catch NT (1.8/2.2/3.0)	Cross-paired wires for increased radial dilating force, basket changes to multiple sizes, rotatable handle
	Sacred Heart	Halo (6 wire) (1.5)	
Tipped	Cogentix Medical/ Laborie	Flat/Helical (2.5)	
	Coloplast	Dormia N.Stone (2.5/3.0/4.0)	
	Cook	NForce (2.2/3.2)	
	Sacred Heart	Apex (2.4)	
Miscellaneous	Bard	EXPAND212 (3)	2-1-2-1 wire design for increased wire coverage over stone
		Dimension (2.4/3.0)	Able to articulate position of basket at handle
	Boston Scientific	Escape (1.9)	2 in 1 basket designed to hold stone and allow simultaneous lithotripsy
		Graspit (2.6/3.3)	Shaped like grasping forceps, has serrated nitinol wire edges
		OptiFlex (1.3)	Rotation control knob on handle, extendable cage diameter
	Cook	NCompass (1.5/2.4)	16 wire meshed construction designed for small stone fragment retrieval
		NTrap (2.8)	Woven meshed wires extend beyond stone preventing retropulsion of fragments

[a] CR Bard, Salt Lake City, UT, USA.
[b] Cogentix Medical/Laborie, Geleen, the Netherlands.
[c] Olympus Medical, Shinjuku, Tokyo, Japan.

Over the past several years, the 4-wire tipless basket has become the primary basket for many urologists. These baskets tend to be highly capable of ensnaring stones in the 4-wire basket shape while at the same time being relatively atraumatic because of the lack of a pointed tip.

They are also typically able to conform to the shape of the calyx and reach stones that may be just out of reach from the tip of the endoscope itself.

Several performance characteristics from 5 commercially available tipless nitinol stone baskets were recently compared.[17] Measured characteristics of each basket included perforation force, radial dilation force, opening dynamics, and resistance toward deflection. Perforation force, a safety metric whereby a high value is indicative of a lesser likelihood of tissue trauma, was measured using a digital force gauge to assess perforation of a piece of aluminum foil with the basket tip. The Sacred Heart Halo 1.5F basket (Sacred Heart, Minnetonka, MN, USA) had the highest mean force required to perforate the foil, whereas the 2.2F Coloplast Dormia (Coloplast, Humlebaek, Denmark) basket required the lowest mean force. The 1.5F Halo also demonstrated the greatest radial dilation force, a metric that can have clinical meaning when attempting to expand the ureter with the basket in the event of an entrapped or impacted stone. This is a feature typically stronger for helical baskets. Opening dynamics of each basket was characterized as either linear or exponential. Linear dynamics are commonly preferred for a basket because it allows for a better hold on the stone, as well better control of the basket and visualization. The Cook 2.2 NCircle (Cook Medical, Bloomington, IN, USA) was the only basket that had a linear opening dynamic. Lastly, the 1.5F Halo had the least effect on ureteroscope deflection; although, of note, the 1.5 baskets from Coloplast and Cook were not assessed in this study.

Small-profile baskets 1.5F or smaller have also been a newer addition to the basket market. As demonstrated in the aforementioned study, small profile baskets interfere with deflection of the ureteroscope to a lesser degree. Another advantage is that they do not occlude as much of the working channel and thus do not result in as great a diminution in irrigation. Magheli and colleagues[18] formally compared 3 popular 1.3 to 1.5F basket models: Boston Scientific OptiFlex (Boston Scientific, Marlborough, MA, USA) 1.3F, Cook NCircle 1.5F, and Halo 1.5F. The smaller 1.3F OptiFlex basket was associated with the least diminution in ureteroscope deflection (7.1°–8.0° with the OptiFlex vs 10.1°–11.4° with the other baskets) and channel flow rate (from 70 mL/min at baseline to 37.9–38.2 mL/min with the OptiFlex compared with 29.1–30.3 mL/min with the other baskets).

Another recent trend in stone baskets has been introduction of end-engaging baskets (**Fig. 3**). These baskets differ from traditional baskets that encompass stones circumferentially and instead engage and release them in a head-on fashion.[19] This mechanism may allow for more precise grasping and disengagement of stones, which can be useful when relocating stones within the kidney or disengaging a stone in the ureter. There

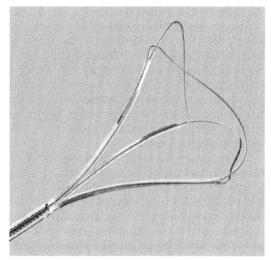

Fig. 3. Cook NGageTM end-engaging basket. (*Courtesy of* Cook, Bloomington, IN, USA; with permission.)

are currently 2 commercially available end-engaging Nitinol basket devices, the Cook NGage and the Boston Scientific Dakota with an Open-Sure handle. The NGage comes as a 1.7 or 2.2F with 8 or 11 mm opening diameters of the baskets. The Dakota is a 1.9F basket with a single basket that is 8 mm at baseline but capable of being expanded to 11 mm if necessary with the Open-Sure handle.

A recent in vitro comparison of the 2 devices (1.7F NGage model) showed comparable durability, but favored the Dakota device in terms of capturing and releasing stones 7 to 8 mm or greater. The Dakota was preferentially able to capture larger stones 11 mm in size and was more effective in releasing larger stones with the Open-Sure feature.[19]

Although the aforementioned baskets have found favor for many as versatile devices generally suitable for most stone procedures, alternative basket designs are still available as well and are particularly useful for specific scenarios. Tipped, stainless steel flat wire baskets are an excellent instrument for obtaining tissue in the event of trying to biopsy upper tract urothelial carcinoma. In 1 study by Kleinmann and colleagues,[20] use of a 2.4F stainless steel flat wire basket was associated with being able to obtain a definitive diagnosis on biopsy in 93% of cases compared with 63% of cases when a 3F cup biopsy forceps was used. Disposable ureteroscopic graspers on the other hand can prove useful in extracting retained foreign bodies such as broken laser fibers or migrated ureteral stents. Flexible 2- and 3-pronged graspers are other suitable disposable retrieval devices that can be used for this purpose.

Efficient stone basketing requires optimal laser lithotripsy into sufficiently small fragments that can be retrieved and pass through the ureter or UAS without resistance. Increasing the internal diameter of a UAS from 10 to 12F can enable a stone fragment with nearly twice the volume to be extracted.[7] Historically, extraction efficiency has focused on the size of the sheath, but recent research efforts have focused instead on optimizing stone fragments.

Cordes and colleagues[21] designed a stone retrieval basket to use as a measurement proxy to estimate stone size. Their initial prototype had a sensitivity of 56% and specificity of 84% for predicting stones greater than 6 mm; however, it was deemed inferior to visual estimation of stone size by the surgeon.[22] In an effort to improve performance, they recently described an updated, all nitinol version, of their tipped, 2.5F basket with a sliding handle. The prototype handle is unique in that it has a standardized scale with a corresponding stone measurement (2, 5, and 8 mm) when the basket is closed around the stone. Ideally, this could provide useful information to the surgeon with regard to whether the stone is appropriate to try to extract or if it requires fragmentation; however, the clinical performance of this prototype basket has not yet been described.

Ziemba and colleagues[23] took a different approach to stone measuring, choosing instead to focus on computer estimates of stone size as opposed to physical measurements. To accomplish this, they developed specialized stone measuring software for use during ureteroscopy. After an initial calibration, their software can take measurements when the stone is engaged in the basket using the distance from the scope tip to help determine size. The authors tested it during 5 procedures and compared stone measurements as obtained using the software to actual measurements using calipers. Among 30 measured stones with a median size of 3.2 × 2.2 mm, the median longitudinal and transverse measurement errors were 0.14 and 0.09 mm, respectively.

Lastly, an inherent limitation of currently available baskets is that they require additional manipulation to open and close. This is most commonly performed by an assistant, but this has been identified to potentially reduce efficiency, particularly in cases where the assistant may not be facile with the basket. One device with the potential to improve on this is the LithoVue Empower retrieval deployment device (Boston Scientific), which is a new accessory that allows the LithoVue ureteroscope and compatible retrieval devices to be used simultaneously with a single hand (**Fig. 4**).

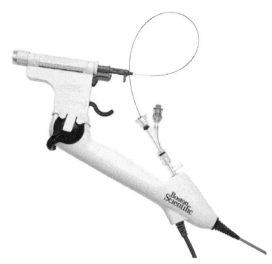

Fig. 4. LithoVue Empower retrieval deployment device (Boston Scientific). (*Courtesy of* Boston Scientific, Marlborough, Massachusetts, USA; with permission.)

Bioadhesives

Despite the significant technical advances in stone basket design, the direct removal of individual stone fragments remains a time-consuming and potentially difficult process. This is often used as rationale for why a dusting approach is preferable; however, even small stones and debris have potential to cause problems later, whether it be ureteral occlusion, stone growth, or infection.[24–26] This limitation has resulted in interest in using bioadhesives to aggregate stone particles and facilitate removal in a more efficient fashion.

The initial adhesive used for this purpose was blood, with the earliest report of "coagulum pyelolithotomy" dating back to open kidney stone surgeries in the 1940s.[27] An application of this technique to ureteroscopic surgery was described more recently, using an autologous venous blood sample taken from the patient intra-op and injected into the renal collecting system to agglutinate all stone fragments resulting from endoscopic lithotripsy.[28,29] A detailed description of the technique was provided by Cloutier and colleagues,[29] using a 10-mL autologous venous blood sample that is then injected slowly (over 5 min) into the renal pelvis after stopping irrigation and removing any residual contrast that may interfere with agglutination. The ureteroscope is then removed and another 5 to 10 minutes are given for further agglutination before returning to the renal pelvis and irrigating any non-coagulated blood, leaving agglutinated stone fragments behind, which are then extracted using a standard nitinol basket.

Concerns with such an approach technique include the added procedure time for blood injection and coagulation, as well as the impaired visibility following blood injection. To manage these issues, Hein and colleagues[30] developed a biocompatible polysaccharide-based adhesive system consisting of 2 substrates that can be applied directly through the ureteroscope working channel onto the stone fragments and debris. In combination, the substrates form a gel at a body temperature of 37°C to create an adhesive lump around the stone fragments without adhering to the renal system or the instruments. The bioadhesive system was also dyed blue for improved visualization (**Fig. 5**). The clinical utility of this novel bioadhesive was tested in a porcine kidney model, in which the authors reported a 100% SFR among 15 cases when using the bioadhesive in combination with basket extraction compared with just 60% SFR with traditional basketing of fragments in an additional 15 cases. In addition, use of the bioadhesive was associated with a reduction of mean retrieval time from 36 minutes 56 seconds to 10 minutes 33 seconds ($P = .001$).[30]

The group then compared performance with the bioadhesive to that of autologous blood using the same model. Although the blood and bioadhesive were effective in enabling high SFRs (both achieved 100% SFR in comparison with only 60% in the control group), the bioadhesive was associated with improved clinical performance, including decreased procedure time and fewer numbers of instrument passes (10:36 vs 26:12 min, $P = .001$; average instrument pass of 8.46 in the bioadhesive group vs 22.30 in the blood group, $P = .001$). The bioadhesive cohort also had a shorter clotting time and better visibility. The viability and biocompatibility system were recently confirmed in vivo with URS and PCNL in a porcine model.[31] The system has not been tested in humans at the time of this review.

Anti-retropulsion devices
Other types of disposables that bear mention in the management of ureteral stones are anti-retropulsion devices (ARDs). These devices are designed to prevent proximal migration of ureteral stones during instrumentation and fragmentation, with the intention to reduce the likelihood of losing a stone in the more complex renal collecting system, or necessitating use of a flexible scope to search for a migrated stone. Several different ARDs are available for use.

The Stone Cone (Boston Scientific)[32] consists of a wire and a radio-opaque carrying catheter. Once deployed beyond the stone, removal of the catheter allows for spiraling of the wire proximal to the stone, preventing proximal migration during lithotripsy. Two other wire-based ARDs include

the PercSys Accordian (Accordian Medical, Indianapolis, IN, USA), which is meant to be passed beyond the stone like a wire and then folded like an accordion beyond it, and the XenX (ROCAMED, Monaco-Monte Carlo), which is passed like a wire but acts as a nitinol ureteral mesh when opened.

Basket type ARDs are also available. The NTrap (Cook Medical) is one such device that is meant to be deployed just beyond the ureteral stone and, when positioned, features a curved wire mesh design to prevent proximal migration and catch small fragments during lithotripsy.[33] Other available basket type ARDs include the LithoCatch and Parachute baskets (Boston Scientific).

Alternative ARDs include inflatable balloons (Passport, Boston Scientific), and viscous lidocaine jelly, each of which has been shown to be feasible for this purpose. One unique type of viscous ARD was Backstop (Boston Scientific), a water-soluble polymer that exists in an aqueous state at cold temperatures but becomes viscous when it reaches body temperature. This allows instillation proximal to the stone and then dissolution when flushed with cool saline on completion of stone treatment. Unfortunately, this product is not commercially available at this time.

Despite the numerous available options, ARD use has not found widespread favor for routine ureteroscopy. A recent analysis from the Clinical Research Office of the Endourological Society Ureteroscopy Global Study found that ARDs were only used worldwide in 14.5% of cases. The most frequently used ARDs in the study were the Stone Cone (Boston Scientific) and the NTrap (Cook Medical). Use of an ARD was associated with a slight decrease in stone migration (2%) and higher SFR (2.8%) without increased risk of complication.[34] The cost-effectiveness of ARD use was not directly measured in this study; however, is recognized to be less expensive than stone retreatment. Whether or not ARD actually decreases the likelihood of secondary procedures for residual fragments remains unanswered.[35]

Percutaneous stone extraction
Many of the aforementioned devices are applicable to PCNL in particular when using a flexible scope through the kidney; however, percutaneous access to the kidney allows for several unique methods of removing stones as well. One of the most effective and widely used methods of stone fragmentation and removal during PCNL is ultrasonic lithotripsy, which will be discussed in Daniel A. Wollin and Michael E. Lipkin's article, "Emerging Technologies in Ultrasonic and Pneumatic Lithotripsy," in this issue. An emerging alternative

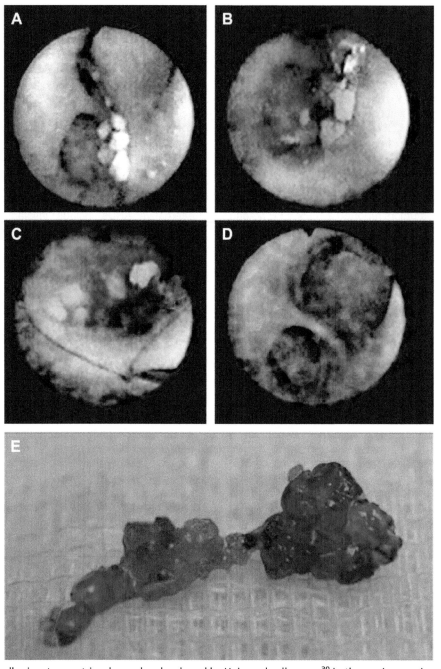

Fig. 5. Bioadhesive stone retrieval complex developed by Hein and colleagues[30] in the ex vivo porcine model. (*A*) residual fragments in 2 calyces. (*B*) Application of components 1 and 2. (*C*) Endoluminal lump retrieval. (*D*) Calyces after retrieval without residual fragments. (*E*) Retrieved lump. (*From* Hein S, Schoenthaler M, Wilhelm K, et al. Novel biocompatible adhesive for intrarenal embedding and endoscopic removal of small residual fragments after minimally invasive stone treatment in an ex vivo porcine kidney model: initial evaluation of a prototype J Urol 2016;196(6); with permission.)

to this is laser lithotripsy with combination suction enabled through disposable handpieces.

Two devices are currently available for this purpose. The LithAssist (Cook Medical) is a disposable device featuring a steel canula 38 cm long and 11.6F in diameter. Within the canula is a separate 5F lumen meant to house a laser fiber. These are attached to an ergonomic handpiece with vacuum suction capabilities in the base controlled by a trigger on the handpiece, allowing for single operator control of suction. In an in vitro comparison, the LithAssist performed favorably with improved efficiency compared with ultrasonic lithotripsy in treating hard stones,[36] but decreased efficiency for soft stones. The other disposable device that has been described is the laser suction handpiece (LSHP) (Lumenis, Israel). This device is similar in design as the LithAssist but features a slightly longer canula (40 cm) 11.3F in diameter. Another difference is the laser location that sits outside of the working cannula and does not occupy any of the lumen, potentially reducing interference with suction efficiency. In a comparison study using the device in a porcine model, the LSHP performed comparably relative to the LithAssist. Surgeons found the LSHP and LithAssist to be similar easy to use and effective, although the LHSP scored higher in regard to laser fiber visibility during use, probably because of the externalized laser pathway, which sits above the device lumen as opposed to within it, making it visible along the entirety of its course.[37] One limitation of these newer devices is a lack of clinical data comparing their efficacy with more established ultrasonic and pneumatic devices for PCNL, with only anecdotal evidence of its efficacy in humans to date.[38]

Another alternative approach to evacuating stones via suction is manual extraction. This can be particularly useful in the event of a hard stone that is resistant to fragmentation with traditional energy sources. Reusable steel devices such as 2- and 3-pronged graspers are effective but can be traumatic and cumbersome. This led to the development of the Perc-NCircle (Cook Medical), which is a 12F, 38-cm-long handheld disposable basket on a spring-loaded handle. In an in vitro comparison between the NCircle and a 3-pronged grasping forceps, the NCircle was found to be associated with faster stone extraction time. It also was associated with a reduced likelihood of dislodging the percutaneous access sheath, which only occurred in 7% of cases compared with 53% of the cases when the 3-pronged grasper was used.[39]

SUMMARY

The optimal method to retrieve upper urinary tract stones continues to evolve. Innovation in disposable retrieval devices has enabled much of this evolution and is partially responsible for the increased utilization of ureteroscopy, now the most common technique used to treat upper urinary stones. Future efforts in disposable retrieval device technology are primarily focused on making ureteroscopy safer and more efficient and are likely to make this procedure an even more popular treatment option for surgical stone management in the coming years.

REFERENCES

1. Oberlin DT, Flum AS, Bachrach L, et al. Contemporary surgical trends in the management of upper tract calculi. J Urol 2015;193(3):880–4.
2. Takayasu H, Aso Y. Recent development for pyeloureteroscopy: guide tube method for its introduction into the ureter. J Urol 1974;112(2):176–8.
3. Schoenthaler M, Buchholz N, Farin E, et al. The Post-Ureteroscopic Lesion Scale (PULS): a multicenter video-based evaluation of inter-rater reliability. World J Urol 2014;32(4):1033–40.
4. Reis Santos JM. Ureteroscopy from the recent past to the near future. Urolithiasis 2018;46(1):31–7.
5. Ng YH, Somani BK, Dennison A, et al. Irrigant flow and intrarenal pressure during flexible ureteroscopy: the effect of different access sheaths, working channel instruments, and hydrostatic pressure. J Endourol 2010;24(12):1915–20.
6. Huang J, Zhao Z, AlSmadi JK, et al. Use of the ureteral access sheath during ureteroscopy: a systematic review and meta-analysis. PLoS One 2018;13(2):e0193600.
7. De Coninck V, Keller EX, Rodríguez-Monsalve M, et al. Systematic review of ureteral access sheaths: facts and myths. BJU Int 2018;122(6):959–69.
8. Kourambas J, Byrne RR, Preminger GM. Does a ureteral access sheath facilitate ureteroscopy? J Urol 2001;165(3):789–93. Available at: http://www.ncbi.nlm.nih.gov/pubmed/11176469. Accessed June 24, 2018.
9. Humphreys MR, Shah OD, Monga M, et al. Dusting versus basketing during ureteroscopy-which technique is more efficacious? a prospective multicenter trial from the EDGE research consortium. J Urol 2018;199(5):1272–6.
10. Zeng G, Wang D, Zhang T, et al. Modified access sheath for continuous flow ureteroscopic lithotripsy: a preliminary report of a novel concept and technique. J Endourol 2016;30(9):992–6.
11. Well Lead Medical Co. ClearPetra. 2018. Available at: http://www.presurgy.com/media/files/ClearPetra/Catalogo ClearPetra Sheath-20160426.pdf. Accessed July 1, 2018.
12. Zhu Z, Cui Y, Zeng F, et al. Comparison of suctioning and traditional ureteral access sheath during flexible ureteroscopy in the treatment of renal stones. World J Urol 2018;1–9. https://doi.org/10.1007/s00345-018-2455-8.
13. Deng X, Song L, Xie D, et al. A novel flexible ureteroscopy with intelligent control of renal pelvic pressure: an initial experience of 93 cases. J Endourol 2016;30(10):1067–72.

14. Rehman J, Monga M, Landman J, et al. Characterization of intrapelvic pressure during ureteropyeloscopy with ureteral access sheaths. Urology 2003; 61(4):713–8.

15. Jung H, Osther PJS. Intraluminal pressure profiles during flexible ureterorenoscopy. Springerplus 2015;4(1):373.

16. Huang J, Xie D, Xiong R, et al. The application of suctioning flexible ureteroscopy with intelligent pressure control in treating upper urinary tract calculi on patients with a solitary kidney. Urology 2018;111: 44–7.

17. Patel N, Akhavein A, Hinck B, et al. Tipless nitinol stone baskets: comparison of penetration force, radial dilation force, opening dynamics, and deflection. Urology 2017;103:256–60.

18. Magheli A, Semins MJ, Allaf ME, et al. Critical analysis of the miniaturized stone basket: effect on deflection and flow rate. J Endourol 2012;26(3): 275–7.

19. Bechis SK, Abbott JE, Sur RL. In vitro head-to-head comparison of the durability, versatility and efficacy of the NGage and novel Dakota stone retrieval baskets. Transl Androl Urol 2017;6(6):1144–9.

20. Kleinmann N, Healy KA, Hubosky SG, et al. Ureteroscopic biopsy of upper tract urothelial carcinoma: comparison of basket and forceps. J Endourol 2013;27(12):1450–4.

21. Cordes J, Nguyen F, Pinkowski W, et al. A new automatically fixating stone basket (2.5 F) prototype with a nitinol spring for accurate ureteroscopic stone size measurement. Adv Ther 2018;35(9):1420–5.

22. Cordes J, Teske L, Nguyen F, et al. A comparison between an in vitro ureteroscopic stone size estimation and the stone size measurement with the help of a scale on stone baskets. World J Urol 2016;34(9): 1303–9.

23. Ziemba JB, Li P, Gurnani R, et al. A user-friendly application to automate CT renal stone measurement. J Endourol 2018;32(8):685–91.

24. Altunrende F, Tefekli A, Stein RJ, et al. Clinically insignificant residual fragments after percutaneous nephrolithotomy: medium-term follow-up. J Endourol 2011;25(6):941–5.

25. Osman MM, Alfano Y, Kamp S, et al. 5-year-follow-up of patients with clinically insignificant residual fragments after extracorporeal shockwave lithotripsy. Eur Urol 2005;47(6):860–4.

26. Ozgor F, Simsek A, Binbay M, et al. Clinically insignificant residual fragments after flexible ureterorenoscopy: medium-term follow-up results. Urolithiasis 2014;42(6):533–8.

27. Dillon MJ. Coagulum pyelolithotomy to remove multiple stones. AORN J 1982;36(4):680–9.

28. Traxer O, Dubosq F, Chambade D, et al. How to avoid accumulation of stone fragments in the lower calix during flexible ureterorenoscopy. Prog Urol 2005; 15(3):540–3 [in French]. Available at: http://www.ncbi.nlm.nih.gov/pubmed/16097170. Accessed July 22, 2018.

29. Cloutier J, Cordeiro ER, Kamphuis GM, et al. The glue-clot technique: a new technique description for small calyceal stone fragments removal. Urolithiasis 2014;42(5):441–4.

30. Hein S, Schoenthaler M, Wilhelm K, et al. Novel biocompatible adhesive for intrarenal embedding and endoscopic removal of small residual fragments after minimally invasive stone treatment in an ex vivo porcine kidney model: initial evaluation of a prototype. J Urol 2016;196(6):1772–7.

31. Hein S, Schoeb DS, Grunwald I, et al. Viability and biocompatibility of an adhesive system for intrarenal embedding and endoscopic removal of small residual fragments in minimally-invasive stone treatment in an in vivo pig model. World J Urol 2018;36(4): 673–80.

32. Desai MR, Patel SB, Desai MM, et al. The Dretler stone cone: a device to prevent ureteral stone migration-the initial clinical experience. J Urol 2002; 167(5):1985–8. Available at: http://www.ncbi.nlm.nih.gov/pubmed/11956424. Accessed September 17, 2018.

33. Wang C-J, Huang S-W, Chang C-H. Randomized trial of NTrap for proximal ureteral stones. Urology 2011;77(3):553–7.

34. Saussine C, Andonian S, Pacík D, et al. Worldwide use of antiretropulsive techniques: observations from the clinical research office of the endourological society ureteroscopy global study. J Endourol 2018;32(4):297–303.

35. Ursiny M, Eisner BH. Cost-effectiveness of anti-retropulsion devices for ureteroscopic lithotripsy. J Urol 2013;189(5):1762–6.

36. Okhunov Z, del Junco M, Yoon R, et al. In vitro evaluation of LithAssist: a novel combined holmium laser and suction device. J Endourol 2014;28(8):980–4.

37. Dauw CA, Borofsky MS, York N, et al. A usability comparison of laser suction handpieces for percutaneous nephrolithotomy. J Endourol 2016;30(11): 1165–8.

38. Ghani KR, Aldoukhi AH, Roberts WW. Dusting utilizing suction technique (DUST) for percutaneous nephrolithotomy: use of a dedicated laser handpiece to treat a staghorn stone. Int Braz J Urol 2018;44(4):840–1.

39. Hoffman N, Lukasewycz SJ, Canales B, et al. Percutaneous renal stone extraction: In vitro study of retrieval devices. J Urol 2004;172(2):559–61.

Laser Fibers for Holmium:YAG Lithotripsy: What Is Important and What Is New

Bodo E. Knudsen, MD, FRCSC

KEYWORDS

- Laser fiber • Holmium:YAG • Lithotripsy • Ureteroscopy • Retrograde intrarenal surgery
- Flexible ureteroscope

KEY POINTS

- The optical laser fibers used for holmium:YAG laser lithotripsy have evolved over the years, but differences in fiber performance continue to exist.
- Reviewing the available data on fiber performance and selecting fibers that are more robust and less likely to fracture during use may lead to lower ureteroscope repair rates.
- Understanding the true fiber diameter and its impact on fiber flexibility and flow rates helps set expectations of performance for the fiber during clinical use.

INTRODUCTION

The holmium:YAG laser has been the gold standard for intracorporeal stone treatment over the past 10 years to 15 years. This is based both on the effectiveness of the holmium:YAG laser to fragment stones of all compositions, a critically important property that limited the adoption of other types of laser for lithotripsy, and on its wide margin of safety. The holmium:YAG laser operates at a wavelength of approximately 2140 nm in the near-infrared spectrum. This results in the laser energy being absorbed in water and thereby is ideal for the aqueous environment in which laser lithotripsy is performed.[1]

To deliver the laser energy to the stone, both the holmium:YAG laser console and a fiber delivery system are needed. A wide range of console options is available, from low-power systems, capable of delivering only 10 W to 20 W of power, to high-powered 120-W to 140-W systems, capable of delivery of both high pulse energy and high frequency. More recently, many consoles now have the additional option of variable pulse duration that can have an impact on the performance of the system. The second critical component is the fiber delivery system that allows for the laser energy to be transmitted from the console, through the endoscope, and then delivered to the target stone.[2] The laser fiber is the focus of this review.

The holmium:YAG laser allows for the use of low-hydroxyl silica optical fibers, which are robust but inexpensive fibers and are available in a variety of diameters and core sizes. Although cosmetically many of the fibers used with the holmium:YAG laser appear similar (**Fig. 1**), their performance characteristics can vary greatly. Understanding the intended, and at times nonintended, properties of the fibers is critical for urologists to maximize the effectiveness and safety of the procedures.[3]

Disclosure Statement: Dr B.E. Knudsen is a Consultant for Boston Scientific, Bard Medical, and Olympus Surgical. He is also a Researcher for Boston Scientific and Cook Urology.
Department of Urology, The Eye and Ear Institute, 915 Olentangy River Road, Third Floor, Columbus, OH 43212, USA
E-mail address: Bodo.Knudsen@osumc.edu

Urol Clin N Am 46 (2019) 185–191
https://doi.org/10.1016/j.ucl.2018.12.004
0094-0143/19/© 2018 Elsevier Inc. All rights reserved.

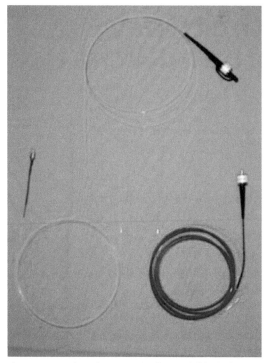

Fig. 1. Examples of commercially available holmium: YAG optical laser fibers.

THE IDEAL FIBER

An ideal fiber for holmium:YAG laser lithotripsy would have a combination of several properties. It would transmit laser energy efficiently and not lose energy through the course of its length. The connector would also need to couple well with the laser console, permitting the laser energy to launch smoothly into the fiber's core. The fiber would be robust and not fail with bending, either mechanically or during energy transmission. The tip of the fiber would be resistant to burn-back during use. The fiber would have a small diameter to limit its impact on reducing irrigation flow rate through the endoscopes and it would be highly flexible for use through flexible endoscopes. The fiber should have low insertion force through the endoscope to minimize the risk of damaging the scope during fiber insertion. Laser fiber manufacturers have attempted to create ideal fibers, but the laws of physics often dictate that compromises must occur. For example, decreasing the diameter of a fiber may result in it being more flexible with improved irrigation flow rates, but the tradeoff may be that the small tip is less resistant to burn-back. Attempting to balance the requirements of an ideal fiber has been a challenge.[3–6]

COMPONENTS OF A LASER FIBER

The laser fiber is constructed of several key components. The fibers have a core, a cladding, and a jacket (**Fig. 2**). Each of the structures plays an important role in the overall performance of the fiber.[3,7]

The silica glass core of the fibers used with the holmium:YAG laser is the laser light–transmitting portion. Ideally, laser energy should travel efficiently through the core through a process termed, *total internal reflection*. Should laser light escape outside of the core into the cladding or worse the jacket, fiber failure can occur. The core is surrounded by the cladding. The cladding may be made of similar material to the core but has a lower index of refraction, which is important for total internal reflection to occur at the boundary of the core and cladding. The jacket, or outer coating, encases the core and cladding and functions to protect the delicate glass components of the fiber. The jackets are often colored, which aids in visualizing the fiber both endoscopically and outside the patient.

LASER FIBER CORE

A range of fiber core sizes is used for holmium:YAG laser lithotripsy, from approximately 150 μm to 1000 μm. The larger 550-μm to 1000-μm core fibers are usually reserved for use through large rigid instruments, such as nephroscopes and cystoscopes, because they lack flexibility and can be too large to fit through the working channel of endoscopes used for ureteroscopy. These large core fibers are most commonly used in a straight configuration and are capable of delivering laser energy at both high–pulse energy and high frequency settings. These 550-μm to 1000-μm core fibers are robust and the basic fiber design has remained relatively static over the past decade. Rather it is with the smaller 365-μm and below core fibers that are used during ureteroscopic procedures where much of the innovation and study has occurred.

The beam profile of the holmium:YAG lasers couples best with core sizes of greater than 200 μm and ideally larger than approximately 240 μm. Smaller core sizes risk launching the laser energy into the cladding, which can damage or destroy the fiber. Manufacturers have designed ferrules that can absorb or redirect laser energy back into the core of the fiber.[3] Such designs, however, increase the complexity of the fiber connector and may be more prone to failures, such as overheating. Prior bench testing of fibers has demonstrated that fibers with core sizes less than 240 μm were more prone to failure.[6]

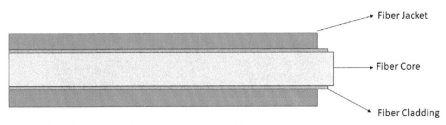

Fig. 2. Longitudinal section demonstrating components of laser fiber.

Therefore, for flexible ureteroscopy with intracorporeal lithotripsy, choosing a fiber with a core size of 240 μm to 270 μm offers a fair tradeoff between durability and size.

FIBER PERFORMANCE: TRUE DIAMETER

Knowing the true measured diameter of a laser fiber is critical in understanding how that fiber might perform. For example, a larger fiber may be less flexible and limit irrigation flow. Unfortunately, the commercial naming of laser fibers has resulted in confusion regarding how large a fiber truly is. Often urologists request a 200-μm laser fiber to use for their procedures, not necessarily understanding that the fibers are not 200 μm in overall diameter. There are few commercially available fibers that can be used for laser lithotripsy that are 200 μm in diameter. The true diameter of most fibers is significantly greater because the diameter must take into account the combination of the fiber's core, cladding, and jacket. For example, the Cook (Spencer, Indiana) HLF-S200 fiber is marketed as having a 200-μm diameter, but it is the fiber core that measures 200 μm and the true diameter of the fiber, when taking the core, cladding, and jacket into account, is approximately 374 μm. Another even more confusing example is the Boston Scientific (Marlborough, Massachusetts) Flexiva 200 fiber. Although the name of the fiber implies it is 200 μm, the core is approximately 240 μm and the true diameter of the fiber 443 μm, so no part of the fiber is 200 μm.[4] These naming schemes unfortunately have led to confusion for end users. It would be helpful for industry to post standardized specifications clearly on the fiber packaging that include fiber diameter, fiber core size, whether a fiber has a tapered or nontapered connection, a description and photo of the tip design (flat, ball, oval, and so forth), and whether it is single use or reusable. This way users could quickly review this information before selecting a fiber and have a better understanding of how it might perform. This would go a long way in lessening the current confusion that surrounds these parameters.

FIBER PERFORMANCE: FLEXIBILITY

The flexibility of a laser fiber is an important performance component for fibers used during retrograde intrarenal surgery (RIRS), especially for stones located in the lower pole. The diameter of the fiber, as well as the components used to construct the fiber, has an impact on the flexibility. A stiffer, less-flexible fiber has the potential to put added strain on the deflection mechanism of a delicate flexible ureteroscope, which could lead to premature failure of the device. Therefore, the author recommends using a fiber with a core size of 270 μm or less for RIRS.

When a selection of fibers with 240-μm to 270-μm core diameters was evaluated for flexibility, approximately 30° to 60° of baseline deflection was lost when inserted into a Stryker (Kalamazoo, Michigan) U-500 flexible ureteroscope that has 275° of baseline deflection. Fibers with a slightly smaller core size of 200 μm had slightly less deflection loss, averaging 20° to 30° of deflection loss in the U-500.[4] Therefore, if maximal deflection is needed to reach a stone, then a 200-μm core fiber may be the best option to reach the target. Prior performance testing has shown, however, that 200-μm core fibers are not as robust as fibers with core sizes of 240 μm to 270 μm, likely secondary to the tapered connectors that are often used with the smaller 200-μm fibers.[6] Therefore, a trade-off occurs, where flexibility and durability must be balanced.

FIBER PERFORMANCE: DURABILITY

Another important performance parameter of laser fibers is the resistance to fracture with bending. When lasing stones with the ureteroscope deflected, there is a potential for fiber failure, with the fiber tip breaking at the point of maximal deflection. Typically, the fibers do not fail with bending alone but rather fail when the laser is activated with the fiber in a deflected position. The concept is that, with bending, there can be a loss of total internal reflection of the laser energy within the fiber core, and, when the energy leaks into the cladding, especially the jacket, the fiber will fail due to thermal damage.[1] Both increasing the pulse energy setting of the laser and the tightness of the fiber bend increase the risk of fiber failure.[5] Should this occur during a clinical case, it could result in catastrophic damage to the flexible ureteroscope secondary to damage from the laser energy. Furthermore, the broken piece of the fiber could fall into the kidney and require extraction, which may be technically difficult. If the broken piece of fiber is not extracted, it has the potential to be a nidus for future stone formation. Prior study has shown that there are significant differences among commercially available fibers in terms of resistance to fracture with bending. As new fibers are introduced into the marketplace, independent performance evaluation is needed to ensure fiber performance can match the demands of lower-pole RIRS. Moving and displacing stones from the lower pole to an easier to access location, such as the renal pelvis or upper pole, is also a prudent strategy to reduce the risk of fiber failure. This decreases the strain on the deflection mechanism of the flexible ureteroscope and may increase the stone-free rates after the procedure.[8,9]

FIBER TIP

Historically, the tips of the laser fibers used in urology have been primarily flat. The fibers either come cleaved and polished in the original packaging from the manufacturer or are recleaved during the procedure if significant burn-back of the tip occurs. For fibers that are reusable, the fibers are cleaved and the jacket stripped from the tip prior to resterilization. The practice of stripping the fiber is to prevent the plastic components of the jacket, which do not conduct laser energy, to melt and hang off the tip of the fiber, leading to difficultly getting the fiber tip in contact with the target stone. At times the jacket can also break off in small pieces during the lithotripsy process. Some investigators, however, have challenged the concept that fiber jackets need to be stripped and that simply cutting the tip of the fiber and the jacket flush results in good performance while providing the added benefit of safer passage through a flexible ureteroscope.[10] Ultimately it may depend on the brand of laser fiber and the fiber tip coating, because, in the author's experience, there have been difficulties at times with some fibers when cut flush and the author still prefers to strip the jacket.

More recently, manufacturers have introduced modifications to the fiber tip. The most common of these is a round tip or ball tip (**Fig. 3**). By placing a ball tip on the end of the fiber, it allows for the

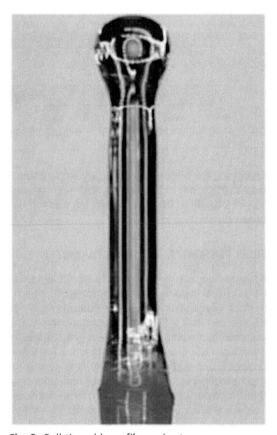

Fig. 3. Ball-tipped laser fiber prior to use.

fiber to be passed with less resistance through a flexible ureteroscope. The concept is that the ball tip slides more freely in the working channel of the ureteroscope and is less likely to dig in or gouge the delicate inner lining. During a procedure, a ball tip allows a fiber to be advanced through the channel with the ureteroscope in a deflected position, something not recommended with a flat tip fiber. This may be helpful when there is a difficult-to-reach lower pole stone and the surgeon does not want to pull the ureteroscope out of the lower pole to advance the fiber once the target is identified. A recent study compared the force needed to insert a series of ball/round tip fibers through a flexible ureteroscope and confirmed that the force needed was significantly less than a traditional flat tip fiber.[11] It is important to understand that the protection the ball tip offers should only be considered present during the first pass of the fiber through the ureteroscopy. Once the laser has been activated and pulses delivered, burn-back of the ball tip fiber is expected to occur. As the ball tip burns back, it loses the protective effect when passed through the ureteroscope working channel.

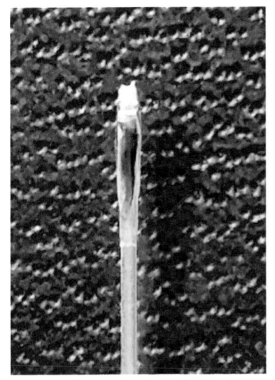

Fig. 4. Laser fiber showing burn-back of the fiber tip and charring of the jacket.

The question has been raised whether changing the tip configuration of a fiber from a flat tip to a ball tip design has an impact on the ablative properties during laser lithotripsy. Several studies have evaluated this and determined that the ablative properties were not impacted positively or negatively.[12,13]

FIBER BURN-BACK

During laser lithotripsy, the tip of the laser fiber burns back variable amounts based on multiple factors (**Fig. 4**). Burn-back during a procedure might result in having to pause the procedure to reprepare the fiber tip or it may lead to more difficulties efficiently ablating the target stone if the burnt-back jacket of the fiber interferes with the fiber core establishing good contact with the target stone. Although all the factors that contribute to fiber burn-back may not yet be fully understood, several factors have been reported to have an impact on the rate that the fiber burns back during the procedure.

Higher pulse energy setting on the holmium:YAG laser results in more rapid burn-back of the fiber tip. Traditional fragmenting settings, where the pulse energy is set at 0.6 J to 1.0 J, results in more rapid deterioration of the fiber tip as opposed to dusting setting using lower pulse energy settings of 0.2 J to 0.3 J. The density or hardness of the stone is also a contributing factor to fiber burn-back. A dense, hard stone has a greater detrimental effect on the fiber tip than a softer stone.[14–16] Another factor that impacts the rate of fiber burn-back is the pulse duration of the holmium:YAG laser. Initially, commercially available holmium:YAG lasers did not have variable pulse duration and were considered to have short pulse duration. Now numerous manufacturers are offering laser consoles with variable pulse duration, where the end user can select the pulse duration. Pulse duration seems to have an impact on the rate of laser fiber burn-back. At the same pulse energy settings, longer pulse duration decreases that rate of burn-back and shorter pulse duration increases the rate burn-back.[15,17]

The clinical relevance of the laser settings having an impact on fiber burn-back may vary depending on the stone size. For example, if a smaller 5-mm stone is rapidly fragmented with several pulses of the laser into 3 to 4 pieces that can be retrieved with a basket, then the burn-back of the fiber might never become a factor. If fragmentation settings are used on a very large hard stone, however, then the fiber might need to be cleaved and/or stripped multiple times during the procedure. To best use a strategy of preservation of the fiber tip and limiting fiber burn-back, a low pulse energy setting (ie, dusting setting) of 0.2 J to 0.3 J is selected, coupled with a higher pulse frequency and a long pulse duration. The author uses these settings at the start of RIRS laser lithotripsy procedures and then adjusts the settings as needed to get the desired clinical effect.

SINGLE USE VERSUS REUSABLE

Currently, there is a wide range of commercially available laser fibers, with both single-use and reusable variants available. Historically, reusable fibers were more costly to purchase, but with repeated use, the cost is amortized over the life of the fiber, and reusable fibers can be more cost-effective than single-use variants.[18] In general terms, performance between single-use and reusable fibers has been similar, although there have been examples where the reusable version from a manufacturer outperformed their single-use version.[5,6] In recent years, a shift has begun to occur, with some laser fiber manufacturers focusing on high-cost, single-use fibers. An example of this is the Boston Scientific Flexiva and Flexiva TracTip 200 fiber line. These fibers have a 240-μm core size, eliminating the need for a taper, and the TracTip variant has a ball tip with a proprietary coating on it. The fibers are single use only and reusable variants are not available. These fibers sit at the high end of the price spectrum for holmium:YAG fibers but have been shown to have excellent performance characteristics.[19] With the increasing focus on cost-effectiveness, the potential for bundled payments, and the ongoing rising costs of health care, it is becoming increasingly challenging to balance costs of flexible ureteroscopy with efficiency and performance. Physicians and administrators need to make difficult decisions in the future. Is it better to use a costly single-use ureteroscope and a less expensive laser fiber because damaging the channel of a single-use scope is less of a concern? Or should a premium single-use fiber be used with a reusable ureteroscope to reduce the risk of fiber damage to the ureteroscope and hence reduce overall repair costs? There may not be one correct answer to these question, but future work likely will help determine which options are both the most efficacious and cost-effective.

OPEN VERSUS CLOSED PLATFORMS

When the holmium:YAG laser was first introduced to clinical practice in urology, a majority of laser platforms were open, meaning that fibers from different manufacturers could be used with different laser consoles. In most circumstances, the fibers were compatible with various consoles, but some exceptions occurred, including an apparent incompatibility of a Trimedyne (Irvine, California) fiber with a Lumenis (Yokneam, Israel) and New Star (Roseville, California) holmium:YAG laser.[20] Although some manufacturers focus on the production and sales of both laser consoles and fibers, other manufacturers have focused strictly on fiber production and sales. This has led to a robust marketplace with numerous innovative designs. More recently there has been a trend of laser console manufacturers to lock down their consoles and only allow use of their own fibers with the platform. This typically is done with radiofrequency identification (RFID) tags embedded into the fiber connector. Without the correct RFID tag, the laser console does not activate. The argument from these manufacturers is that it ensures a consistent level of performance from their system and that the fiber performance can be internally validated by the manufacturer with its own console. It also ensures, however, that the manufacturer of the console can profit from the lucrative laser fiber sales, especially with the trend toward higher-priced single-use fibers. From a consumer standpoint, locking down consoles may stifle innovation, given that the smaller fiber-only manufacturers may become locked out of the business completely. This would lead to less competition, less bargaining power, less innovation, and likely higher prices.

MULTIPULSE TECHNOLOGY

Recently multipulse holmium:YAG systems have been introduced. Lumenis is the first platform to the market and has dubbed this technology, Moses. Although the exact details of the mechanism have not been fully reported, it seems to work by using a double pulse of the laser. The first pulse is delivered to create a vapor channel to the stone and then the second pulse contacts the target stone and provides the lithotripsy effect. Reports demonstrate the potential for reduced retropulsion and greater ablation efficiency compared with standard short-pulse modes.[21] Currently, Moses technology is available only on the top-tier MOSES Pulse™ 120H (Lumenis, Yokneam, Israel)" laser, which requires 50-amp electrical service. In addition, to use the Moses mode, a proprietary fiber is needed. These fibers contain an RFID transmitter in the connector that permits activation of the Moses mode. It is unclear at this time if the Moses mode would function with other fibers because an unlocked Moses platform is not commercially available. The cost of the Moses fiber is at the high end of the pricing spectrum and investigators have questioned the cost-effectiveness of the system.[22] This is an area to follow closely over the next several years as other manufacturers inevitably enter the market.

SUMMARY

The optical laser fibers used for holmium:YAG laser lithotripsy have evolved over the years but differences in fiber performance continue to exist. Reviewing the available data on fiber performance and selecting fibers that are more robust and less likely to fracture during use may lead to lower ureteroscope repair rates. Understanding the true fiber diameter and its impact on fiber flexibility and flow rates helps set expectations of performance for the fiber during clinical use. The introduction of ball-tipped laser fibers does not seem to have improved the ablation efficiency of the fiber, but it provides an important benefit of smooth passage through a ureteroscope channel with a lower propensity to damage the channel. Fiber burn-back can occur during laser lithotripsy, but by using a strategy of lower pulse energy settings coupled with long pulse duration, the degree of burn-back can be minimized. A trend toward single-use laser fibers and RFID-equipped fibers that lock out competitors' fibers from holmium:YAG laser consoles is occurring.

REFERENCES

1. Marks AJ, Teichman JM. Lasers in clinical urology: state of the art and new horizons. World J Urol 2007;25(3):227–33.
2. Kronenberg P, Somani B. Advances in lasers for the treatment of stones-a systematic review. Curr Urol Rep 2018;19(6):45.
3. Nazif OA, Teichman JM, Glickman RD, et al. Review of laser fibers: a practical guide for urologists. J Endourol 2004;18(9):818–29.
4. Akar EC, Knudsen BE. Evaluation of 16 new holmium:yttrium-aluminum-garnet laser optical fibers for ureteroscopy. Urology 2015;86(2):230–5.
5. Knudsen BE, Glickman RD, Stallman KJ, et al. Performance and safety of holmium: YAG laser optical fibers. J Endourol 2005;19(9):1092–7.
6. Mues AC, Teichman JM, Knudsen BE. Evaluation of 24 holmium:YAG laser optical fibers for flexible ureteroscopy. J Urol 2009;182(1):348–54.
7. Fried NM, Irby PB. Advances in laser technology and fibre-optic delivery systems in lithotripsy. Nat Rev Urol 2018;15(9):563–73.
8. Auge BK, Dahm P, Wu NZ, et al. Ureteroscopic management of lower-pole renal calculi: technique of calculus displacement. J Endourol 2001;15(8):835–8.
9. Wolf JS Jr. Ureteroscopic treatment of lower pole calculi: comparison of lithotripsy in situ and after displacement. Int Braz J Urol 2002;28(4):367–8.
10. Kronenberg P, Traxer O. Are we all doing it wrong? Influence of stripping and cleaving methods of laser fibers on laser lithotripsy performance. J Urol 2015;193(3):1030–5.
11. Nguyen A, Jain, R, Rose, E, et al. PD46-06 Mechanical, physical and performance characteristics of Holmium:YAG optical fibers for flexible ureteroscopy. Paper presented at: AUA Annual Meeting. San Francisco, CA May 18–21, 2018.
12. Kronenberg P, Traxer O. Lithotripsy performance of specially designed laser fiber tips. J Urol 2016;195(5):1606–12.
13. Shin RH, Lautz JM, Cabrera FJ, et al. Evaluation of novel ball-tip holmium laser fiber: impact on ureteroscope performance and fragmentation efficiency. J Endourol 2016;30(2):189–94.
14. Haddad M, Emiliani E, Rouchausse Y, et al. Impact of the curve diameter and laser settings on laser fiber fracture. J Endourol 2017;31(9):918–21.
15. Kronenberg P, Traxer O. Update on lasers in urology 2014: current assessment on holmium:yttrium-aluminum-garnet (Ho:YAG) laser lithotripter settings and laser fibers. World J Urol 2015;33(4):463–9.
16. Mues AC, Teichman JM, Knudsen BE. Quantification of holmium:yttrium aluminum garnet optical tip degradation. J Endourol 2009;23(9):1425–8.
17. Wollin DA, Ackerman A, Yang C, et al. Variable pulse duration from a new holmium:YAG laser: the effect on stone comminution, fiber tip degradation, and retropulsion in a dusting model. Urology 2017;103: 47–51.
18. Knudsen BE, Pedro R, Hinck B, et al. Durability of reusable holmium:YAG laser fibers: a multicenter study. J Urol 2011;185(1):160–3.
19. Khemees TA, Shore DM, Antiporda M, et al. Evaluation of a new 240-mum single-use holmium:YAG optical fiber for flexible ureteroscopy. J Endourol 2013; 27(4):475–9.
20. Marks AJ, Mues AC, Knudsen BE, et al. Holmium:yttrium-aluminum-garnet lithotripsy proximal fiber failures from laser and fiber mismatch. Urology 2008; 71(6):1049–51.
21. Elhilali MM, Badaan S, Ibrahim A, et al. Use of the moses technology to improve holmium laser lithotripsy outcomes: a preclinical study. J Endourol 2017;31(6):598–604.
22. Stern KL, Monga M. The Moses holmium system - time is money. Can J Urol 2018;25(3):9313–6.

Emerging Laser Techniques for the Management of Stones

Ali H. Aldoukhi, MBBS, MS[a],*, Kristian M. Black, BS[a],
Khurshid R. Ghani, MBChB, MS, FRCS[b]

KEYWORDS

- Ureteroscopy • Laser • Dusting • Fragmentation • Holmium • Moses

KEY POINTS

- Modern holmium lasers allow the selection of multiple parameters, such as pulse energy, frequency, pulse width, and modulation, that can help optimize lithotripsy efficiency.
- Dusting uses settings of low pulse energy and high frequency to break down stones using dancing, painting, and chipping strategies.
- Fragmentation and retrieval uses settings of high pulse energy and low frequency to break stones into extractable fragments.
- Noncontact laser lithotripsy (popcorn technique) is used to pulverize stones into very small fragments; optimal parameters include high frequency, keeping the fiber in close proximity to the stone, and performing it in a small calyx.
- The Moses technology is a pulse modulation method for the holmium laser that delivers energy over 2 pulses in order to reduce retropulsion and increase fragmentation.

INTRODUCTION

Treatment of kidney stones has developed over the years from open lithotomy to minimally invasive endoscopic lithotripsy.[1] Because of advances in endoscope design and miniaturization, along with the development of highly effective surgical lasers, ureteroscopy (URS) and laser lithotripsy has become the predominant method for urinary stone treatment in North America.[2] The holmium:yttrium-aluminum-garnet (Ho:YAG) laser is the most widely used laser for URS, with modern systems providing users with a range of settings and parameters that have numerous effects on stone fragmentation. In particular, next-generation Ho:YAG systems have led to the development and widespread adoption of techniques such as dusting whereby fragments are left in situ for spontaneous passage, in contrast with the conventional method of fragmentation and active fragment retrieval.[3] Advanced Ho:YAG technologies have been introduced, such as the Moses technology, a pulse modulation mode that improves holmium laser energy transmission through water.[4] In addition, the thulium fiber laser (TFL) is a new, solid-state, diode-pumped laser that may provide urologists with increased options for stone treatment.[5] This review article discusses the technical parameters and methods for laser lithotripsy, outlines strategies and settings for different scenarios, and introduces the new technologies in this rapidly evolving field.

Disclosure: K.R. Ghani is a consultant for Boston Scientific and Lumenis; K.R. Ghani has a scientific investigator grant from Boston Scientific.
[a] Department of Urology, University of Michigan, Medical Sciences Unit I, 1301 Catherine Street, Room 4432, Ann Arbor, MI 48109, USA; [b] Department of Urology, University of Michigan, NCRC Building 16, Room 114W, 2800 Plymouth Road, Ann Arbor, MI 48109, USA
* Corresponding author.
E-mail address: ahaldouk@med.umich.edu

Urol Clin N Am 46 (2019) 193–205
https://doi.org/10.1016/j.ucl.2018.12.005

HOLMIUM LASER

The Ho:YAG laser is a solid-state, flashlamp-pumped pulsed laser, and is the current standard for lithotripsy during URS, partly because of its excellent safety profile, its ability to fragment stones of any composition, and use of small laser fibers that permit endoscope irrigation and flexibility.[6,7] Because its wavelength is 2120 nm, it is highly absorbed in water, with a low penetration depth that limits the amount of energy reaching surrounding tissue.[8] Laser activation causes the release of energy from the fiber tip, creating a vapor channel allowing for direct absorbance of radiation by the stone. This direct irradiance leads to a photothermal reaction that causes chemical decomposition of the calculus.[6] Although collapse of the cavitation bubble has been noted to generate shockwaves, they do not significantly contribute to total fragmentation.[6]

The process of ablation and fragmentation are highly dependent on the total power (Watts) delivered to the stone, which is a product of the pulse energy (PE) and frequency (**Fig. 1**). Although original Ho:YAG lasers were low-power systems (15–20 W), modern systems can accommodate greater power. To achieve higher power, the systems require multiple laser rods and cavities, giving rise to the term multicavity laser. Initially developed for prostate surgery, which requires increased energy for cutting and coagulation, these systems permit higher frequencies. As a result, the use of high-power systems for laser lithotripsy has increased, with one recent survey showing that 41% of endourologists used 100-W machines.[3] At present, the highest power available is the 120-W system.[9] Next-generation systems also allow pulse width (PW) manipulation to either short-pulse (SP) or long-pulse (LP) modes. Altering the PE, frequency, and PW, in addition to new parameters related to pulse modulation, can affect stone ablation, retropulsion, and laser fiber tip degradation.[10] Adjusting these parameters can optimize lithotripsy and improve the efficiency of fragmentation.

Pulse Energy

PE, measured in joules (J), is the total optical energy emitted from the laser fiber tip in 1 pulse. The amount of PE available depends on the power of the holmium system, with ranges from 0.2 to 6.0 J. For URS, PE typically ranges from 0.2 to 2.0 J depending on the technique and stone durility. Stone ablation volume and fragment size increase proportionally to the PE setting.[11,12] Higher PE (>0.5 J) produces larger fragments that are ideal for removal using retrieval devices.

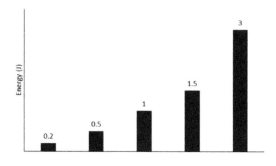

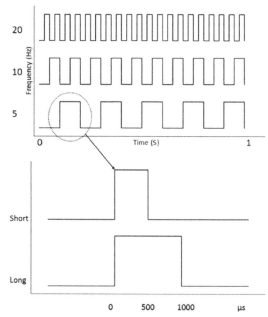

Fig. 1. Holmium laser settings that are adjusted during laser lithotripsy: pulse frequency, PE, and pulse width. (*From* Aldoukhi AH, Roberts WW, Hall TL, et al. Holmium laser lithotripsy in the new stone age: dust or bust? Front Surg 2017;4:57; with permission.)

Higher PE may have more impact on ablation volume than increasing the total power, although this relationship has only been shown in a single study.[13] Low-PE (LoPE) settings produce smaller fragments and are optimal for techniques such as dusting, a method that relies on breaking stones into tiny fragments. In an evaluation of multiple stone types, using a PE of 0.2 J to break the stone led to less than 1-mm fragments most of the time.[12]

There are several drawbacks to using higher PE, including greater laser fiber tip degradation[14] and stone retropulsion,[12,15] which can hinder ablation efficiency and procedure time. Retropulsion decreases efficiency by increasing the distance between the fiber tip and stone, resulting in less energy reaching the stone.[16] Time is also lost trying to maintain contact with the stone as it moves.

Frequency

Frequency, measured in hertz (Hz), is the number of pulses emitted from the laser fiber per second. If the PE is kept constant and the frequency increases, fragmentation rates can increase.[17,18] Studies assessing the effect of increasing frequency on retropulsion but where power remains constant, are limited. In one recent study, increasing the frequency from 15 to 50 Hz when using LoPE at 0.2 J had a negligible effect on retropulsion.[18] Another study also noted that frequency had a minimal effect on net retropulsion when PE and fiber diameter were kept constant.[19] High-power holmium lasers can now achieve frequencies up to 80 Hz, supporting techniques such as high-frequency dusting.[9]

Pulse Width

PW, also described as pulse duration or length, is defined as the duration of the single optical pulse emitted from the fiber tip. Ho:YAG systems have traditionally used a single fixed SP mode ranging from 150 to 350 μs. Next-generation systems are equipped with LP modes ranging from 500 to 1300 μs. Compared with SP, LP delivers the same amount of total energy but it is delivered over a longer period of time (see **Fig. 1**).

A major advantage of using LP is decreased retropulsion of the stone, which can offset the negative effects higher PE may have on retropulsion.[20–22] Reductions in retropulsion of 30% to 50% have been reported when using LP.[22] This reduction is partly caused by the geometry of the ablation crater, because LP mode creates deeper, more narrow craters that cause less retropulsion.[22] In addition, LP reduces laser fiber tip degradation, also known as burnback,[10,21] which is a result of thermal shock, and chemical and mechanical breakdown of the silica fiber.[23] Burnback decreases fiber length and energy delivered to the stone, thus decreasing lithotripsy efficiency. Most studies have not reported a difference in ablation when comparing SP with LP.[21,24,25] Although a few studies have shown that SP is superior, this may be attributed to differences in experimental setup; even so, the differences are small.[22,26] **Table 1** summarizes the different effects of changing these parameters on outcomes.

Other Technical Parameters Affecting Laser Lithotripsy

Two other factors that affect fragmentation are the laser fiber size, and the fiber tip to stone working distance. Smaller core diameter fibers are associated with more retropulsion compared with larger core fibers. This difference is caused by the small recoil momentum for the small fibers.[15,22] Fragmentation is similar among the fiber sizes when using low pulse energies ($\leq$1.0 J) but greater for larger fibers when using higher pulse energies.[23,27]

The fiber tip to stone working distance has implications on lithotripsy efficiency because energy from the holmium laser is highly absorbed in water.[6–8] The greatest fragmentation occurs when the laser is activated while in contact with the stone, and, if the fiber tip distance increases, it reduces fragmentation efficacy because the energy reaching the stone diminishes as the distance between the laser fiber and stone increases.[8] The authors have found that fragmentation volume is reduced by as much as 40% when 1 J is applied with the laser fiber positioned just 1 mm away from the stone, with no fragmentation occurring at 3 mm.[28]

TECHNIQUES FOR URETEROSCOPIC STONE SURGERY

The goal of laser lithotripsy during URS is to either break stones into smaller fragments that can be retrieved with ancillary devices, commonly known

---

Table 1
Relationship of changing pulse energy, frequency, and pulse width on laser lithotripsy outcomes

Parameter	Definition	Unit	Parameter Change	Ablation Volume	Retropulsion	Fiber Tip Degradation
Pulse energy	Total laser energy content emitted in a single optical pulse	Joules	Increase	↑	↑	↑
			Decrease	↓	↓	↓
Frequency	Number of pulses emitted per second	Hertz	Increase	↑	=/↑	↑ (if power increased)
			Decrease	↓	No Effect	No effect
PW	Length of 1 emitted pulse	Microseconds	SP	=	↑	↑
			LP	=	↓	↓

as fragmentation and basketing or active retrieval, or into very fine fragments that are left in situ for spontaneous passage. The latter technique is termed dusting. The strategy used depends on stone and patient characteristics, anatomic location, available equipment, and surgeon experience and preference. Although there may be a dichotomy in strategy, modern urologists need to be facile in both methods. When treating larger renal stones, an approach that initially uses dusting followed by retrieval of larger fragments may be necessary. A hybrid technique consisting of both strategies may provide the greatest versatility for the range of scenarios commonly encountered during laser lithotripsy.

Fragmentation and Retrieval

Fragmentation uses low-frequency and high-PE (LoFr-HiPE) settings (eg, 0.8–1.2 J × 6–10 Hz) to break stones into fragments small enough to be extracted until no extractable fragments remain. When selecting PE, it is common to start at a setting between 0.6 and 1.0 J, increasing as necessary for harder stones.[29] This method optimizes lithotripsy efficiency by discovering the lowest effective PE setting for that particular stone and size, especially because fiber tip

burnback and retropulsion increase with higher PE.[12,14,15] To perform this technique, the laser fiber tip should be kept at the center of the stone, pinning it against the urothelial wall, while firing intermittently.[30] This positioning allows the stone to break into equal-sized fragments and also decreases the risk of damage to the urothelial wall (**Fig. 2**).

Stone location, density, and volume are factors to consider when selecting a fragmentation and retrieval method. For nonimpacted mobile stones in the lower ureter, fragmentation may be a better option, because this location easily permits retrieval of fragments with a basket. The density of the stone may be calculated on a computed tomography (CT) scan (Hounsfield units), which can act as a guide in the selection of lithotripsy technique and whether a ureteral access sheath (UAS) to facilitate retrieval will be required. Hard stones may be difficult to ablate using a dusting technique. Stone volume dictates the number of repeated passages of the ureteroscope to remove a stone, whereas the size of the UAS influences the maximum size of the fragment that can be extracted in a basket (**Fig. 3**). For large stones, the number of scope passages needed for complete active retrieval can be daunting.

Painting

When: Best for softer stones

How: Place fiber in contact with stone, brush back and fourth across stone, ablating layer by layer

Chipping

When: Best for harder stones

How: Place fiber in contact with edge of stone and hold steady as small chips fragment off

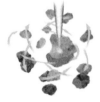

Popcorning

When: Best for group of 3–4 mm fragments in a nondilated calyx

How: Place fiber near stone, but not in contact with the urothelium. Deliver intermittent laser bursts causing movement of stones and fine fragmentation

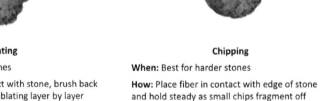

Fragmenting

When: Best for single stones

How: Place fiber in contact with stone and pin against the urothelium. Focus fiber on one point until the stone breaks

Fig. 2. Laser lithotripsy technique options during retrograde intrarenal surgery.

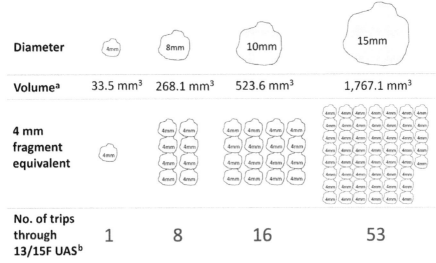

Diameter	4mm	8mm	10mm	15mm
Volume[a]	33.5 mm³	268.1 mm³	523.6 mm³	1,767.1 mm³
4 mm fragment equivalent				
No. of trips through 13/15F UAS[b]	1	8	16	53

Fig. 3. The effect of stone size on stone volume on retrieval, and estimated number of trips needed to remove fragments through a 13/15-Fr UAS. [a] Spherical stone volume $V = \frac{4}{3}\pi r^3$. [b] 13/15-Fr UAS can accommodate a 4-mm stone.

Dusting Technique

Dusting uses high-frequency and low-PE (HiFr-LoPE) settings (eg, 0.2–0.5 J × 20–80 Hz) to break stones into submillimeter fragments. With this strategy, tiny stone particles are ejected that float in the irrigating fluid,[31] as well as dependent fragments of various sizes. The aim when executing a dusting technique is to incorporate a setting parameter so that most of the fragments breaking off the stone are as small as possible, thereby maximizing the goal of complete passage of fragments. The development of Ho:YAG systems with HiFr-LoPE settings has made dusting a popular technique. Dusting settings were used by 67% of endourologists in a recent survey of Endourology Society members.[3] The benefits and drawbacks of dusting compared with fragmentation and retrieval are listed in **Table 2**.

Table 2
Advantages and disadvantages of dusting and retrieval techniques for ureteroscopic laser lithotripsy

Method	Advantages	Disadvantages
Dusting	• Produces smaller fragments • Avoids routine use of UAS, and thus reduces risk of ureteral trauma • Shorter operation time • No need for assistant • Avoids routine postoperative stenting • Able to offer treatment in cases of failed UAS insertion	• Requires next-generation laser system (high capital equipment cost) • May not be suitable for hard stones (eg, calcium oxalate monohydrate) • Stone-free rate may depend on surgeon skill • Concern for fragment drainage in certain patients (eg, spinal cord injury) • May result in no fragment for analysis
Fragmentation and basket retrieval	• Uses low-power laser system (low capital equipment cost) • Ability to extract complete stone in noncomplicated cases • Suitable for hard stones • Able to send fragments for composition analysis	• Produces larger fragments • Longer operation time • Higher disposable costs • Need for assistant • Risk of ureteral injury from using UAS • Routine ureteral stenting if using access sheath

Adapted from Aldoukhi AH, Roberts WW, Hall TL, et al. Holmium laser lithotripsy in the new stone age: dust or bust? Front Surg 2017;4:57; with permission.

When treating renal stones, a complete dusting technique consists of 2 phases: contact laser lithotripsy, followed by noncontact laser lithotripsy. Contact laser lithotripsy is the initial debulking step, in which the laser fiber tip is placed on the stone surface and fired, keeping the stone intact and reducing its overall size by ejecting tiny fragments. Later, it is inevitable that the stone will end up breaking into smaller fragments. These pieces can then be dealt with using noncontact laser lithotripsy, also known as popcorning, which is achieved by firing the fiber tip away from the stone surface in an enclosed area such as the renal calyx.

Contact laser lithotripsy

Dancing and chipping are techniques used during the contact phase of dusting (see **Fig. 2**).[30] Dancing is accomplished by sweeping the laser fiber tip horizontally across the face of the stone in a painting motion while firing continuously. Ideally, ablation of the stone surface should be uniform, with the goal to interrogate parts of the stone that project forward, so that it is debulked and shaved in a careful manner taking extra precaution in the center of the stone to avoid it fracturing and breaking into large chunks. For hard stones, a chipping technique can be used by constantly firing with the laser tip positioned at the outer edge of the stone. As small chips (usually measuring <1 mm) break off, they expose new surfaces. Targeting these surfaces allows the stone to rotate in a pottery wheel–like fashion until the bulk of the stone has been reduced in size. An important principle when undertaking contact phase dusting is that the initial laser setting may need to be modified as the stone is dusted and decreases in size. If the stone begins to wobble, reducing the PE or frequency can improve lithotripsy efficiency.[9] Once the stone breaks into smaller fragments, they are extracted or undergo noncontact laser lithotripsy to become even smaller fragments, which are left in situ for spontaneous passage.[30]

Noncontact laser lithotripsy

During this phase, stone fragments are pulverized in a calyx with the laser activated in bursts away from the stone, resulting in a whirlpool-like effect and stone disintegration as the fragments come into direct contact with the laser tip (see **Fig. 2**). The technique allows the surgeon to not spend time repositioning the laser on the stone between pulses. Described as the popcorn effect because of the chaotic and noisy movement of fragments, it was first studied by Chawla and colleagues.[32] The optimal settings for popcorning have been studied by multiple investigators.[32–36] In general, studies show a trend of superior fragmentation when using settings with higher power output. Chawla and colleagues[32] reported that 1.5 J × 40 Hz (60 W) resulted in a 63% decrease in stone mass compared with 42% when using 1.0 J × 20 Hz (20 W). Emiliani and colleagues[33] showed that the most significant predictors of efficiency were higher frequencies (40 Hz vs 20 Hz), higher PE (1.5 J vs 0.5 J), and longer time (4 minutes vs 2 minutes). Klaver and colleagues[34] confirmed that popcorning is more effective if performed with more fragments. Recently, Wollin and colleagues[35] showed that settings of 0.5 J × 40 Hz (20 W) and 0.5 J × 80 Hz (40 W) performed best for popcorning.

The authors have investigated parameters that influence outcomes during popcorning and found several important factors. First, using settings with higher pulse frequencies results in better fragmentation outcomes. For example, popcorning for 3 minutes at a setting of 0.5 J × 80 Hz (on SP) resulted in significantly greater submillimeter fragmentation compared with popcorning for 6 minutes at a setting of 1 J × 20 Hz (on either SP or LP).[36] In our clinical experience with the 120-W system, we use 0.5 J × 80 Hz as our default setting for popcorning, which we have called popdusting.[9,37] We have also found that fragmentation improves when the laser fiber is positioned closer to the stone surface compared with the traditional method of placing the fiber away from the stone. Furthermore, popcorning is more effective if performed in a small calyceal model compared with a larger one (**Fig. 4**).[36] However, one important factor to consider when popcorning is heat generation. Several studies have reported that temperatures can increase to high levels when using high power settings and low irrigation rates.[38–41] Temperature increases are mitigated if measures such as intermittent laser firing, higher irrigation rates, or use of cooled irrigation are incorporated. A guide to laser settings for the various techniques of dusting and fragmentation based on Ho:YAG power parameters is provided in **Table 3**.

DUSTING VERSUS RETRIEVAL: OUTCOMES

There are limited clinical data comparing fragmentation and retrieval with dusting techniques for URS. In the only randomized study, Schatloff and colleagues[42] compared the two techniques for treating ureteral stones and did not find a significant difference in stone-free rates (SFRs) between the two groups. However, unplanned visits were higher in the group that were left with ureteral fragments for spontaneous passage. A critique of this

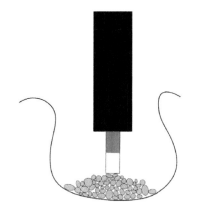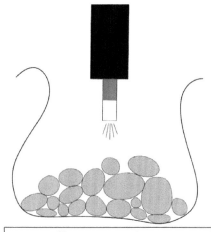

Effective technique	Ineffective technique
• Fiber in contact with stones	• Fiber away from stones (>2 mm)
• Higher frequency (>40 Hz)	• Lower frequency (≤20 Hz)
• Small calyx	• Large calyx

Fig. 4. Factors that should be considered when performing the popcorn technique.

early study is that the technique did not incorporate LoPE dusting settings with fragments broken down to 2 mm in size, and not fine fragments. Also, there may be limited advantages to dusting ureteral stones because this is a location that easily permits basket retrieval.

More recently, the Endourology Disease Group For Excellence (EDGE) research consortium conducted a multi-institutional prospective study comparing fragmentation and retrieval with the dusting technique for renal stones treated at high-volume centers in North America.[43] Patients with radiopaque renal stones measuring 5 to 20 mm were recruited, with 68 in the dusting group

and 82 in the retrieval group. Patients received postprocedural ureteral stents and α-blockers for 30 days. The primary outcome was no residual fragments (RFs) on radiographs and/or ultrasonography at 4 to 6 weeks postoperatively. The SFR was higher for the retrieval group (74.7% vs 58.1%); however, this difference was not significant on multivariate analysis. Although operative time was significantly longer for the retrieval group, there were no differences in symptomatic RFs, complications, or reintervention rates.

Limitations of the EDGE study included significantly larger stones in patients undergoing dusting, which may confound the SFR results. Also,

Table 3
Dusting and fragmentation settings for ureteroscopy based on holmium:yttrium-aluminum-garnet power

Ho:YAG System Power	Low 20 W	Medium 30–60 W	High 80–100 W	High 120 W Moses
Fragmenting	0.8–1.2 J × 6–8 Hz SP	1.0–1.2 J × 6–8 Hz LP[a]	1.0–1.2 J × 6–8 Hz LP	1.0–1.4 J × 8 Hz MC
Dusting (ureteral stone)	0.5 J × 10 Hz SP	0.2 J × 15–20 Hz LP[a]	0.2–0.3 J × 30 Hz LP	0.2–0.3 J × 30 Hz MC
Dusting (renal stone)	0.5 J × 15 Hz SP	0.2 J × 20–25 Hz LP[a]	0.2–0.3 J × 50 Hz LP	0.3–0.4 J × 50–70 Hz MD
Popcorning	1 J × 15 Hz SP	1 J × 15–20 Hz LP[a]	0.5 J × 50 Hz SP or 1 J × 30 Hz LP	0.5 J × 80 Hz SP

Abbreviations: LP, long pulse; MC, Moses contact; MD, Moses distance; SP, short pulse.
[a] If variable PW selection available, use LP. Some medium-power systems are unable to go lower than 0.5 J.

the laser specifications for the dusting technique were not specified and it is not clear whether it was performed with the HiFr-LoPE technique. The investigators concluded that retrieval results in a higher SFR at the expense of longer procedure time and greater use of the UAS (100% vs 16% for dusting), which may increase total procedural cost.

Tracey and colleagues[9] recently reported a retrospective series on outcomes of dusting technique using HiFr-LoPE settings in 71 patients. PE setting in this study ranged between 0.2 and 0.5 J with frequency between 50 and 80 Hz. Stone clearance with less than 2-mm RFs was 74% and the zero-fragment rate was 62%. A limitation of this study, as well as the EDGE study, is that CT was not exclusively used to determine the SFR. When using CT, studies assessing fragmentation and retrieval techniques have reported zero-fragment rates between 55% and 60%.[44] More recently, Canvasser and colleagues[45] showed the limitations of basketing, obtaining a complete SFR of only 55% after fastidious retrieval in a prospective cohort of 104 patients in a high-volume center. The limited data comparing dusting and basketing techniques so far do not suggest superiority for any method.[9,43,46] Each technique has its advantages and disadvantages, and modern stone surgeons should be familiar with both methods. In select cases, a dusting technique offers the option of stentless URS, whereas retrieval with a UAS often necessitates a ureteral stent. The decision as to which strategy is used should be made based on the clinical scenario and the available resources.[47] A combination of the two techniques may be needed to optimize outcomes, cost, time, and morbidity. Regardless of technique, CT-based studies have shown that complete SFRs are suboptimal and future directions will focus on suction or stabilization devices that can enhance laser strategies.

LASER TECHNIQUES FOR ENDOSCOPIC BLADDER STONE SURGERY

Ho:YAG lasers are commonly used as an energy source for bladder stone fragmentation during transurethral surgery and several studies have reported on treatment results.[48–51] Teichman and colleagues[51] reported the first series of the Ho:YAG laser for the cystoscopic treatment of large bladder calculi greater than 4 cm using settings of 0.6 to 1.4 J and 6 to 15 Hz. Since these early reports, high-power Ho:YAG systems have been introduced, which have improved the setting options for fragmentation. The use of higher frequencies can help reduce the procedure time compared

with low-watt systems in which frequency is limited to 15 to 20 Hz. Because of the large size of these stones, and the larger outflow channel and irrigation with the cystoscope, higher PE and power can be used to fragment stones and still achieve a dusting effect. Although fragmentation of large and hard stones may have been arduous with the Ho:YAG, we have found these stones can now be tackled safely as an ambulatory procedure in a single stage with high-power systems.

LASER TECHNIQUES FOR PERCUTANEOUS RENAL STONE SURGERY

For patients with stone burdens greater than 2 cm or those with staghorn calculi, percutaneous nephrolithotomy (PCNL) is the gold standard treatment.[52,53] Although the workhorse for lithotripsy during PCNL has been the ultrasonic and/or pneumatic device, an early handpiece proved the utility of combined suction with a holmium laser fiber to permit simultaneous lithotripsy and suction of fragments.[54] Since then, the introduction of dedicated laser suction devices has made the holmium laser a viable energy source for fragmentation during PCNL.

The LithAssist (Cook Medical, Bloomington, IN) is a disposable handheld suction device with an 11.6-Fr dual-lumen stainless steel cannula. The laser fiber can be passed through a 5-Fr inner lumen with the remaining space used for suction. In an in vitro study comparing this device with the Swiss LithoClast Ultra, it was found to work especially well for harder-composition stones.[55] The laser suction handpiece (LSHP; Lumenis, San Jose, CA) is specifically designed for the 120-W holmium laser and can be used to fragment and suck stones using laser fiber sizes ranging from 200 to 550 μm.[56] It has a 12-Fr suction channel and the fiber is held in a separate working channel, in contrast with the dual-lumen configuration of the LithAssist. The feasibility of the LSHP and a dusting technique to treat staghorn calculi using both rigid and flexible endoscopy with the same laser fiber has been shown.[57] More clinical studies are needed to evaluate the full potential of laser suction devices for PCNL. For centers with limited resources, the Ho:YAG can serve as the energy source for all types of stone surgery.

NEW TECHNOLOGY
Moses Platform for Holmium Laser Lithotripsy

One of the recent advances in holmium lasers is the Moses technology. The term Moses in relation to laser ablation was first used when investigating the interaction between laser energy and fluid medium.[58] Isner and colleagues[58] described the bubble that forms when laser energy is transmitted through fluid. The energy causes a "vapor tunnel [that] serves as a pathway permitting transmission of radiation between the parted seas of blood or water" hence the term the Moses effect[58,59] Holmium laser energy is highly absorbed in water and most of the energy goes to form the vapor bubble through which the energy is transmitted to the stone.[60] For SP or LP modes, all the energy is delivered in 1 pulse, which causes most of the energy to be lost in forming the vapor bubble.

In contrast, the Moses technology changes how the energy is delivered to the stone, a process called pulse modulation. The energy is delivered over 2 pulses.[4,61] The first pulse delivers part of the energy to form the vapor bubble. Once the bubble is formed, the second pulse delivers the rest of the energy through the already-formed vapor channel (**Fig. 5**). This method ensures that more energy is delivered to the stone compared with the regular pulse mode. The Moses platform has 2 settings: the Moses contact (MC) mode, intended for operation at a close distance, and Moses distance (MD) mode, which is designed for lithotripsy at a distance of 1 to 2 mm.[4]

Elhilali and colleagues[4] were the first to investigate this technology. They found that retropulsion distance was significantly lower for both Moses modes compared with the regular pulse mode for all tested laser settings. Moses mode also resulted in significantly greater ablation volume compared with SP mode.[4] In a follow-up study by the same group, they assessed fragmentation efficiency using either SP or Moses mode in an in vitro simulation model.[62] Procedure time was significantly shorter when using Moses mode compared with SP mode. The shorter procedure

time was attributed to a reduction in stone retropulsion decreasing the time needed to reposition the laser fiber. However, they only compared it with SP, and not the LP mode, which also has advantages in reducing stone retropulsion. It is not yet clear how the Moses mode compares with the LP mode. In our in vitro assessment of the technology, we compared fragmentation of a large artificial stone model over 3 minutes using Moses modes and LP. Although we did not find differences in fragmentation comparing MC with LP mode, we showed significantly greater fragmentation when using MD mode compared with LP.[63]

Cost is an important factor that needs to be considered when using newer technologies like the Moses platform. A recent study by Stern and Monga[64] assessed whether the time saved during the procedure can translate into cost savings. They estimated that the Moses technology would result in a cost increase of approximately $292 and $253 compared with using the regular mode for stones that are less than or equal to 10 mm and greater than 10 mm in size respectively. They concluded that the Moses technology can be cost-effective if the laser fiber cost can be reduced or if the procedure time is reduced by at least 4 minutes.[64]

EMERGING TECHNOLOGY
Thulium Fiber Laser

In the TFL, the energy is generated in a chemically doped small laser fiber, hence the term fiber laser.[65] The energy generated is transferred to another laser fiber, which is then delivered to the target tissue. TFL operates at wavelengths of either 1908 or 1940 nm.

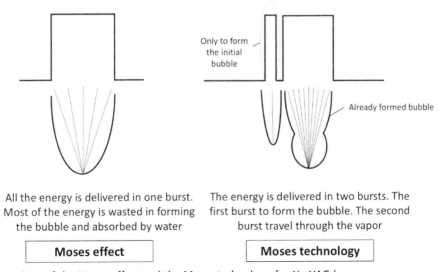

All the energy is delivered in one burst. Most of the energy is wasted in forming the bubble and absorbed by water

Only to form the initial bubble

Already formed bubble

The energy is delivered in two bursts. The first burst to form the bubble. The second burst travel through the vapor

| Moses effect | Moses technology |

Fig. 5. Comparison of the Moses effect and the Moses technology for Ho:YAG laser.

There are major technical differences between the TFL and Ho:YAG lasers. First, TFL operates at a wavelength that has a higher absorption peak in water compared with Ho:YAG, which operates at 2120 nm. For this reason, it has been hypothesized that increased water absorption leads to better fragmentation.[66,67] Second, the energy for TFL is generated in a small fiber so it can be coupled to laser fibers with core diameters as small as 100 μm. For the Ho:YAG laser, the energy is generated from a larger crystal and can only be coupled to fibers larger than 200 μm.[65] For TFL, the smaller fibers allow higher irrigation rates and better ureteroscope maneuverability. Third, the range of settings available on the two laser systems are different. TFL has pulse energies as small as 33 mJ and frequency as high as 2000 Hz, compared with the holmium laser in which 200 mJ is the lowest PE and 80 Hz is the highest currently achievable frequency.[5,9,37] This difference could be an advantage when using the dusting technique for URS. In terms of stone fragmentation, when the bubble dynamics are compared between the two laser systems, TFL produces a smaller bubble profile with lower collapse pressure than the Ho:YAG laser pulse.[68] Furthermore, PW is longer and more uniform in shape for the TFL. **Table 4** summarizes the

differences between the TFL and holmium laser for lithotripsy.

There are several in vitro studies comparing the 2 laser systems with only 1 clinical study.[5,66] Blackmon and colleagues[66] compared uric acid (UA) and calcium oxalate monohydrate (COM) stone fragmentation using TFL and Ho:YAG. Compared with Ho:YAG, TFL resulted in 4 and 8 times greater fragmentation for UA and COM stones respectively. Furthermore, assessment of crater ablation using optical coherence tomography showed that TFL resulted in deeper craters compared with the Ho:YAG laser. In a clinical evaluation of the TFL, Traxer and colleagues[69] found it to be safe and effective for treating renal and ureteral stones for all stone compositions during URS. Although the TFL is a promising technology, more clinical studies are needed to better understand the use of TFL for lithotripsy in comparison with the holmium laser.

SUMMARY

Laser techniques during endoscopic stone surgery can result in fragments that are small enough for retrieval or small enough for spontaneous passage. Getting it just right requires an understanding of setting parameters in order to improve lithotripsy efficiency and stone clearance. In general, high PE is used for active retrieval, whereas low PE is used for dusting technique. LP mode results in less stone retropulsion and fiber tip degradation. The popcorn technique is used to pulverize stones into fine fragments and is an important endgame strategy for dusting. Optimal parameters for popcorning include high frequency, keeping the fiber in contact with the stone, and performing it in a small calyx. The Moses technology for the holmium laser is a pulse modulation method that delivers energy over 2 pulses in order to reduce retropulsion and increase fragmentation. The TFL is an emerging laser technology, and future research will help clinicians understand how to incorporate these technologies and techniques with the aim of improving patient outcomes.

Table 4
Comparison of holmium:yttrium-aluminum-garnet and thulium fiber laser platforms for laser lithotripsy

Characteristic	Ho:YAG	TFL
Wavelength (nm)	2120	1940
Optical pumping	Flash lamp	Laser diode
PE (J)	0.2–6	0.033–6
Pulse frequency (Hz)	5–80	1–2000
PW (μs)	350–1300	200–1200
Temporal pulse profile	Peak initially and taper toward the end "shark fin"	Uniform shape
Core laser fiber size (μm)	>200	>100
Maximum power output (W)	120	50
Availability	In clinical use for >20 y	Preclinical data but limited clinical experience

REFERENCES

1. Shah J, Whitfield HN. Urolithiasis through the ages. BJU Int 2002;89(8):801–10.
2. Ordon M, Urbach D, Mamdani M, et al. The surgical management of kidney stone disease: a population based time series analysis. J Urol 2014;192(5):1450–6.
3. Dauw CA, Simeon L, Alruwaily AF, et al. Contemporary practice patterns of flexible ureteroscopy for treating renal stones: results of a worldwide survey. J Endourol 2015;29(11):1221–30.

4. Elhilali MM, Badaan S, Ibrahim A, et al. Use of the Moses technology to improve holmium laser lithotripsy outcomes: a preclinical study. J Endourol 2017;31(6):598–604.

5. Hardy LA, Gonzalez DA, Irby PB, et al. Fragmentation and dusting of large kidney stones using compact, air-cooled, high peak power, 1940-nm, thulium fiber laser. Paper presented at: SPIE BiOS2018. San Francisco, February 7, 2018.

6. Chan KF, Vassar GJ, Pfefer TJ, et al. Holmium:YAG laser lithotripsy: a dominant photothermal ablative mechanism with chemical decomposition of urinary calculi. Lasers Surg Med 1999;25(1):22–37.

7. Leveillee RJ, Lobik L. Intracorporeal lithotripsy: which modality is best? Curr Opin Urol 2003;13(3):249–53.

8. van Leeuwen TG, van der Veen MJ, Verdaasdonk RM, et al. Noncontact tissue ablation by holmium:YSGG laser pulses in blood. Lasers Surg Med 1991;11(1):26–34.

9. Tracey J, Gagin G, Morhardt D, et al. Ureteroscopic high-frequency dusting utilizing a 120-W holmium laser. J Endourol 2018;32(4):290–5.

10. Kronenberg P, Traxer O. Update on lasers in urology 2014: current assessment on holmium:yttrium-aluminum-garnet (Ho:YAG) laser lithotripter settings and laser fibers. World J Urol 2015;33(4):463–9.

11. Shin RH, Lautz JM, Cabrera FJ, et al. Evaluation of novel ball-tip holmium laser fiber: impact on ureteroscope performance and fragmentation efficiency. J Endourol 2016;30(2):189–94.

12. Sea J, Jonat LM, Chew BH, et al. Optimal power settings for holmium:YAG lithotripsy. J Urol 2012;187(3):914–9.

13. Kronenberg P, Traxer O. In vitro fragmentation efficiency of holmium: yttrium-aluminum-garnet (YAG) laser lithotripsy–a comprehensive study encompassing different frequencies, pulse energies, total power levels and laser fibre diameters. BJU Int 2014;114(2):261–7.

14. Mues AC, Teichman JMH, Knudsen BE. Quantification of holmium:yttrium aluminum garnet optical tip degradation. J Endourol 2009;23(9):1425–8.

15. Lee H, Ryan RT, Teichman JM, et al. Stone retropulsion during holmium:YAG lithotripsy. J Urol 2003;169(3):881–5.

16. Jansen ED, van Leeuwen TG, Motamedi M, et al. Temperature dependence of the absorption coefficient of water for midinfrared laser radiation. Lasers Surg Med 1994;14(3):258–68.

17. Spore SS, Teichman JM, Corbin NS, et al. Holmium:YAG lithotripsy: optimal power settings. J Endourol 1999;13(8):559–66.

18. Li R, Ruckle D, Keheila M, et al. High-frequency dusting versus conventional holmium laser lithotripsy for intrarenal and ureteral calculi. J Endourol 2017;31(3):272–7.

19. White MD, Moran ME, Calvano CJ, et al. Evaluation of retropulsion caused by holmium: YAG laser with various power settings and fibers. J Endourol 1998;12(2):183–6.

20. Kamal W, Kallidonis P, Koukiou G, et al. Stone retropulsion with Ho: YAG and Tm: YAG lasers: a clinical practice-oriented experimental study. J Endourol 2016;30(11):1145–9.

21. Sroka R, Pongratz T, Scheib G, et al. Impact of pulse duration on Ho:YAG laser lithotripsy: treatment aspects on the single-pulse level. World J Urol 2015;33(4):479–85.

22. Kang HW, Lee H, Teichman JM, et al. Dependence of calculus retropulsion on pulse duration during Ho: YAG laser lithotripsy. Lasers Surg Med 2006;38(8):762–72.

23. Vassar GJ, Teichman JM, Glickman RD. Holmium:YAG lithotripsy efficiency varies with energy density. J Urol 1998;160(2):471–6.

24. Bader MJ, Pongratz T, Khoder W, et al. Impact of pulse duration on Ho:YAG laser lithotripsy: fragmentation and dusting performance. World J Urol 2015;33(4):471–7.

25. Bell JR, Penniston KL, Nakada SY. In vitro comparison of holmium lasers: evidence for shorter fragmentation time and decreased retropulsion using a modern variable-pulse laser. Urology 2017;107:37–42.

26. Wezel F, Hacker A, Gross AJ, et al. Effect of pulse energy, frequency and length on holmium:yttrium-aluminum-garnet laser fragmentation efficiency in non-floating artificial urinary calculi. J Endourol 2010;24(7):1135–40.

27. Kuo RL, Aslan P, Zhong P, et al. Impact of holmium laser settings and fiber diameter on stone fragmentation and endoscope deflection. J Endourol 1998;12(6):523–7.

28. Aldoukhi AH, Roberts WW, Hall TL, et al. Watch your distance: The role of laser fiber working distance on fragmentation when altering pulse width or modulation. J Endourol 2018. [Epub ahead of Print].

29. Matlaga BR, Chew B, Eisner B, et al. Ureteroscopic laser lithotripsy: a review of dusting vs fragmentation with extraction. J Endourol 2018;32(1):1–6.

30. Hecht SL, Wolf JS Jr. Techniques for holmium laser lithotripsy of intrarenal calculi. Urology 2013;81(2):442–5.

31. Doizi S, Keller EX, De Coninck V, et al. Dusting technique for lithotripsy: what does it mean? Nat Rev Urol 2018;15(11):653–4.

32. Chawla SN, Chang MF, Chang A, et al. Effectiveness of high-frequency holmium:YAG laser stone fragmentation: the "popcorn effect". J Endourol 2008;22(4):645–50.

33. Emiliani E, Talso M, Cho SY, et al. Optimal settings for the noncontact holmium:YAG stone fragmentation popcorn technique. J Urol 2017;198(3):702–6.

34. Klaver P, de Boorder T, Rem AI, et al. In vitro comparison of renal stone laser treatment using fragmentation and popcorn technique. Lasers Surg Med 2017;49(7):698–704.

35. Wollin DA, Tom WR, Jiang R, et al. An in vitro evaluation of laser settings and location in the efficiency of the popcorn effect. Urolithiasis 2018. https://doi.org/10.1007/s00240-018-1066-6.

36. Aldoukhi AH, Roberts WW, Hall TL, et al. Understanding the popcorn effect during holmium laser lithotripsy for dusting. Urology 2018;122:52–7.

37. Aldoukhi AH, Roberts WW, Hall TL, et al. Holmium laser lithotripsy in the new stone age: dust or bust? Front Surg 2017;4:57.

38. Aldoukhi AH, Ghani KR, Hall TL, et al. Thermal response to high-power holmium laser lithotripsy. J Endourol 2017;31(12):1308–12.

39. Buttice S, Sener TE, Proietti S, et al. Temperature changes inside the kidney: what happens during holmium:yttrium-aluminium-garnet laser usage? J Endourol 2016;30(5):574–9.

40. Molina WR, Silva IN, Donalisio da Silva R, et al. Influence of saline on temperature profile of laser lithotripsy activation. J Endourol 2015;29(2):235–9.

41. Wollin DA, Carlos EC, Tom WR, et al. Effect of laser settings and irrigation rates on ureteral temperature during holmium laser lithotripsy, an in vitro model. J Endourol 2018;32(1):59–63.

42. Schatloff O, Lindner U, Ramon J, et al. Randomized trial of stone fragment active retrieval versus spontaneous passage during holmium laser lithotripsy for ureteral stones. J Urol 2010;183(3):1031–5.

43. Humphreys MR, Shah OD, Monga M, et al. Dusting versus basketing during ureteroscopy–which technique is more efficacious? A prospective multicenter trial from the EDGE research consortium. J Urol 2018;199(5):1272–6.

44. Ghani KR, Wolf JS Jr. What is the stone-free rate following flexible ureteroscopy for kidney stones? Nat Rev Urol 2015;12(5):281–8.

45. Canvasser N, Lay A, Kolitz E, et al. MP75-12 prospective evaluation of stone free rates by computed tomography after aggressive ureteroscopy. J Urol 2017;197(4):e1007–8.

46. Portis AJ, Rygwall R, Holtz C, et al. Ureteroscopic laser lithotripsy for upper urinary tract calculi with active fragment extraction and computerized tomography followup. J Urol 2006;175(6):2129–33 [discussion: 2133–4].

47. Weiss B, Shah O. Evaluation of dusting versus basketing - can new technologies improve stone-free rates? Nat Rev Urol 2016;13(12):726–33.

48. Bagley D, Erhard M. Use of the holmium laser in the upper urinary tract. Tech Urol 1995;1(1):25–30.

49. Grasso M. Experience with the holmium laser as an endoscopic lithotrite. Urology 1996;48(2):199–206.

50. Matsuoka K, Iida S, Nakanami M, et al. Holmium:yttrium-aluminum-garnet laser for endoscopic lithotripsy. Urology 1995;45(6):947–52.

51. Teichman JM, Rogenes VJ, McIver BJ, et al. Holmium:yttrium-aluminum-garnet laser cystolithotripsy of large bladder calculi. Urology 1997;50(1):44–8.

52. Assimos D, Krambeck A, Miller NL, et al. Surgical management of stones: American Urological Association/Endourological Society guideline, part I. J Urol 2016;196(4):1153–60.

53. Preminger G, Assimos D, Lingeman J, et al. Chapter 1: AUA guideline on management of staghorn calculi: diagnosis and treatment recommendations. J Urol 2005;173(6):1991–2000.

54. Cuellar DC, Averch TD. Holmium laser percutaneous nephrolithotomy using a unique suction device. J Endourol 2004;18(8):780–2.

55. Okhunov Z, del Junco M, Yoon R, et al. In vitro evaluation of LithAssist: a novel combined holmium laser and suction device. J Endourol 2014;28(8):980–4.

56. Dauw CA, Borofsky MS, York N, et al. A usability comparison of laser suction handpieces for percutaneous nephrolithotomy. J Endourol 2016;30(11):1165–8.

57. Ghani KR, Aldoukhi AH, Roberts WW. Dusting utilizing suction technique (DUST) for percutaneous nephrolithotomy: use of a dedicated laser handpiece to treat a staghorn stone. Int Braz J Urol 2018;44(4):840–1.

58. Isner JM, DeJesus SR, Clarke RH, et al. Mechanism of laser ablation in an absorbing fluid field. Lasers Surg Med 1988;8(6):543–54.

59. Isner JM, Clarke RH. Cardiovascular laser therapy. New York: Raven Press; 1989.

60. Jansen ED, Asshauer T, Frenz M, et al. Effect of pulse duration on bubble formation and laser-induced pressure waves during holmium laser ablation. Lasers Surg Med 1996;18(3):278–93.

61. Trost D, Inventor; ESC medical systems Inc Lumenis Ltd assignee. Laser pulse format for penetrating an absorbing fluid. US patent US5321715A. June 6, 1994.

62. Ibrahim A, Badaan S, Elhilali MM, et al. Moses technology in a stone simulator. Can Urol Assoc J 2018;12(4):127–30.

63. Aldoukhi AH, Roberts WW, Hall TL, et al. Watch your distance: The role of laser fiber working distance on fragmentation when altering pulse width or modulation. J Endourol 2018. https://doi.org/10.1089/end.2018.0572.

64. Stern KL, Monga M. The Moses holmium system - time is money. Can J Urol 2018;25(3):9313–6.

65. Fried NM, Irby PB. Advances in laser technology and fibre-optic delivery systems in lithotripsy. Nat Rev Urol 2018;15(9):563–73.

66. Blackmon RL, Irby PB, Fried NM. Holmium:YAG (lambda = 2,120 nm) versus thulium fiber (lambda = 1,908 nm) laser lithotripsy. Lasers Surg Med 2010; 42(3):232–6.

67. Majaron B, Plestenjak P, Lukač M. Thermo-mechanical laser ablation of soft biological tissue: modeling the micro-explosions. Appl Phys B 1999;69(1): 71–80.

68. Hardy LA, Kennedy JD, Wilson CR, et al. Analysis of thulium fiber laser induced bubble dynamics for ablation of kidney stones. J Biophotonics 2017; 10(10):1240–9.

69. Traxer O, Rapoport L, Tsarichenko D, et al. V03-02 First clinical study on superpulse thulium fiber laser for lithotripsy. J Urol 2018;199(4): e321–2.

Emerging Technologies in Ultrasonic and Pneumatic Lithotripsy

Daniel A. Wollin, MD[a,b],*, Michael E. Lipkin, MD, MBA[a]

KEYWORDS

• Pneumatic • Ultrasonic • Percutaneous • Lithotripsy • Devices

KEY POINTS

• Pneumatic and ultrasonic lithotripsy methods form the backbone of percutaneous stone fragmentation.
• Various combination devices have been developed to use the benefits of each fragmentation method.
• Novel devices use single-probe construction to allow for a maximal lumen size and improve suction capabilities.

INTRODUCTION

Percutaneous nephrolithotomy remains the treatment of choice for staghorn renal calculi, renal stones greater than 2 cm, and lower pole renal stones greater than 1 cm.[1,2] Through its years of development, percutaneous nephrolithotomy stone fragmentation technology has improved from simple grasping removal to single-energy lithotripsy and eventually the combination ultrasonic/pneumatic lithotrites currently in use. Through the advanced technologies developed, more efficient fragmentation has become possible, also allowing for a variety of treatment options depending on stone location, size, and composition. This article discusses the basics of pneumatic and ultrasonic lithotripsy, with attention paid to current and future generations of percutaneous lithotripsy devices.

PERCUTANEOUS LITHOTRIPSY MECHANISMS

In this section, we discuss the basic mechanisms of pneumatic and ultrasonic lithotripsy, with additional focus on historical and currently used single-energy devices.

Pneumatic Lithotripsy

Pneumatic or ballistic lithotripsy uses the rapid forward motion of a rigid projectile to produce a jackhammer effect on the target stone. Multiple mechanisms exist to produce the ballistic effect, from compressed air and carbon dioxide cartridges to electrokinetic energy generation. The Swiss Lithoclast (EMS, Nyon, Switzerland), which was developed in the 1990s, was the first clinically available percutaneous pneumatic lithotripsy device. This technology uses a tank of compressed air or hospital air lines to fire a projectile against a metal probe with a pressure of 3 atm with foot-pedal control. The probe, which ranges from 2.4F to 9.6F catheter, is solid, fires at 12 cycles/second, and requires stone contact to produce stone fragmentation. This device, since its initial clinical evaluation in 1991, has become the basis for future pneumatic lithotripter devices, with alterations in energy source, compactness, and method of control.[3]

Disclosure: Dr M.E. Lipkin serves as a consultant for Boston Scientific. Dr D.A. Wollin has nothing to disclose.
[a] Division of Urologic Surgery, Duke University Medical Center, 40 Medicine Circle, Durham, NC 27710, USA;
[b] Division of Urologic Surgery, VA Boston Healthcare System, 1400 VFW Parkway, West Roxbury, MA 02132, USA
* Corresponding author. Duke University Medical Center, Room 1573, White Zone, Box 3167, Durham, NC 27710.
E-mail address: daniel.wollin@gmail.com

To improve the portability and ease-of-use of the Swiss Lithoclast, the LMA StoneBreaker (Cook Medical, Bloomington, IN) was developed (**Fig. 1**A).[4] This device is a self-contained handheld pneumatic lithotripter that uses small cartridges of carbon dioxide gas at high pressure for the ballistic energy source. Each cartridge contains enough gas for approximately 80 to 100 discharges, although studies have shown that the device's efficacy decreases as the gas within the cartridge diminishes.[5] The initial clinical experience with this device showed similar fragmentation efficiency compared with the Lithoclast, with improved maneuverability, portability, and ease-of-use.[6,7] Given the simpler and quicker setup of this device, it also serves as an excellent backup when other, more complicated, technologies may fail.

A similar portable ballistic lithotripter, the Swiss LithoBreaker (EMS), uses a battery-operated electrokinetic mechanism to fire a rigid probe toward the target stone. This handheld device, which runs on rechargeable batteries, was found to deliver more consistent shocks than the StoneBreaker with similar fragmentation efficiency, likely because of gas depletion in the latter lithotrite.[5,8] Although the hand positioning was noted to be slightly more uncomfortable for the Swiss LithoBreaker for percutaneous procedures, the portability of both handheld devices greatly simplifies their use.[5]

The ballistic method of stone fragmentation, with its high-energy and low-frequency jackhammer effect, produces large stone fragments for easy removal. Pneumatic lithotripsy has been shown in numerous studies to be a safe and efficacious method of stone removal, with greater success seen with harder stone compositions.[9–11] Compared with other methods of lithotripsy, the pneumatic technologies are low-cost and low-maintenance.

Given the rigid nature of the pneumatic probe and the need for direct energy transfer from the source to the probe and stone, these devices are most efficient when the probe remains completely undeflected. For this reason, pneumatic lithotripsy performs best when used through the rigid nephroscope with minimal deflection of the probe. An additional concern with pneumatic lithotripsy is the solid nature of the probe, which does not allow for concurrent suction; a combination suction-pneumatic probe setup (LithoVac) was developed for the Swiss Lithoclast with improvements in stone retropulsion, although frequent clogging decreased the potential for widespread clinical utility.[9,12]

Ultrasonic Lithotripsy

Ultrasonic lithotripsy was first reported for treatment of renal calculi by Mulvaney in 1953.[13] Since that time, the technology has significantly improved, although the basic concepts remain constant. The mechanism of ultrasonic stone fragmentation involves an electric current passing through a piezoceramic plate; this piezoelectric apparatus produces ultrasonic vibrations at a frequency from 23 to 25 kHz, which are transmitted to a metal probe that contacts the stone. The rapid vibrations of this method produce small stone fragments that are suctioned through the lumen of the larger probes, which are often hollow to

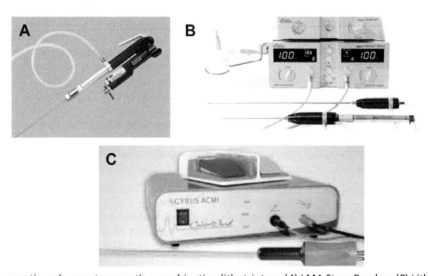

Fig. 1. Pneumatic and current-generation combination lithotripters. (*A*) LMA StoneBreaker. (*B*) Lithoclast Master. (© 2018 Boston Scientific Corp.) (*C*) CyberWand. (*Courtesy of* [*A*] Cook Medical, Bloomington, IN; and [C] Olympus, Tokyo, Japan; with permission.)

allow for concurrent suction. The suction capability is also used to cycle irrigation to avoid thermal tissue injury and cool the piezoelectric elements within the handpiece and prevent overheating.[14] Given the direct mechanical transfer of energy from the vibrating probe to the stone, contact must be applied for fragmentation to occur. Similar to pneumatic lithotrites, the direct mechanical transfer of energy along the probe requires that ultrasonic probes are maintained with minimal deflection to maximize fragmentation. Also, a larger probe diameter (up to 12F catheter) allows for improved irrigation cycling and stone fragment removal with the suction mechanism. For these reasons, ultrasonic devices are most often used during percutaneous procedures where large, straight access tracts are available.

Karl Storz (Tuttlingen, Germany), along with several other device manufacturers, created early ultrasonic lithotripters with similar functionality. With improvements in probe size, suction capability, device stability, and varying ultrasonic frequencies, there have been enhancements in ultrasonic stone fragmentation, although the basic mechanisms remain unchanged. Varying devices have been tested against each other in laboratory settings, suggesting that the Storz Calcuson was the most efficient first-generation ultrasonic lithotrite, whereas more recent testing documented the superiority of the LUS-2 (Olympus, Tokyo, Japan) and USL-2000 (Circon-ACMI, Southborough, MA).[15,16]

Ultrasonic lithotripsy is an inexpensive method of stone fragmentation given the low-cost generator and reusable ultrasound probes. The ultrasonic mechanism of lithotripsy produces fragmentation through rapid vibration of the rigid stone material; as such, vibration against tissue produces minimal tissue injury and is safe.[17–19] The efficacy of this method is incredibly high in the proper stone type, with a success rate of up to 98.3% in a percutaneous setting.[20]

Despite its efficacy, ultrasonic fragmentation remains a faster method of lithotripsy for softer stones, whereas certain stones (including cystine composition and smoother stones) may be more difficult to fragment with this technology.[11,21] Thermal injury is feasible given the potential for temperature rise at the end of the probe, although adequate irrigation (at least 30 mL/min) significantly reduces this potential.[21] To prevent this thermal injury or device malfunction, care must be taken to ensure working suction and avoid occlusion of the suction setup. Some devices have been outfitted with a foot pedal for intermittent suction control to allow for more granular manipulation of this feature, although this same method is accomplished by wall suction and intermittent tube clamping by an assistant. However, smaller ultrasonic probes do not boast a hollow lumen and lose the benefits gained by concurrent suction. Lastly, given the method of energy generation and suction capabilities, this technology by definition remains tethered to the generator and vacuum setup, preventing the portability seen with the handheld pneumatic devices.

CURRENT-GENERATION COMBINATION LITHOTRIPSY DEVICES
Lithoclast Master

A significant technologic development in intracorporeal percutaneous lithotripsy occurred when the two previously discussed techniques were combined in a single device, producing a dual-probe lithotrite. This was first performed by EMS to create the Lithoclast Master, which has since been improved on and marketed under various names (Lithoclast Ultra, Lithoclast Select in conjunction with Boston Scientific, Marlborough, MA), and was first used clinically in 2001 (**Fig. 1**B).[22] In this device, a pneumatic air-driven probe is attached coaxially within a hollow ultrasound probe with suction capability, allowing for individual or combination energy discharge. Because of several studies demonstrating the improved efficacy of these devices, especially their ability to fragment a large variety of stone types, they have since become the gold standard for percutaneous lithotripsy.[23–27] In initial *in vitro* studies, the combination Lithoclast was compared with pneumatic and ultrasonic single-energy devices in either a hands-free or hands-on lithotripsy model with substantial improvement in fragmentation efficiency.[23–25] In the clinical realm, the combination Lithoclast has shown similar superiority, with studies suggesting at worst a clinical equivalence with ultrasonic fragmentation and at best a 200% improvement in lithotripsy speed.[26,27] Studies specifically noted an improvement in fragmentation with harder stone composition, likely caused by the addition of pneumatic capabilities to the ultrasonic foundation of the device.[26]

Although the combination of pneumatic and ultrasonic energy sources allowed for a marriage of each method's advantages, the placement of a pneumatic probe within the lumen of the ultrasonic device has been noted to reduce suction capacity. Even with a large probe size (eg, 11.4F catheter), the pneumatic probe presence decreases the lumen that is used for suction purposes. Similarly, although the concurrent suction may reduce its effect, the retropulsion associated with pneumatic lithotripsy remains an issue because the ballistic motion may push the stone away from the ultrasonic probe, preventing continuous contact and energy delivery. Finally, this device is unwieldy to manage because of the sheer size and weight of the multipart handpiece, the complexity of setup, and multiple connections to the suction and multifunction generator, although these factors were improved with later versions of these devices.

CyberWand

The CyberWand (Olympus) is a similar dual-energy device, but one that produces the ballistic motion using a different method (**Fig. 1**C). The device uses a dual-probe coaxial system, but both probes are hollow. The inner 8.3F catheter probe is connected to the handpiece, which produces an ultrasonic vibration at 21 kHz, whereas the outer 11.3F catheter probe is allowed to move freely, pushed distally by a sliding piston on the inner probe and brought back into position with a spring coil; this produces a lower-frequency ballistic motion of the outer probe. Concurrent suction occurs through the common lumen of the dual probes. The CyberWand was compared with the Lithoclast combination device through *in vitro* tests, which showed improved stone penetration time for the dual-ultrasonic technology, although these results were not supported when clinical studies began to examine this device.[28]

Through two large multicenter trials, the CyberWand was compared with other contemporaneous lithotrites; a first study compared it with the Olympus LUS-2, which showed no significant differences in stone clearance time or stone-free rate.[29] Similarly, a more recent multicenter trial showed no significant differences in stone clearance rates among the CyberWand, the Lithoclast Select, and the LMA StoneBreaker (used in concert with the LUS-2 for suction).[7] Together, these data show that the clinical efficacy of the CyberWand is likely not as promising as initially believed from the benchtop studies, potentially because of probe failures, suction clogging, or the smaller inner lumen reducing suction capabilities. Additionally, the CyberWand was noted to be significantly louder than other percutaneous lithotripsy technologies, with one study suggesting that greater than 90 minutes of device activation daily would require hearing protection to prevent long-term hearing loss.[30]

NEXT-GENERATION LITHOTRIPSY DEVICES

Since the initial use of large rigid ultrasonic and pneumatic devices for percutaneous nephrolithotomy, many improvements have been made to reach the current-generation technology. These advancements have continued such that several newer devices have become available in recent years, all of which have returned to a single-probe solution. In this section, we discuss three novel lithotrites, their mechanisms of action and details, and review the available data on these devices.

UreTron

The first novel device is the UreTron (Med-Sonics, Erie, PA), which, unlike the other novel devices in this review uses a single-probe ultrasonic mechanism. The UreTron attempts to improve on previous single-probe ultrasonic devices by featuring a unique vibration and control theory to improve stone fragmentation across stone types. The largest probe size has a 10.5F catheter outer diameter and the vibration, which is controlled by a foot pedal, is comparable with other ultrasonic devices at 21 kHz. The foot pedal has hard and soft stone mode activation, with these options producing different pulse patterns aimed to optimize fragmentation of each particular stone type.

This device was approved by the Food and Drug Administration (FDA) for use in 2012, and a clinical study was performed between 2012 and 2014 on 31 patients to evaluate its efficacy in percutaneous nephrolithotomy; in this article, the UreTron results were compared with other device cohorts from a concurrent study.[31] The device was found to be safe for use with similar rates of complications to the CyberWand, Lithoclast Select, and LUS-2/StoneBreaker combination. Importantly, the UreTron was found to have the highest stone clearance rate, with a stone removal speed greater than 10 mm^2/min faster than the other cohorts. Additionally, when comparing the UreTron with all other devices, the novel lithotrite exhibited more efficient stone clearance with comparable stone-free rates and need for secondary procedures. This superiority remained when isolating the patients with "hard" stones, or those with predominantly calcium oxalate, brushite, cystine, or uric acid.

The authors of the UreTron study suggest two main reasons for the improvement in clinical efficacy over current devices. They first offer that enhancements in pulse management and vibration control allow for more targeted ultrasonic fragmentation based on stone type, specifically allowing for improved lithotripsy of hard stones, which has historically been difficult with ultrasonic methods. Secondly, they suggest that improved suction management with the UreTron and lower risk of suction clogging benefited the newer device; they believe the probe size difference served to produce this benefit because the inner diameter of the UreTron probe size used was 7.5F catheter compared with the inner lumen of the CyberWand (6.3F catheter). Still, additional clinical testing is required to determine the true superiority of this single-probe, ultrasound-only device.

ShockPulse

The following next-generation device is the Shock-Pulse (Olympus), which uses a single-probe ultrasonic mechanism with free mass elements and a return spring to produce concurrent ballistic movements of the probe (**Fig. 2**A). In a similar method to the CyberWand, the piezoelectric elements within the handpiece produce 21-kHz vibrations of the probe with the free mass and spring producing ballistic energy of the same probe at a rate of 300 Hz. The combination of energies theoretically allows for ultrasonic fragmentation of softer stone components, and the intermittent mechanical energy from the free mass movements along the probe is able to fragment the harder portions of the target stone. Unlike the other devices discussed, the device is controlled by buttons on the handpiece instead of a foot pedal, with standard and high-intensity settings available; suction intensity is also controlled through a dial on the handpiece. Importantly, the ShockPulse probes are as large as 11.3F catheter, with an inner lumen diameter of 9.6F catheter, which was the largest lumen of the currently available devices. The ShockPulse probes are also available in smaller sizes, including 10.2F, 5.5F, 4.5F, and 2.91F catheter.

The ShockPulse was FDA approved in 2014 and a single *in vitro* study exists comparing the device with current-generation lithotrites with a small clinical cohort tested concurrently.[32] In this study, the authors evaluated multiple technologies (LUS-2, Lithoclast Select, CyberWand) compared with the ShockPulse, with hands-on and hands-free *in vitro* assessments. The hands-on setup involved a single operator performing lithotripsy on a stone phantom made from either Ultracal-30 or plaster of Paris in a rubberized container within a water tank; time to retrievable fragments and time to complete fragment evacuation was recorded by an observer for each device and stone six times. The hands-free setup involved a fixed-force downward drill test through a large stone phantom or group of small stone phantoms, with time to complete drilling recorded by an electronic timer.

Time to retrievable fragments was similar among all devices; although the time to complete evacuation was fastest for the ShockPulse, when comparing individually, the only statistically significant difference was that the CyberWand was outperformed by all other devices. In the drill test, the ShockPulse and CyberWand were significantly faster when testing large stones, whereas the ShockPulse was superior to all other systems when multiple small stones were tested. Clinically, the authors performed six cases using the new device and claimed excellent usability, with no difficulties, complications, or clogging of the suction; they also noted a significant noise reduction compared with the CyberWand. They achieved stone-free status in five of the six patients by computed tomography and suggest this device is an effective, and potentially superior, tool for percutaneous lithotripsy. It remains to be seen if the improved results of benchtop testing for this device translate to improved clinical efficacy.

Lithoclast Trilogy

The final novel lithotrite to be discussed is the Lithoclast Trilogy (EMS and Boston Scientific). This device, which is the newest model in the Lithoclast

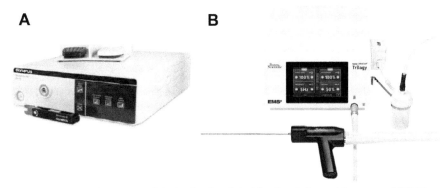

Fig. 2. Novel combination lithotripters. (*A*) ShockPulse. (*B*) Lithoclast Trilogy. (*Courtesy of* [*A*] Olympus, Tokyo, Japan; with permission. and [*B*] © 2018 Boston Scientific Corp.)

line of percutaneous lithotripsy technology, similarly returns to a single-probe design, although the mechanism uses ultrasonic and electromagnetic energy to create a combination ultrasonic/ballistic energy delivery (**Fig. 2**B). The probe, which is RFID tagged to ensure the generator can interpret the probe size, attaches to the handpiece and is oscillated with a piezoelectric ultrasonic generator at a rate of 24 kHz. Concurrently, an electromagnetic generator produces a ballistic motion of the entire probe at an adjustable rate up to 12 Hz.

As with other ultrasonic-based devices, suction is available through the hollow probe, with the foot pedal controlling suction and lithotripsy activation. The strength of ultrasonic vibration, suction, and frequency of ballistic energy discharge are adjustable through a touch screen on the generator. Several probe sizes are available (3.3F, 4.5F, 5.7F, 10.2F, and 11.7F catheter), with the smallest probe sizes abandoning the hollow lumen and associated suction capabilities. To allow for the ultrasonic and electromagnetic energies, the cord for the handpiece includes a separate hydrocooling system that pumps through the generator. This requirement does add weight to the handpiece and associated cord.

The Lithoclast Trilogy, which was FDA approved in early 2018, has only been studied in an *in vitro* setting, although a handful of clinical cases have been performed with this device at select locations. The solitary published study regarding this device attempted to evaluate the Trilogy compared with the ShockPulse and Lithoclast Select in a similar fashion to the ShockPulse study mentioned previously.[33] In this study, the authors used a hands-on stone evacuation test performed by a single operator, with 10 runs completed for each device. They also performed a hands-free fixed-weight drill test as described previously, with 10 trials completed for each device (five trials with 1 lb of weight, five trials with 2 lb of weight). Of note, given the retropulsion occasionally seen when the Lithoclast Select pneumatic energy is continuously activated alongside the ultrasonic vibration, the Select was compared in two different manners: one set of trials was performed with continuous pneumatic activation and one set was performed with ultrasonic energy alone. Lastly, a high-speed camera was used to evaluate the probe tip dynamics of the two novel devices to determine any potential differences that may explain variability in device efficiency.

In the clearance trial, the Lithoclast Trilogy was significantly faster than all other devices. In this study, the ShockPulse and Lithoclast Select (with ultrasonic energy alone) were not significantly different. In the hands-free drill testing, the Lithoclast Select (with pneumatic and ultrasonic energy), ShockPulse, and Lithoclast Trilogy were all significantly faster than the Lithoclast Select with ultrasonic energy alone. As such, the authors concluded that the Lithoclast Trilogy is a potentially useful tool for percutaneous lithotripsy and seems to be superior to other standard devices with regard to stone clearance. Of note, the high-speed camera analysis of the ShockPulse and Lithoclast Trilogy disclosed that both devices have minimal probe tip excursion with ultrasonic oscillation, although the Lithoclast Trilogy ultrasonic movement was approximately 16 times greater in magnitude than that of the ShockPulse. Similarly, the Lithoclast Trilogy impactor movement seemed to be 25 times greater in magnitude than that of the ShockPulse. The authors suggest that these larger movements, and the larger probe diameter of the Lithoclast Trilogy, may generate the improved results seen in their study. Still, further clinical studies are needed to evaluate the true nature of this novel device.

SUMMARY

Pneumatic and ultrasonic lithotripsy devices have become the backbone of percutaneous nephrolithotomy and subsequent intracorporeal lithotripsy, with newer devices combining multiple energy sources and balancing features with maneuverability. As novel methods of lithotripsy enter the clinical sphere, it is a requirement that the operating urologist understand the available surgical options and the associated mechanisms used to best treat their patients. Constant experimentation and innovation allow for improved testing of available devices and produce newer technologies to further urology.

REFERENCES

1. Assimos D, Krambeck A, Miller NL, et al. Surgical management of stones: American Urological Association/Endourological Society Guideline, PART I. J Urol 2016;196(4):1153–60.
2. Assimos D, Krambeck A, Miller NL, et al. Surgical management of stones: American Urological Association/Endourological Society Guideline, PART II. J Urol 2016;196(4):1161–9.
3. Wisard M, Jichlinski P, Languetin JM, et al. First clinical evaluation of the CHUV ballistic lithoclast. Helv Chir Acta 1991;58(3):319–21 [in French].
4. Rane A, Kommu SS, Kandaswamy SV, et al. Initial clinical evaluation of a new pneumatic intracorporeal lithotripter. BJU Int 2007;100(3):629–32.

5. Wang AJ, Baldwin GT, Gabriel JC, et al. In-vitro assessment of a new portable ballistic lithotripter with percutaneous and ureteroscopic models. J Endourol 2012;26(11):1500–5.

6. Chew BH, Arsovska O, Lange D, et al. The Canadian StoneBreaker trial: a randomized, multicenter trial comparing the LMA StoneBreaker and the Swiss LithoClast(R) during percutaneous nephrolithotripsy. J Endourol 2011;25(9):1415–9.

7. York NE, Borofsky MS, Chew BH, et al. Randomized controlled trial comparing three different modalities of lithotrites for intracorporeal lithotripsy in percutaneous nephrolithotomy. J Endourol 2017;31(11):1145–51.

8. Khoder WY, Bader MJ, Haseke N, et al. In vitro comparisons of retropulsion and fragmentation efficacy of 2 cordless, handheld pneumatic and electromechanical lithotripsy devices. Urology 2014;83(4):726–31.

9. Delvecchio FC, Kuo RL, Preminger GM. Clinical efficacy of combined lithoclast and lithovac stone removal during ureteroscopy. J Urol 2000;164(1):40–2.

10. Denstedt JD, Razvi HA, Rowe E, et al. Investigation of the tissue effects of a new device for intracorporeal lithotripsy: the Swiss Lithoclast. J Urol 1995;153(2):535–7.

11. Radfar MH, Basiri A, Nouralizadeh A, et al. Comparing the efficacy and safety of ultrasonic versus pneumatic lithotripsy in percutaneous nephrolithotomy: a randomized clinical trial. Eur Urol Focus 2017;3(1):82–8.

12. Haupt G, Pannek J, Herde T, et al. The Lithovac: new suction device for the Swiss Lithoclast. J Endourol 1995;9(5):375–7.

13. Mulvaney WP. Attempted disintegration of calculi by ultrasonic vibrations. J Urol 1953;70(5):704–7.

14. Lowe G, Knudsen BE. Ultrasonic, pneumatic and combination intracorporeal lithotripsy for percutaneous nephrolithotomy. J Endourol 2009;23(10):1663–8.

15. Kuo RL, Paterson RF, Siqueira TM Jr, et al. In vitro assessment of ultrasonic lithotriptors. J Urol 2003;170(4 Pt 1):1101–4.

16. Liatsikos EN, Dinlenc CZ, Fogarty JD, et al. Efficiency and efficacy of different intracorporeal ultrasonic lithotripsy units on a synthetic stone model. J Endourol 2001;15(9):925–8.

17. Grocela JA, Dretler SP. Intracorporeal lithotripsy. Instrumentation and development. Urol Clin North Am 1997;24(1):13–23.

18. Howards SS, Merrill E, Harris S, et al. Ultrasonic lithotripsy: laboratory evaluation. Invest Urol 1974;11(4):273–7.

19. Piergiovanni M, Desgrandchamps F, Cochand-Priollet B, et al. Ureteral and bladder lesions after ballistic, ultrasonic, electrohydraulic, or laser lithotripsy. J Endourol 1994;8(4):293–9.

20. Segura JW, Patterson DE, LeRoy AJ, et al. Percutaneous removal of kidney stones: review of 1,000 cases. J Urol 1985;134(6):1077–81.

21. Marberger M. Disintegration of renal and ureteral calculi with ultrasound. Urol Clin North Am 1983;10(4):729–42.

22. Haupt G, Sabrodina N, Orlovski M, et al. Endoscopic lithotripsy with a new device combining ultrasound and lithoclast. J Endourol 2001;15(9):929–35.

23. Auge BK, Lallas CD, Pietrow PK, et al. In vitro comparison of standard ultrasound and pneumatic lithotrites with a new combination intracorporeal lithotripsy device. Urology 2002;60(1):28–32.

24. Hofmann R, Weber J, Heidenreich A, et al. Experimental studies and first clinical experience with a new Lithoclast and ultrasound combination for lithotripsy. Eur Urol 2002;42(4):376–81.

25. Kuo RL, Paterson RF, Siqueira TM Jr, et al. In vitro assessment of lithoclast ultra intracorporeal lithotripter. J Endourol 2004;18(2):153–6.

26. Lehman DS, Hruby GW, Phillips C, et al. Prospective randomized comparison of a combined ultrasonic and pneumatic lithotrite with a standard ultrasonic lithotrite for percutaneous nephrolithotomy. J Endourol 2008;22(2):285–9.

27. Pietrow PK, Auge BK, Zhong P, et al. Clinical efficacy of a combination pneumatic and ultrasonic lithotrite. J Urol 2003;169(4):1247–9.

28. Kim SC, Matlaga BR, Tinmouth WW, et al. In vitro assessment of a novel dual probe ultrasonic intracorporeal lithotriptor. J Urol 2007;177(4):1363–5.

29. Krambeck AE, Miller NL, Humphreys MR, et al. Randomized controlled, multicentre clinical trial comparing a dual-probe ultrasonic lithotrite with a single-probe lithotrite for percutaneous nephrolithotomy. BJU Int 2011;107(5):824–8.

30. Soucy F, Ko R, Denstedt JD, et al. Occupational noise exposure during endourologic procedures. J Endourol 2008;22(8):1609–11.

31. Borofsky MS, El Tayeb MM, Paonessa JE, et al. Initial experience and comparative efficacy of the uretron: a new intracorporeal ultrasonic lithotriptor. Urology 2015;85(6):1279–83.

32. Chew BH, Matteliano AA, de Los Reyes T, et al. Benchtop and initial clinical evaluation of the shock-pulse stone eliminator in percutaneous nephrolithotomy. J Endourol 2017;31(2):191–7.

33. Carlos EC, Wollin DA, Winship BB, et al. In vitro comparison of a novel single probe dual-energy lithotripter to current devices. J Endourol 2018;32(6):534–40.

Emerging Technologies in Lithotripsy

Tim Large, MD, Amy E. Krambeck, MD*

KEYWORDS

• Lithotripsy • Urinary calculi • Histotripsy • Burst wave lithotripsy • Fragmentation • Urolithiasis

KEY POINTS

- Appropriate patient selection is key to success with shockwave lithotripsy.
- Slow rate, ramping of energy, appropriate coupling, and frequent imaging are important for successful shockwave lithotripsy.
- Burst wave lithotripsy demonstrates successful fragmentation and limited tissue damage of in vivo stones by delivering a 1:1 high-to-low-amplitude burst of ultrasound energy over a short segment of time.
- Histotripsy is capable of fragmenting stones but current success is limited by cavitation bubbles at the stone–fluid interface.
- Infused microbubble technology may be a future adjunct to improve efficiency and safety of all lithotripsy technologies.

INTRODUCTION

Extracorporeal treatment of nephrolithiasis has been a mainstay surgical therapy for the treatment of nephrolithiasis since the original experience with the HM-3 lithotripter was reported in 1984.[1] Multiple new iterations of the original external shockwave lithotripter have emerged over the last 30 years. Reduction in the size of new lithotripters has improved the mobility and the ease with which shockwave treatments can be delivered to patients with nephrolithiasis.[2] Additionally, through elucidation of optimal shockwave generators, advances in stone-tracking software and identification of ideal patients and stone compositions, the success rate of extracorporeal shockwave lithotripsy (ESWL) has been optimized.[3] Despite these improvements, ESWL is slowly being supplanted by endoscopic surgical treatments such as ureteroscopy (URS) and percutaneous

nephrolithotomy (PCNL). This trend has been reported in a recent European study evaluating the utilization of ESWL compared with alternative surgical options for the treatment of nephrolithiasis.[4] The study reported that ESWL usage peaked in 2006 with progressive decline since then. In the United States, ESWL accounts for 36.3% of surgical interventions for nephrolithiasis based on American Board of Urology Case logs in 2013; which is less than URS (59.6%) and a significant decline from 2003 when ESWL accounted for 54% of stone procedures.[5] This trend is driven by multiple factors, including the increased health care cost associated with ESWL compared with URS, the evolution of training programs toward endoscopy, and the objective finding that ESWL has lower stone-free rates (SFRs) and higher retreatment rates compared with URS and PCNL.[6] Nevertheless, with appropriate patient selection and continued improvements in

Disclosures: Dr A.E. Krambeck is a consultant for Boston Scientific and Lumenis. She is also an advisor at Cook Medical. Dr T. Large has nothing to disclose.
Department of Urology, Indiana University, Methodist Hospital, 1801 Senate Boulevard, Suite 220, Indianapolis, IN 46202, USA
* Corresponding author.
E-mail address: gecoots@gmail.com

Urol Clin N Am 46 (2019) 215–223
https://doi.org/10.1016/j.ucl.2018.12.012

shockwave technology it is unlikely that extracorporeal stone interventions will become obsolete. In fact, advances in the understanding of stone comminution have resulted in a novel application of focused ultrasound (US) to propel and fragment kidney stones.[7] This platform, called burst wave lithotripsy (BWL), has the potential to revolutionize the treatment of nephrolithiasis. Early clinical successes with BWL are promising and indicate that symptomatic patients with nephrolithiasis will be treated immediately in an outpatient clinic setting using standard US equipment.[8] Improvements in current, as well as emerging, technologies in stone fragmentation are reviewed with the intent of providing an update on the advances in extracorporeal lithotripsy.

EXTRACORPOREAL SHOCKWAVE LITHOTRIPSY

ESWL is among of the most frequently used treatment modalities for nephrolithiasis in the United States.[3] The principles of stone comminution secondary to external shockwaves remain unchanged; however, the technology has undergone several modifications and understanding of the optimal patient or stone for successful ESWL has improved. The current American Urological Association (AUA) guidelines state that ESWL should be offered for mid and upper pole kidney stones less than 20 mm.[9,10] Additionally, patients with ureteral stones should be informed that ESWL has the lowest morbidity and complication rate but it is associated with a lower SFR with a higher potential for retreatment compared with URS.[9] If patients prefer to undergo ESWL therapy instead of URS, ESWL is appropriate for the treatment of mid and proximal ureteral stones. Based on the metaanalysis performed in the AUA guidelines, ESWL seems to have minimal benefit for stones greater than 1 cm in the lower pole of the kidney or stones in the distal ureter.[10]

Additional efforts to predict positive outcomes after ESWL, other than stone location, have been published. Early studies have demonstrated that the larger stones or larger total stone volumes increase the likelihood of residual fragments after ESWL.[11,12] Kanao and colleagues[11] found that SFRs ranged from 94% for a solitary 5 mm stone to as low as 11% for multiple stones totaling 2 cm or greater stone burden.[12] Previous studies have demonstrated that certain stone compositions, such as brushite, cystine, and calcium oxalate monohydrate (COM) stones, are fairly resistant to ESWL[13,14]; however, current era computed tomography scanning techniques can only reliably differentiate stones into uric acid and nonuric acid stone compositions,[15] leading clinicians to rely more on stone density measurements. El-Assmy and colleagues[16] looked at 103 stones treated with ESWL and found that those greater than 1000 HU required more shocks at 80 and even 120 kV to comminute than stones less than 1000 HU. Wang and colleagues[17] performed a multivariate analysis of comminution factors for ESWL and found that HU greater than 900 was a significant predictor of ESWL failure. Patient size also influences ESWL success. Skin-to-stone distance (SSD), which is an average of 3 measurements from the skin to the stone at 90° and 45° angles, has been found to also influence stone fragmentation (**Fig. 1**). Cutoff points for success vary but some of the earlier studies noted distances greater 10 cm[18,19] or 9 cm[20] as predictors of failure.

One group, attempting to improve patient selection using an algorithmic approach that incorporated all the aforementioned variables, created the Triple D scoring system. The Triple D system can stratify ESWL success based on favorable factors, including stone density (<600 HU), stone dimension (volume <150 mL), and SSD (<12 cm) (**Table 1**).[21] Patients are awarded points for having favorable properties in each category. Follow-up imaging after ESWL with renal US and kidney, ureter, bladder (KUB) radiograph has demonstrated that patients with a Triple D score of 3 demonstrate a 96% SFR after ESWL compared with 21.4% for a score of 0.

A variety of innovations in ESWL technology continue to occur with the goals of improving equipment mobility, reducing patient discomfort,

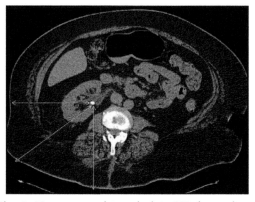

Fig. 1. Measures used to calculate SSD (*arrows*) are incorporated into the Triple D score and have been used to predict success rates of extracorporeal shockwave lithotripsy. Patients who are stone-free after ESWL have an average SSD of 11.3 cm compared with those who are not stone-free with an average SSD of 12.4 cm (*P*<.05).

Table 1
Adaptation of the Triple D score, which elegantly predicts the success rate of ESWL based on stone size, skin-to-stone distance, and stone density

Variable	Points: Yes = 1; No = 0	Success Rate
SSD	SSD <12 cm	—
Stone density	<600 HU	—
Ellipsoid stone volume	<150 mL	—
Total	0	21.4%
	1	41.3%
	2	78.7%
	3	96.1%

Data from Tran TY, McGillen K, Cone EB, et al. Triple D score is a reportable predictor of shockwave lithotripsy stone-free rates. J Endourol 2014;29(2):226–30.

and minimizing renal tissue injury. Unfortunately, these improvements have resulted in a general reduction in the comminution efficiency of the newer generation lithotripters compared with the original Dornier HM-3 lithotripter (Dornier Med-Tech, Webling, Germany). Multiple studies have demonstrated that the wider expanding shockwave focus (F2), impacting the stone, characteristic of the HM-3 lithotripter is more effective than lithotripters with intermediate and narrow F2 focal zones.[22,23] In cases with multiple stones, Zehnder and colleagues[23] showed a 20% higher SFR (P = .003) at 3 months with an 8% lower retreatment rate (P = .003) when comparing the HM-3 with the Storz Modulith SLX-F2 lithotripter (STORZ MEDICAL AG, Tägerwilen, Switzerland). The reduction in fragmentation of the newer lithotripters is thought to be a result of a narrower focal zone at F2, which is characteristic of smaller more mobile lithotripters.[24] The focal zone was narrowed to decrease pain associated with the procedure and allow ESWL to be performed without the need of general anesthesia. With a smaller focal zone, fewer shocks are successfully delivered to the stone during respiratory movement and instead are deposited into the surrounding tissue. Using US to monitor for stone motion in 10 subjects undergoing ESWL, Sorensen and colleagues[25] found that 40% of shocks did not come in contact with the stone and likely damaged the surrounding tissue. To overcome the limitation of the smaller F2 device, manufacturers increased the energy delivered in hopes of improving stone fragmentation. Despite higher peak pressures delivered at F2 with second-generation and third-generation lithotripters, the efficiency of stone

fragmentation has reduced.[26] A wider F2 encases the stone within the shockwave and increases the sheer, compression, and spalling stresses on the stone.[2] Additionally, a broader focal zone increases the likelihood that shockwave energy contacts a stone during respiratory-induced stone movement. Efforts have been made to widen the F2 of newer generation lithotripters without losing the benefits of limited skin contact and pain. Through the use of modified acoustic lenses that widen the F2 focal zone, Neisius and colleagues[27] were able to show improved stone comminution efficiency in a third-generation electromagnetic lithotripter. The modified lens and wider F2 focal zone used to fragment synthetic BegoStones implanted in the urinary system of sedated pigs increased reduction in stone mass from 54% plus or minus 23% to 88% plus or minus 11% (P = .01) after 3000 shocks.

In addition to the F2 focal zone characteristics, the source of shockwave energy can improve stone fragmentation efficiency. Novel lithotripters tend to be powered by electromagnetic, piezoelectric, and electroconductive generators rather than the electrohydraulic (spark gap) generator used in the HM-3. The spark gap generator of the HM3 degrades with use and becomes less efficient during its lifetime. Thus the generator requires frequent changes to obtain maximal results.[28] In a recent in vitro study comparing 3 novel lithotripters (Sonolith electroconductive i-sys EDAP TMS, Vaulx-en-Velin, France, Stortz electromagnetic Modulith SLX F2 STORZ MEDICAL AG, Tägerwilen, Switzerland, Wolf Piezolith 3000 Richard Wolf GmbH, Knittlingen, Germany) delivering 1000 shocks to 300 mg gypsum stones reduced the stone size by approximately 45 mg (15%), 210 mg (70%), and 260 mg (86%), respectively (P<.05).[24] This led the investigators to conclude that lithotripters powered by electromagnetic and piezoelectric generators are more efficient. Comparative studies looking at electromagnetic-powered, or piezoelectric-powered, and electrohydraulic-powered lithotripters demonstrate mixed results but tend to favor the electrohydraulic-powered HM-3. One study compared an electrohydraulic (HM-3) and a piezoelectric-powered (EDAP LT01) lithotripter and found a 77.2% versus 42.5% SFR, respectively, 3 months after lithotripsy for stones greater than 30 mm.[29] There are multiple confounding variables within these studies but, ultimately, the improved durability of the electromagnetic and piezoelectric generators has resulted in their proliferation compared with the spark gap generators for novel external shockwave lithotripters.

Coupling is essential to deliver maximal shock-wave energy to the stone. The original HM3 required the patient be fully submerged in a water bath, resulting in the ultimate coupling conditions. However, the HM3 required the dedication of an entire operating room for 1 procedure, and it was difficult for the anesthesiologist to safely manage the anesthetized patient while submerged. Thus, subsequent-generation lithotripters have relied on the coupling medium instead of the water bath. The optimal agent to couple the patient to the lithotripter is a water-soluble gel rather than a petroleum jelly. Anesthetic creams, such as EMLA (Aspen Pharma Trading Limited, Dublin, Ireland), have also been tested and do not seem to be appropriate for coupling. A study by Cartledge and colleagues[30] found no reduction in procedural morbidity or pain with using EMLA cream for coupling and showed no improvement compared with US jelly for stone comminution efficiency. When using a water-based coupling agent, all efforts should be made to limit air pockets because they are a significant deterrent to coupling and can occur spontaneously or with movement. Air pockets covering as little as 2% of the coupling area will diminish stone comminution by 20% to 40%.[31] To date, there are no commercially available monitoring tools to detect and prevent bubbles in the coupling media; however, the technology exists. Bohris and colleagues[32] used video cameras placed in the head of a Dornier Doli SII lithotripter (Dornier MedTech, Webling, Germany) to detect air pockets in the coupling gel. The investigators found that air bubbles could be actively monitored and the presence of air bubbles affected the number of shockwave needed for stone fragmentation.

Shockwave delivery rate and shockwave power modifications have been a focus for potential modifications to maximize stone fragmentation and minimize tissue injury during ESWL.[33] Slower rates were originally unfavorable because the prolonged operating times limited the number of patients who could be treated in a day and were thought to delay the delivery of required shocks to achieve stone comminution. A better understanding of cavitation bubble characteristics, including the ability for cloud bubbles to attenuate subsequent shockwaves and bubble dissipation rates, has provided a rationale of the observation that increasing rates does not equate to quicker stone comminution.[34] In 2016, Kang and colleagues[35] performed a metaanalysis that included 13 randomized controlled trials of subjects with stones ranging in size from 5 to 30 mm. The definition of successful lithotripsy varied but was largely defined as stone fragments less than 4 mm up to 3 months after ESWL. The investigators demonstrated an odds ratio between 2.2 and 2.7 (95% CI 1.3–4.6) for success when comparing low (60–70 shocks/min) and intermediate (80–90 shocks/min) to high (120 shocks/min) shockwave rates. These findings were affirmed in previous metaanalysis that showed better success with a low shock rate, with an average of approximately 500 fewer shocks and 23 minutes less of operating room time ($P = .1$ and $P<.001$, respectively).[36] In addition to shock rate, power-ramping protocols have been explored in depth. SFRs, defined as less than 2 mm fragments on KUB at 1 and 3 months, were superior (81% vs 48%, $P<.03$) with a ramping protocol compared with fixed shocking of 18 kV for 2500 shocks. Based on delayed resolution of elevated levels of urinary microalbumin and β2-microglobulin after fixed ESWL compared with the ramping protocol ($P<.05$), the investigators concluded that ramping may be protective against tissue injury. These findings were reiterated in a study by Connors and colleagues[33] in which anesthetized pigs underwent 300 pretreatment shockwaves followed by 2000 standard shocks at 24 kV compared with fixed-energy ESWL. Renal lesions caused by local hemorrhage were measured as a percentage of functional renal volume (FRV) loss. Pretreated pigs, on average, had less than 1% FRV compared with 3.5% FRV loss with fixed-energy ESWL. This led the investigators to conclude that pretreatment and ramping allows for vascular constriction during ramping pauses, which reduces hemorrhage and tissue injury.

Finally, improvements in stone-imaging technology used during ESWL have been somewhat stagnant and most devices still rely on original fluoroscopic technology introduced with the first generation of lithotripters. Despite efforts to reduce radiation exposure to patients and providers, fluoroscopy continues to be the preferred image-guidance modality. Advantages of fluoroscopy include familiarity, ease of interpretation, and reliability irrespective of patient characteristics (eg, a large body habitus). Alternatively, US can provide real-time feedback on radiolucent stones without radiation exposure to the surgeon or patient. Unfortunately, the technical challenges of identifying stones and tracking stone fragments during lithotripsy have limited the application of US in ESWL. One area of interest is the combination of US and fluoroscopy to improve the accuracy of shocks delivered to urinary stones. In 1 study, a LiteMed LM-9200 electromagnetic lithotripter (LITEMED Inc., Taipei City, Taiwan) with fluoroscopic and a real-time US-based tracking system were used to treat 1332 subjects with average stone burden of 12.3 cm (59.5% <10 mm, 23.2% 10–20 mm, 17.3% >20 mm). The investigators reported an 80% SFR at 3 months based on KUB or US with only 1716 shocks and an average treatment time of 23.8 minutes.[37] Similar outcomes were reported by Abid and colleagues[38] using a Sonolith i-sys lithotripter with a handheld 3-dimensional US stone locking system called Visio-Tracking (VT). Compared with fluoroscopy alone, the VT-enhanced system showed significantly lower intra-operative radiation exposure of 163 (0–13,926) versus 10,597 (0–54,843) mGy·cm² (P<.001) and improved SFRs of 79.5% versus 54.5% (P = .001). The investigators mention that success with the VT system was user-dependent and acknowledged the learning curve associated with this technology was difficult to overcome, which is a common complaint about US imaging. However, improved outcomes after ESWL can be achieved by learning and integrating real-time US data to enhance ESWL, an advancement that will be even more important as novel US lithotripters emerge.

BURST WAVE LITHOTRIPSY

Focused US technology is nearing clinical application and has generated significant interest in its capacity to propel renal stones. However, another exciting application of focused US is its use as a burst wave lithotripter. Comminution of renal stones is a product of direct energy from the shockwave and indirect energy from collapsing cavitation bubbles that apply stress at the surface and within the stone. With traditional shockwave lithotripsy there is a 5:1 ratio of positive (high-amplitude compressive) to negative (low-amplitude tensile) energy delivered over 4 microseconds.[39] By comparison, BWL delivers a sinusoidal burst of waves with a 1:1 ratio over 0.5 microseconds.[7] The amplitude of the burst waves is a fraction (6.5 MPa vs 40.0 MPa) of that seen with standard ESWL (**Fig. 2**). The initial interest in lower energy amplitudes originated from the observation that the original Dornier HM3 lithotripter is a superior lithotripter compared with newer lithotripters because it delivers shocks with relatively lower pressure amplitudes to a broader focal zone. A burst of low-amplitude, rather than a single high-amplitude shock, is thought to reduce excessive bubble production that occurs during cavitation.[40] Excessive bubbles can shield subsequent waves from making contact with the stone. By minimizing excessive bubble production, BWL vastly increases the efficiency of the shockwave delivered. A single

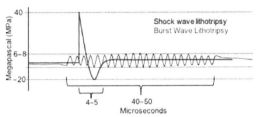

Fig. 2. Difference between a single shockwave versus a burst wave complex used to fracture stones. The lower amplitude of the burst wave has less potential for surrounding tissue damage, avoids serial wave attenuation by residual cavitation bubbles, and can be delivered with a modified US transducer. (*Data from* Matlaga BR, Krambeck AE, Lingeman JE. Surgical management of upper urinary tract calculi. Campbell-Walsh Urology 2016;11:1260–90; and Maxwell AD, Cunitz BW, Kreider W, et al. Fragmentation of urinary calculi in vitro by burst wave lithotripsy. J Urol 2015;193(1):338–44).

burst of low-amplitude shockwaves characteristic of BWL is highly efficient at stone comminution and tends to fragment the stone at the working face, much like a laser rather than the block fragmentation seen with ESWL.

Initial in vitro studies evaluating BWL used artificial stones with characteristics similar to COM stones, as well as naturally occurring uric acid, struvite, and cystine stone from human subjects. Stones ranged in size from 5 to 15 mm in the largest diameter and were mounted to acoustically permeable membranes between 0.5 and 1.4 cm away from 3 US transducers.[7] When exposed to a burst of 50 sinusoidal waves with an amplitude energy of 6.5 MPa, both synthetic and naturally occurring stones fractured. The treatment duration required for stone fragmentation and the size of posttreatment stone fragments were most affected by stone type. Treatment duration ranged from 4 seconds in struvite stones to 21.3 minutes with cystine stones. COM and artificial stones fractured at 120 kHz had the largest portion of fragments, ranging from 3 to 4 mm (**Table 2**). From their initial trials, the investigators concluded that BWL, unlike ESWL, could be applied to all stone types, including cystine stones. They hypothesized, based on these preliminary data, that a frequency between 400 and 500 kHz at 6.5 MPa would be optimal to achieve 1 mm stone fragments.

In 2017, results from BWL application in a porcine model were released. The study had several goals, including (1) to evaluate the extent of renal trauma (focal tubular damage, microscopic hemorrhage, cellular fragmentation, and necrosis) BWL could induce and (2) to assess if

Table 2
The efficiency in stone comminution by burst wave lithotripsy using various transducers, stone types, and energy frequencies

Stone Type	Treatment Duration (range of minutes)	Burst No. (× 1000)	Largest Fragment Size (range mm)	Most Common Fragment Size mm (%)
Artificial at 170 kHz	—	—	3–4	1–2 (40)
Artificial at 285 kHz	—	—	1–2	<1 (80)
Artificial at 800 kHz	—	—	<1	<1 (100)
Struvite at 170 kHz	0.07–2.02	.8–24.24	2–3	<1 (60)
Uric Acid at 170 kHz	0.17–1.4	2.04–16.	3–4	1–2 (40)
COM at 170 kHz	8.0–18.1	96–271.2	3–4	2–3 (75)
Artificial at 335 kHz	—	0.8	<2	<2 (18)
Artificial at 335 kHz + UP	—	0.8	<2	<2 (28)
COM at 335 kHz + UP	—	0.8	<2	<2 (36)
Cystine at 170 kHz	10.3–21.3	123–255	2–3	<1 (60)

UP was imbedded with the standard burst waves every 6 seconds to assist with comminution. COM and cystine stones were efficiently fractured using BWL.

real-time US and/or posttreatment MRI could identify BWL-induced renal injury.[40] Anesthetized supine pigs underwent a laparotomy, followed by direct coupling of the BWL treatment probe (housing 170 and 335 kHz transducers) to the renal capsule. The lower, mid, and upper pole regions of 8 renal units were exposed to BWL with burst amplitudes ranging from 5.8 to 8.1 MPa. Each region (except 3 regions that received no exposure and served as controls) experienced between 5 and 21 minutes of BWL, during which tissue cavitation was monitored with B-mode US. After BWL exposure to each region was complete, the kidneys were fixed in situ and underwent MRI and histomorphometric evaluation. The investigators found that tissue cavitation seen on US during BWL treatment perfectly predicted tissue injury. Posttreatment MRI missed 1 area of injury but demonstrated 100% specificity for injured tissue. Of the 21 treatment sites, 10 had evidence of renal trauma on histomorphometric analysis. The largest percentages of functional tissue damage (2.5% and 5%) occurred with the 170 kHz transducer with a burst wave amplitude of 6.5 MPa for 5 and 17 minutes, respectively. In all other instances of tissue injury, there was less than 0.1% of functional tissue loss. By comparison, early studies with the HM3 lithotripter, delivering standard doses of ESWL (2000 shocks at 24 kV and 2 Hz) resulted in 5% to 6% of functional tissue loss, respectively.[41] The investigators concluded that real-time monitoring for tissue injury is possible during BWL treatments. Additionally,

they thought that in the rare instances that tissue cavitation was missed on US during treatment, the resulting injury was clinically insignificant and no worse than injury seen with ESWL.

In early 2018, having demonstrated both the safety and feasibility of BWL, Maxwell and colleagues[42] sought to improve the efficiency of BWL. In prior studies, the group had observed that BWL expeditiously fractured artificial stones but that the dispersion of fragment was often delayed. Additionally, prior studies had demonstrated that ultrasonic propulsion (UP) could delineate a cluster of stones from a single stone with a strong low-amplitude pulse.[43] A potential solution to expedite BWL was to couple UP with BWL, thus allowing for full delineation of residual fragments and determination if further BWL is needed before the treatment is discontinued. Human COM and artificial stones with similar characteristics to COM stones were exposed to a 20-cycle burst wave with a peak pressure of 8 MPa via a 335 kHz transducer at 40 Hz. The transducer was coupled with a Philips P4-2 (Philips North America Corp, MA, USA) diagnostic US probe with both B-mode imaging for stone targeting and single propulsion pulse of 0.15 MPa. The investigators trialed a variety of different settings but found that the most efficient algorithm included 60 propulsion pulses per minute with BWL. After 5 minutes of treatment on COM stones, BWL alone was compared with BWL and UP for percent of stone reduced to 2 mm or less fragments. There was a 2-fold increase in fragmentation efficiency seen with BWL plus UP (36% $\pm$ 28%) versus BWL (17% $\pm$ 11%) (P = .014). Similar outcomes were observed with artificial stones, which led the investigators to conclude that BWL with interleaved UP is more effective than BWL alone.[42]

Clinical trials evaluating BWL are still lacking but the potential to revolutionize extracorporeal lithotripsy seems to lie with the future development of focused US technology. The first commercial UP unit made by (SonoMotion Inc. San Francisco, CA, USA) is set to debut in 2019. However, there is no indication of when BWL will be available for clinical application.

HISTOTRIPSY

Histotripsy, like BWL, uses focused pulsed US energy to fracture stones. It was originally designed to fractionate tissue structures though extremely precise liquefaction, resulting in tissue defects with sharp demarcated boarders. Histotripsy has been used to perforate cardiac tissue in animal models to create a shunt, and for ablation of benign and malignant tissue lesions.[44] Histotripsy can be regarded as a specific type of high-intensity focused US (HIFU) technology.[45] HIFU technology requires a fluid–tissue interface to work effectively, which prompted some investigators to question its capacity in lithotripsy given the abundant fluid–stone interface within the urinary collecting system. A group from Michigan reported the initial experience with urinary calculi cavitation and fragmentation using US histotripsy. The investigators used gypsum stones with an average mass of 900 mg with largest diameter of 10 mm. Using a 750 kHz transducer delivering a 5-cycle pulse with repetition frequency of 1 kHz, gypsum stones were fractioned for 5 minutes. After treatment, average stone mass was 509 plus or minus 95 mg, representing a 53.4% reduction. Stone fragments were all 100 μm compared with 1 to 2 mm with standard ESWL delivered using the Wolf Piezolith 3000. An optimal stone erosion rate of 85 plus or minus 12 mg/min was achieved with histotripsy at 19 MPa of negative pressure. Standard ESWL with peak positive or negative pressure of 76 or 14 MPa generated a stone erosion rate of 110 plus or minus 27 mg/min.[46] Despite promising preliminary results, HIFU-histotripsy erosion efficiency was limited. Remnant cavitation bubbles that linger on the stone surface for approximately 100 μs shielded the stone from subsequent US pulses and further cavitation. Attempts by Duryea and colleagues[47] to incorporate low-amplitude acoustic pulses for bubble removal did improve in vitro stone erosion;

however, subsequent progression of the technology has been limited and further outcomes are pending.

MICROBUBBLE LITHOTRIPSY

Microbubble technology is emerging as a potential adjunct to ESWL. Targeted microbubbles contain perfluorinated carbon gas centers with phospholipid surfaces that can be modified to have binding domains. In the preliminary application of microbubble lithotripsy for use in stone disease, 1 group modified the surface phospholipid, dipalmitoylphosphatidylcholine, by attaching a bisphosphonate binding domain. They were able to demonstrate in vitro attachment of the microbubble to the surface of a calcium-based stone.[48] The investigators then used a porcine animal model with endoscopically implanted synthetic hydroxyapatite and human stones to evaluate the safety and effectiveness of microbubble lithotripsy. Using a 5 F ureteral catheter, targeting microbubbles were introduced in a retrograde fashion every 90 seconds. A 300 to 1000 kHz US transducer delivering 1.2 plus or minus 0.2 MPa was able to fragment 5 mm stones into 2 mm fragments in less than 30 minutes. Histologic evaluation of renal and ureteral parenchyma and urothelium showed no evidence of hemorrhage or tissue injury.[49] Bubble cavitation is the major mechanism for stone erosion identified in BWL and HIFU-histotripsy. The efficiency of these novel extracorporeal lithotripters is limited by the erosion potential of each shock pulse and the clearance rate of cloud cavitation bubbles. Microbubble technology has the potential to augment both novel platforms by enhancing the erosion efficiency of urinary stones. Furthermore, microbubble technology has the potential to improve the safety of all lithotripsy devices by lowering the required energy being delivered by the external lithotripter.

SUMMARY

Since the original introduction of the HM-3 shockwave lithotripter, knowledge of how stones fragment and what measures can be taken to optimize outcomes has greatly improved. Device-related alterations, such as changes in focal zone area, energy, and delivery rate, as well as imaging modalities for monitoring stone fragmentation, can vastly improve results. The future of lithotripsy seems to be moving toward adjuncts to improve safety and fragmentation, such as microbubble technology. Newer technology lithotripters, such as histotripsy and BWL, work by varying the delivery of US waves to the stone. These technologies seem to hold the key to a future of successful, minimally invasive, bedside treatments for symptomatic stone disease.

REFERENCES

1. Chaussy C, Schüller J, Schmiedt E, et al. Extracorporeal shock-wave lithotripsy (ESWL) for treatment of urolithiasis. Urology 1984;23(5):59–66.
2. Matlaga BR, Krambeck AE, Lingeman JE. Surgical management of upper urinary tract calculi. Campbell-walsh Urology 2016;11:1260–90.
3. Pearle MS, Calhoun EA, Curhan GC. Urologic diseases in America project: urolithiasis. J Urol 2005; 173(3):848–57.
4. Garcia-Galisteo E, Sánchez-Martínez N, Molina-Díaz P, et al. Invasive treatment trends in urinary calculi in a third level hospital. Actas Urol Esp 2015;39(1):32–7.
5. Oberlin DT, Flum AS, Bachrach L, et al. Contemporary surgical trends in the management of upper tract calculi. J Urol 2015;193(3):880–4.
6. Ziemba JB, Matlaga BR. Epidemiology and economics of nephrolithiasis. Investig Clin Urol 2017; 58(5):299–306.
7. Maxwell AD, Cunitz BW, Kreider W, et al. Fragmentation of urinary calculi in vitro by burst wave lithotripsy. J Urol 2015;193(1):338–44.
8. Janssen KM, Brand TC, Bailey MR, et al. Effect of stone size and composition on ultrasonic propulsion ex vivo. Urology 2018;111:225–9.
9. Assimos D, Krambeck A, Miller NL, et al. Surgical management of stones: American Urological Association/Endourological Society Guideline, part I. J Urol 2016;196(4):1153–60.
10. Assimos D, Krambeck A, Miller NL, et al. Surgical management of stones: American Urological Association/Endourological Society Guideline, part II. J Urol 2016;196(4):1161–9.
11. Kanao K, Nakashima J, Nakagawa K, et al. Preoperative nomograms for predicting stone-free rate after extracorporeal shock wave lithotripsy. J Urol 2006; 176(4 Pt 1):1453–6 [discussion: 1456–7].
12. Abdel-Khalek M, Sheir KZ, Mokhtar AA, et al. Prediction of success rate after extracorporeal shock-wave lithotripsy of renal stones—a multivariate analysis model. Scand J Urol Nephrol 2004;38(2):161–7.
13. Segura JW, Preminger GM, Assimos DG, et al. Ureteral stones clinical guidelines panel summary report on the management of ureteral calculi. J Urol 1997;158(5):1915–21.
14. Klee LW, Brito CG, Lingeman JE. Clinical implications of Brushite Calculi. J Urol 1991;145(4):715–8.
15. Leng S, Shiung M, Ai S, et al. Feasibility of discriminating uric acid from non–uric acid renal stones using consecutive spatially registered low-and high-energy scans obtained on a conventional CT scanner. AJR Am J Roentgenol 2015;204(1):92–7.
16. El-Assmy A, Abou-el-Ghar ME, el-Nahas AR, et al. Multidetector computed tomography: role in determination of urinary stones composition and disintegration with extracorporeal shock wave lithotripsy—an in vitro study. Urology 2011;77(2): 286–90.
17. Wang LJ, Wong YC, Chuang CK, et al. Predictions of outcomes of renal stones after extracorporeal shock wave lithotripsy from stone characteristics determined by unenhanced helical computed tomography: a multivariate analysis. Eur Radiol 2005; 15(11):2238–43.
18. Pareek G, Hedican SP, Lee FT Jr, et al. Shock wave lithotripsy success determined by skin-to-stone distance on computed tomography. Urology 2005; 66(5):941–4.
19. Patel T, Kozakowski K, Hruby G, et al. Skin to stone distance is an independent predictor of stone-free status following shockwave lithotripsy. J Endourol 2009;23(9):1383–5.
20. Perks AE, Schuler TD, Lee J, et al. Stone attenuation and skin-to-stone distance on computed tomography predicts for stone fragmentation by shock wave lithotripsy. Urology 2008;72(4):765–9.
21. Tran TY, McGillen K, Cone EB, et al. Triple D score is a reportable predictor of shockwave lithotripsy stone-free rates. J Endourol 2014;29(2):226–30.
22. Dhar NB, Thornton J, Karafa MT, et al. A multivariate analysis of risk factors associated with subcapsular hematoma formation following electromagnetic shock wave lithotripsy. J Urol 2004;172(6, Part 1): 2271–4.
23. Zehnder P, Roth B, Birkhäuser F, et al. A prospective randomised trial comparing the modified HM3 with the MODULITH® SLX-F2 lithotripter. Eur Urol 2011; 59(4):637–44.
24. Faragher SR, Cleveland RO, Kumar S, et al. In vitro assessment of three clinical lithotripters employing different shock wave generators. J Endourol 2016; 30(5):560–5.
25. Sorensen MD, Bailey MR, Shah AR, et al. Quantitative assessment of shockwave lithotripsy accuracy and the effect of respiratory motion. J Endourol 2012;26(8):1070–4.
26. Sapozhnikov OA, Maxwell AD, MacConaghy B, et al. A mechanistic analysis of stone fracture in lithotripsy. J Acoust Soc Am 2007;121(2):1190–202.
27. Neisius A, Smith NB, Sankin G, et al. Improving the lens design and performance of a contemporary electromagnetic shock wave lithotripter. Proc Natl Acad Sci U S A 2014;111(13):E1167–75.
28. Lingeman JE. Extracorporeal shock wave lithotripsy. Development, instrumentation, and current status. Urol Clin North Am 1997;24(1):185–211.

29. Sofras F, Karayannis A, Kastriotis J, et al. Extracorporeal shockwave lithotripsy or extracorporeal piezoelectric lithotripsy? Comparison of costs and results. Br J Urol 1991;68(1):15–7.

30. Cartledge JJ, Cross WR, Lloyd SN, et al. The efficacy of a range of contact media as coupling agents in extracorporeal shockwave lithotripsy. BJU Int 2001;88(4):321–4.

31. Pishchalnikov YA, Neucks JS, VonDerHaar RJ, et al. Air pockets trapped during routine coupling in dry head lithotripsy can significantly decrease the delivery of shock wave energy. J Urol 2006;176(6):2706–10.

32. Bohris C, Roosen A, Dickmann M, et al. Monitoring the coupling of the lithotripter therapy head with skin during routine shock wave lithotripsy with a surveillance camera. J Urol 2012;187(1):157–63.

33. Connors BA, Evan AP, Handa RK, et al. Using 300 pretreatment shock waves in a voltage ramping protocol can significantly reduce tissue injury during extracorporeal shock wave lithotripsy. J Endourol 2016;30(9):1004–8.

34. Nguyen DP, Hnilicka S, Kiss B, et al. Optimization of extracorporeal shock wave lithotripsy delivery rates achieves excellent outcomes for ureteral stones: results of a prospective randomized trial. J Urol 2015;194(2):418–23.

35. Kang DH, Cho KS, Ham WS, et al. Comparison of high, intermediate, and low frequency shock wave lithotripsy for urinary tract stone disease: systematic review and network meta-analysis. PLoS One 2016;11(7):e0158661.

36. Li K, Lin T, Zhang C, et al. Optimal frequency of shock wave lithotripsy in urolithiasis treatment: a systematic review and meta-analysis of randomized controlled trials. J Urol 2013;190(4):1260–7.

37. Chen C-J, Hsu HC, Chung WS, et al. Clinical experience with ultrasound-based real-time tracking lithotripsy in the single renal stone treatment. J Endourol 2009;23(11):1811–5.

38. Abid N, Ravier E, Promeyrat X, et al. Decreased radiation exposure and increased efficacy in extracorporeal lithotripsy using a new ultrasound stone locking system. J Endourol 2015;29(11):1263–9.

39. Coleman A, Saunders JE, Preston RC, et al. Pressure waveforms generated by a Dornier extracorporeal shock-wave lithotripter. Ultrasound Med Biol 1987;13(10):651–7.

40. Janssen KM, Brand TC, Cunitz BW, et al. Safety and effectiveness of a longer focal beam and burst duration in ultrasonic propulsion for repositioning urinary stones and fragments. J Endourol 2017;31(8):793–9.

41. Connors BA, Evan AP, Willis LR, et al. The effect of discharge voltage on renal injury and impairment caused by lithotripsy in the pig. J Am Soc Nephrol 2000;11(2):310–8.

42. Zwaschka TA, Ahn JS, Cunitz BW, et al. Combined burst wave lithotripsy and ultrasonic propulsion for improved urinary stone fragmentation. J Endourol 2018;32(4):344–9.

43. Harper JD, Cunitz BW, Dunmire B, et al. First in human clinical trial of ultrasonic propulsion of kidney stones. J Urol 2016;195(4, Part 1):956–64.

44. Xu Z, Ludomirsky A, Eun LY, et al. Controlled ultrasound tissue erosion. IEEE Trans Ultrason Ferroelectr Freq Control 2004;51(6):726–36.

45. Yoshizawa S, Ikeda T, Ito A, et al. High intensity focused ultrasound lithotripsy with cavitating microbubbles. Med Biol Eng Comput 2009;47(8):851–60.

46. Duryea AP, Hall TL, Maxwell AD, et al. Histotripsy erosion of model urinary Calculi. J Endourol 2010;25(2):341–4.

47. Duryea AP, Roberts WW, Cain CA, et al. Removal of residual cavitation nuclei to enhance histotripsy erosion of model urinary stones. IEEE Trans Ultrason Ferroelectr Freq Control 2015;62(5):896–904.

48. Ramaswamy K, Marx V, Laser D, et al. Targeted microbubbles: a novel application for the treatment of kidney stones. BJU Int 2015;116(1):9–16.

49. Mellema M, Behnke-Parks W, Luong A, et al. PD22-11 absence of ureteral/renal injury following low intensity extracorporeal acoustic energy lithotripsy with stone-targeting microbubbles in an in vivo swine model. J Urol 2018;199(4, Supplement):e479.

New Technologies to Aid in Percutaneous Access

Mohammad Hajiha, MD, D. Duane Baldwin, MD*

KEYWORDS

- Percutaneous nephrolithotomy • Staghorn calculus • Kidney calculi • Radiation • Fluoroscopy
- Interventional ultrasonography • Image-guided surgery

KEY POINTS

- The success of percutaneous nephrolithotomy (PCNL) depends on the quality of the renal access.
- The technical difficulty and risk associated with PCNL access discourage urologists from obtaining their own access.
- Increased awareness of the risks of ionizing radiation has placed an emphasis on novel renal access techniques requiring less radiation exposure.
- Each of the novel techniques presented here has unique advantages and disadvantages, and the best approach may combine features of several different techniques.
- The optimal PCNL access technique should be easy to learn; require minimal radiation; and be safe, economical, efficient, and effective.

 Video content accompanies this article at http://www.urologic.theclinics.com.

INTRODUCTION

Since the original description of percutaneous nephrolithotomy (PCNL) by Fernström and Johansson[1] in 1976, the techniques used for PCNL have evolved significantly. Advances in PCNL have resulted in improved safety and efficacy, and reduced morbidity.

Although advances in PCNL have occurred, the initial renal access remains a challenging and high-risk step. The risk and technical difficulty have resulted in a minority of urologists (<20%) in the United States placing their own access.[2,3] The potential reasons for this trend include the technical difficulty, lack of equipment or necessary skills, hospital politics, the increases in operative time that are not adequately compensated by reimbursement, risk for patient complications, and the risk of radiation exposure to the patient and surgeon.[2] These trends are problematic because

evidence indicates that stone-free rates are higher, whereas complications and hospital stay are lower, with urologist-obtained access.[4,5]

Therefore, continued innovation in access techniques that simplifies the procedure, lowers risk, and reduces radiation exposure is needed. This article provides a high-level overview of recent advances in percutaneous renal access. The techniques are organized based on approach (antegrade or retrograde) and the imaging modality used, such as fluoroscopy, ultrasonography (US), computed tomography (CT), and other novel techniques (laser, electromagnetic, and robotics) (**Table 1**).

TECHNIQUES
Fluoroscopy Guided

The most common imaging modality used by urologists to obtain renal access is biplanar

Disclosure: Dr D.D. Baldwin is consultant for BARD and Olympus. He is speaker for Cook Medical. He is chief science officer for DARRT Medical. Dr M. Hajiha has nothing to disclose.
Department of Urology, Loma Linda University Health, Loma Linda University Medical Center, 11234 Anderson Street, Room A560, Loma Linda, CA 92354, USA
* Corresponding author.
E-mail address: DBaldwin@llu.edu

Table 1
Summary of novel renal access techniques

Approach	Imaging	Technique	Advantages	Disadvantages	Radiation	Study
Antegrade	Fluoro	iPAD assisted	• Clear 3D image of surrounding structures for assistance with needle insertion • Short learning curve • Portable fusion technology	• Radiation use • No real-time 3D image and therefore minimal adjustment of needle path allowed • Requires specialized equipment resulting in additional cost and setup time	High	Rassweiler et al,[47] 2012
Antegrade	Fluoro/robot	PAKY-RCM	• Remotely controlled needle insertion reduces surgeon radiation exposure • Needle can be inserted with surgeon in remote location • Potential reduction in human error	• Requires specialized equipment resulting in additional cost and setup time • Absence of tactile feedback at time of needle insertion • Steep learning curve	High	Su et al,[43] 2002
Antegrade	Fluoro/robot	ANT-X	• Potential reduction in human error • Automated needle trajectory • Some tactile feedback as surgeon inserts needle	• Radiation use • Requires specialized equipment resulting in additional cost and setup time	Moderate	Oo et al,[42] 2018
Antegrade	US/EM	SonixGPS US	• No radiation for access • Computer-generated needle trajectory • Able to follow the location of needle in real time • Facilitates use of US by tracking the needle in and out of US plane	• Requires additional equipment, which can add cost and complexity • Like all US, more difficult in obese patients • Requires correct catheter placement internally, cumbersome	Very low	Li et al,[32] 2015
Antegrade	US/fluoro	All-seeing needle	• Needle image confirms successful puncture of collecting system • Easy to learn	• Unable to redirect needle if in wrong trajectory • Needle images not helpful to guide insertion, only confirm final destination • Increased difficulty in obese patients • Requires specialized needle	Moderate	Bader et al,[36] 2011

Antegrade	US/fluoro	Virtual projection of US onto fluoro	• Combines benefits of US and fluoro • Reduced radiation exposure • Computer-generated needle trajectory	• Requires additional equipment, which can add cost and complexity • Cumbersome calibration steps are necessary	Moderate	Mozer et al,[37] 2007
Antegrade	CT	C-arm CT 3D virtual syngo iGuide navigation	• Provides best visualization of surrounding structures with 3D anatomy • Real-time images to guide trajectory • High success for cases where conventional renal puncture methods have failed	• High radiation dose to patient and surgeon • Reduced accuracy with increased renal mobility • Requires specialized equipment resulting in additional cost and setup time	Very high	Jiao et al,[44] 2018
Retrograde	Fluoro/URS	Lawson retrograde puncture wire	• Select optimal calyx for access using URS • Reduced use of fluoroscopy because starts in the collecting system • Shorter time to establish access • Second viewpoint for calyceal mapping	• Potential for errant path of stylet, especially in obese patients, resulting in: longer length of access sheath and potential injury to surrounding structures (spleen, liver, bowel, vessels) • More difficult in the lower pole	Low/ moderate	Kawahara et al,[14] 2012; Wynberg et al,[15] 2012
Combined antegrade/ retrograde	US/fluoro/URS	Combined US/fluoro/retrograde URS	• Reduced radiation for access • Removes ambiguity for balloon dilation and sheath placement under direct vision • Use of US to localize adjacent organs • Select optimal calyx for access using URS • Second viewpoint for calyceal mapping	• Difficult to perform with single surgeon • Risk of damaging URS with needle • More difficult in the lower pole	Low	Alsyouf et al,[39] 2016

(continued on next page)

Table 1
(continued)

Approach	Imaging	Technique	Advantages	Disadvantages	Radiation	Study
Combined antegrade/ retrograde	Laser/US/ fluoro/URS	Laser DARRT	• Very low use of radiation • Avoids radiating surgeon's hand while providing tactile feedback • Removes ambiguity for balloon dilation and sheath placement • Use of US to localize adjacent organs • Select optimal calyx for access using URS • Second viewpoint for calyceal mapping	• Requires attachable C-arm laser aiming beam, is not present at some centers • More difficult in the lower pole	Very low	Khater et al,[38] 2016
Combined antegrade/ retrograde	EM/URS	EM	• No radiation • Real-time 3D images guiding needle path • Easy to learn	• Requires specialized equipment, resulting in additional cost and setup time • Need specialized needle and ureteric catheter with EM sensor • No visualization of surrounding structures (US not used) • Special EM ureteric catheter can be difficult to maneuver into calyx full of stones	Very Low	Lima et al,[31] 2017

Abbreviations: ANT-X, automated needle targeting with x-ray; 3D, three-dimensional; DARRT, direct alignment radiation reduction technique; EM, electromagnetic; Fluoro, fluoroscopy; PAKY-RCM, percutaneous renal access to the kidney with a remote center of motion device; URS, ureteroscope.

fluoroscopy (86.3%).[6] Patients with large stones represent a vulnerable population because they receive ionizing radiation during the diagnosis, treatment, and follow-up imaging. There is no safe lower limit for radiation exposure. The risks of radiation, including malignancy, increase in direct proportion to exposure.[7,8] The US Food and Drug Administration has called for a reduction in radiation exposure. They specifically targeted CT, fluoroscopy, and nuclear medicine studies as part of an as low as reasonably achievable (ALARA) protocol.[9] Therefore, all PCNL access technique should implement ALARA.

Traditional fluoroscopy
Fluoroscopic-guided access has traditionally been performed in an antegrade fashion using either the bull's-eye or triangulation techniques.[10] In the bull's-eye technique, the needle tip and hub are aligned so that they appear as a dot overlying the target calyx before insertion using continuous fluoroscopy (**Fig. 1**).[1,10] In the triangulation technique, the needle is tracked in multiple planes using fluoroscopy to direct the needle into the desired calyx (**Fig. 2**). Both the bull's-eye and triangulation techniques use continuous fluoroscopy and expose the patient and surgeon to ionizing radiation. Although these

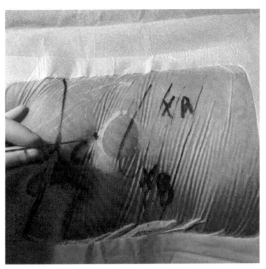

Fig. 2. Triangulation technique.

techniques have not changed drastically, there have been some modifications to the techniques, such as the use of pulsed and low-dose fluoroscopy. Use of low-dose fluoroscopy reduces radiation exposure by half, whereas use of 1 pulse per second decreases the radiation dose by 64% compared with continuous automatic exposure control settings.[11] Specialized needles are being independently developed that allow easier targeting under low-dose and pulsed fluoroscopy using the bull's-eye technique (**Fig. 3**) (Video 1).[12]

Retrograde fluoroscopic-guided technique
Lawson and colleagues[13] described the original retrograde passage of a stylet from the kidney to the skin using fluoroscopy guidance (**Fig. 4**). More recently a technique has been described in which a small needle is advanced in a retrograde fashion through the working port of a flexible ureteroscope.[14,15] Once the desired calyx is visualized, the needle is advanced out of the ureteroscope through the papillae and out from the skin (**Fig. 5**). This newer approach can use direct ureteroscopic vision to select the optimal calyx for access and requires less radiation exposure because of this ability to directly visualize the anatomy.[16] The biggest limitation of the retrograde technique is the potential for an errant path for the track, especially in obese patients because small variations in exit angle from the papillae may lead to needle exit remote from the intended site.[14]

Combined antegrade/retrograde fluoroscopic-guided technique
Grasso and colleagues[17] described the initial use of a combined simultaneous above and

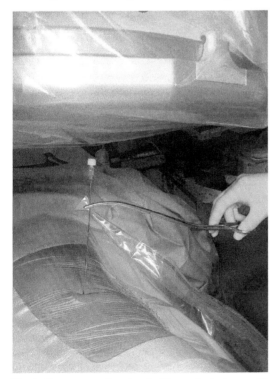

Fig. 1. Surgeon performing bull's-eye technique with the image intensifier of the C-arm rotated 20° toward the surgeon in order to target a posterior calyx.

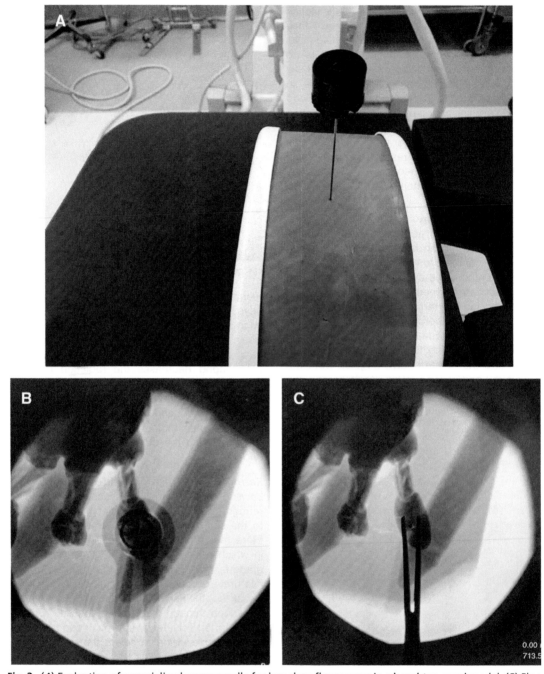

Fig. 3. (*A*) Evaluation of a specialized access needle for low-dose fluoroscopy in a benchtop renal model. (*B*) Fluoroscopic image of specialized needle with radiolucent handle and ring targeting system allows easier visualization of the needle hub compared with (*C*) regular needle with radiopaque metal clamp.

below approach in patients in whom a conventional antegrade fluoroscopic access had failed. Later, Khan and colleagues[16] realized that direct retrograde ureteroscopic vision was beneficial in all cases, not just the complicated ones. They reported using direct ureteroscopic visualization to identify the optimal access calyx, similar to other retrograde techniques, but inserted the needle in a more conventional antegrade approach. In this manner, they avoided the complication of having the skin site remote to the renal exit site. They also were able to directly visualize balloon dilation and sheath insertion.[16]

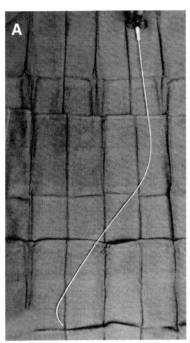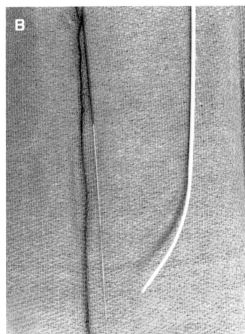

Fig. 4. Generic retrograde renal access device, (*A*) Tip deflecting wire guide. (*B*) Wire stylet, which can be passed through the wire guide.

With the downsizing of flexible ureteroscopes and improved optics over the last 3 decades, the combined PCNL access has been further simplified. Use of the endoscope to directly visualize the papillae and to correctly locate the renal access has been shown to dramatically lower fluoroscopy time (3.2 vs 16.8 minutes; $P<.001$), reduce the number of access tracts (1.01 vs 1.22; $P = .002$), and reduce the need for auxiliary procedures (3.2 vs 12.6%; $P = .04$).[18]

In the combined antegrade and retrograde technique, the ureteroscope can be directed into the desired calyx with the widest and shortest infundibulum offering direct stone access. Gentle ureteroscope irrigation hydrodistends the calyx even in nondilated systems. In addition, the tip of the ureteroscope can be targeted using fluoroscopy. The wire can be grasped ureteroscopically and then pulled past impacted stones into the ureter with minimal fluoroscopy. The surgeon has the option of establishing through-and-through access if desired. Balloon dilation and access sheath placement can be done with direct ureteroscopic visualization without use of fluoroscopy or US (**Fig. 6**).

Ultrasonography Guided

US has seen a new emphasis for PCNL access in the last decade because it allows imaging of adjacent organs while targeting the needle with reduced radiation exposure.[19] In experienced hands, US-guided renal access has similar outcomes to fluoroscopic-guided PCNL.[6] US-guided access is underused in North America,[20] likely because of a decreased familiarity with renal US combined with the larger patient size compared with Asia and Europe.[21] There are 2 techniques for US-guided needle insertion: longitudinal and transverse needle insertion (**Fig. 7**) (Video 2).[22]

Although US-guided needle insertion is increasing, other steps, such as tract dilation, access sheath insertion, and assessment for residual stones, represent an added level of complexity. Subsequently, most users use a combination of fluoroscopy and US for these steps,[23–26] although rarely fluoroless US-guided PCNL has been reported.[22] In a review of 96 US-guided PCNL patients, tract dilation, sheath insertion, and nephrostomy placement were challenging under US alone. The ideal patient for complete US-guided PCNL is thin, has hydronephrosis, and does not have a complex staghorn stone.[23]

The most important advantage of US for renal access is the reduction/elimination of radiation.[27] US allows access even where there is no ability to inject retrograde contrast (impacted ureteral stones or ileal conduits).[19] Other advantages include the ability to image adjacent structures

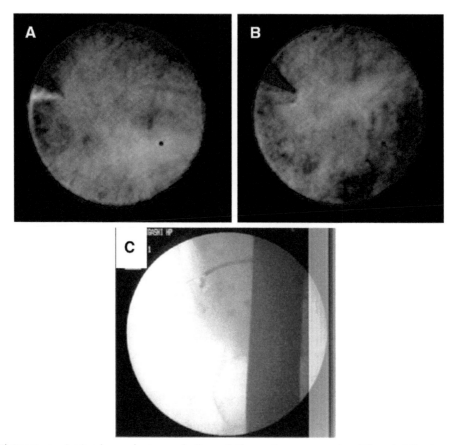

Fig. 5. (*A*) Puncture wire is advanced retrograde through the ureteroscope and positioned at the target papilla. (*B*) Puncture wire is advanced into the papilla. (*C*) Fluoroscopic image of puncture wire exiting ureteroscope. (*From* Kawahara T, Ito H, Terao H, et al. Ureteroscopy assisted retrograde nephrostomy: a new technique for percutaneous nephrolithotomy (PCNL). BJU Int 2012;110(4):588–90; with permission.)

(spleen, liver, colon, and pleura). The main limitations of US are the steep learning curve,[28] difficulty in obtaining high-quality images in the setting of obesity or nondilated systems,[29] and the potential for less-than-ideal access[25] with subsequent lower stone-free rates in large or complex stones.[30]

Modifications to facilitate ultrasonography-guided renal access

Tracking the needle tip can be challenging using US and a variety of approaches have been developed to facilitate this step.[24,31,32] One of the simplest solutions is to increase the visibility of the needle tip through etching, roughening, or polymeric coatings.[33] In addition, minimizing noise by avoiding air bubbles, use of adequate US gel, and imaging before placement of patient drapes improve the US image quality. Recently, contrast-enhanced US has been used to improve renal imaging, and access time has been reduced by 59% when contrast is injected in the collecting system (**Fig. 8**).[34]

Clear guide ultrasonography access A computer-assisted stereoscopic camera system (Clear Guide ONE, Clear Guide Medical, Baltimore, MD) has been designed to improve US-guided renal access. This device contains a 2-camera system that attaches to any commercially available US probe (**Fig. 9**). This system tracks the external portion of the needle and projects its course on the US monitor with guidance lines that change color to indicate the position of the needle. Green lines indicate that the needle trajectory will pass through the plane of the US beam, whereas blue lines project the needle's path outside the US beam (**Fig. 10**) (Video 3). In a prospective benchtop comparison (n = 71), the Clear Guide system was more successful (96% vs 56%; *P*<.001) and faster (114.6 vs 179.5 seconds; *P* = .02) than conventional US in obtaining renal access.[24]

The advantages of this device include easier needle tracking, ability to insert the needle from outside the US plane (particularly beneficial for

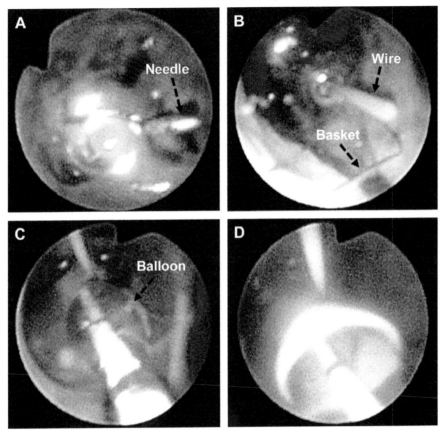

Fig. 6. Ureteroscopic view of (A) access needle insertion, (B) antegrade insertion of wire through the needle lumen with retrograde insertion of a generic retrograde renal access device to establish through and through access. (C) balloon dilation under direct ureteroscopic visualization, (D) access sheath insertion under direct ureteroscopic visualization.

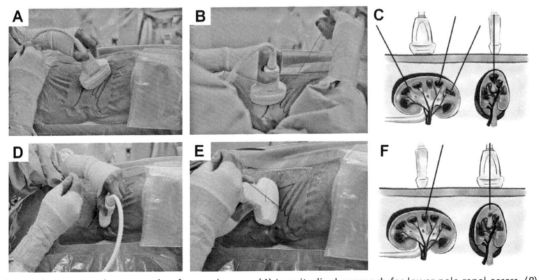

Fig. 7. Ultrasonography approaches for renal access. (A) Longitudinal approach for lower pole renal access. (B) Longitudinal approach for upper pole renal access. (C) Coronal and axial views of the kidney and needle in longitudinal approach. (D) Transverse approach for lower pole renal access. (E) Transverse approach for upper pole renal access. (F) Coronal and axial views of the kidney and needle in transverse approach. (*From* Chu C, Masic S, Usawachintachit M, et al. Ultrasound-guided renal access for percutaneous nephrolithotomy: a description of three novel ultrasound-guided needle techniques. J Endourol 2016;30(2):153–8; with permission.)

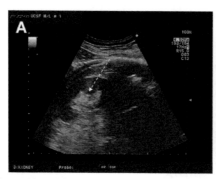 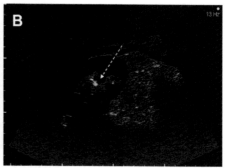

Fig. 8. (*A*) B-mode US shows the nondilated renal collecting system as a central hyperechoic area (*dashed arrow*). (*B*) One minute after retrograde US contrast injection, contrast-enhanced US imaging shows the renal collecting system as an extremely bright echogenic area (*dashed arrow*) facilitating clear differentiation of the urinary space from renal parenchyma and peripelvic fat. (*Courtesy of* Thomas Chi and colleagues.)

upper pole access), and that it is easier to learn. The primary device limitations are the added cost and complexity; the potential for visual interference from the surgeon's hand or other objects; and that smaller-caliber needles may deflect or bend internally, creating a discrepancy between the projected and the actual needle path.

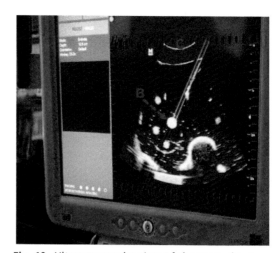

Fig. 9. Clear Guide dual-camera system attached to US transducer used in bench top model. (*Courtesy of* Clear Guide ONE; Clear Guide Medical, Baltimore, MD. www.clearguidemedical.com.)

SonixGPS ultrasonography access Another potential solution designed to simplify localization of the needle with US is the SonixGPS system (SonixGPS, Ultrasonic Medical Corporation, Canada) (**Fig. 11**).[35] This device uses electromagnetic tracking to provide the needle location and the projected path of the needle.[32] In a prospective randomized comparison of 97 PCNL patients, the SonixGPS required significantly fewer puncture attempts (1.33 vs 3.16; *P*<.001). The SonixGPS tracks the needle tip location even when out of plane of the US but does add additional cost and complexity.[32]

All-seeing needle In 2006, the concept of direct ureteroscopic visualization of the renal puncture

Fig. 10. Ultrasonography view of the mass phantom: A is simulated vertebra, B target mass, and C represents a top-down view of the US transducer. The green lines indicate that the needle is in plane with the US beam, blue lines indicate that needle's path is outside the US beam.

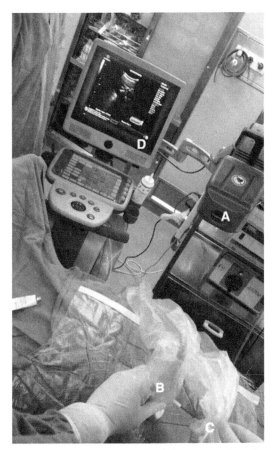

Fig. 11. Percutaneous nephrolithotomy using SonixGPS. A, electromagnetic transmitter; B, US probe; C, SonixGPS proprietary needle; D, needle insertion with electromagnetic guidance on screen in real time. (*From* Li R, Li T, Qian X, et al. Real-time ultrasonography-guided percutaneous nephrolithotomy using SonixGPS navigation: clinical experience and practice in a single center in China. J Endourol 2015;29(2):158–61; with permission.)

needle entering the target calyx was initially described under the term "seeing is believing."[16] The all-seeing needle described by Bader and colleagues[36] introduced another technique to directly visualize needle placement. In this device, a sterilizable 0.9-mm optic (PolyDiagnost, Pfaffenhofen, Germany) is placed as the inner stylet of a modified 16-gauge needle that displays on a conventional monitor (**Fig. 12**). The initial description of this needle included 15 patients undergoing US-guided access (**Fig. 13**).[36] The advantage of the all-seeing needle is direct needle placement confirmation without the need for retrograde ureteroscopy. Limitations include inability to correct the needle trajectory visually within the tissue, especially in obese patients, and inability to visually select the optimal calyx for access.

Combined Fluoroscopy and Ultrasonography

Because both US and fluoroscopy have different potential advantages, optimal outcomes might be achieved by combining the best of both approaches. Several centers have reported their experiences with combined US and fluoroscopic approaches.[20,24,26] Chi and colleagues[26] reviewed 562 PCNL patients performed with combined US and fluoroscopy, finding high stone-free rates (90.5%) and low complications (transfusion, 2.2%; pleural effusion, 0.5%). Novel techniques for combining fluoroscopy and US to achieve renal access are described here.

Virtual projection of ultrasonography onto fluoroscopy

Mozer and colleagues[37] performed renal puncture by virtual projection of a US puncture tract onto the fluoroscopic images obtained at the beginning of the procedure. Because these saved

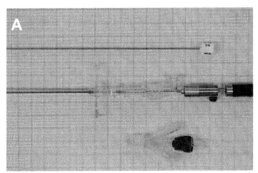
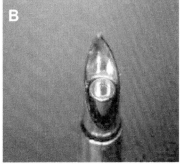

Fig. 12. The all-seeing needle. (*A*) The optical system inserted into the needle shaft and additional adapters. (*B*) Tip of the needle with optical system inserted. (*From* Bader MJ, Gratzke C, Seitz M, et al. The "all-seeing needle": initial results of an optical puncture system confirming access in percutaneous nephrolithotomy. Eur Urol. 2011;59(6):1054–9; with permission.)

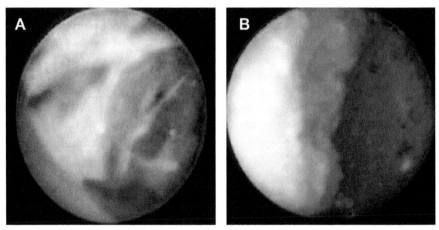

Fig. 13. The endoscopic view of the all-seeing needle. (*A*) Fatty tissue before entering the collecting system. (*B*) View of the needle inside the collecting system showing the stone before dilation and placement of PCNL access sheath for stone treatment. (*From* Bader MJ, Gratzke C, Seitz M, et al. The "all-seeing needle": initial results of an optical puncture system confirming access in percutaneous nephrolithotomy. Eur Urol 2011;59(6):1054–9; with permission.)

fluoroscopic images are used to project the US-guided tract over them, this allows the reduction of radiation exposure. This system was tested in a phantom model and a successful clinical PCNL (0.8 minute of fluoroscopy) (**Fig. 14**).[37]

Laser direct alignment radiation reduction technique

The laser direct alignment radiation reduction technique (DARRT) is a combined fluoroscopy/US technique designed to maximize the benefits of each approach. The surgeon uses a laser emanating from the image intensifier to direct needle placement. The procedure starts with US to ensure there is no lung or visceral structures overlying the kidney. Next, during end-expiration, the surgeon positions a clamp on the flank targeting the opacified calyx with the image intensifier rotated 10° to 30° toward the surgeon. Using fluoroscopy set to fixed, low-dose settings at 1 pulse per second, the surgeon positions the clamp tip and the laser beam over the target calyx. The needle tip and hub are then aligned with the laser and inserted. The C-arm is then rotated 45° in the opposite direction to judge needle depth or alternatively a ureteroscope directly visualizes the needle in the calyx (Video 4).

The procedure can be performed using a conventional needle, although it is difficult to localize

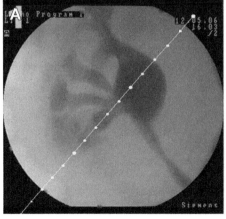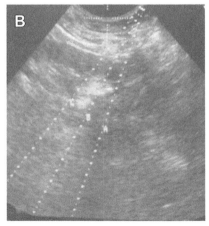

Fig. 14. Virtual projection of US puncture tract onto fluoroscopic images using Polaris infrared camera system and surgical navigation system. (*A*) Fluoroscopic images of the target lower pole calyx with US puncture tract projected onto it. (*B*) US images of the puncture tract. (*From* Mozer P, Conort P, Leroy A, et al. Aid to percutaneous renal access by virtual projection of the ultrasound puncture tract onto fluoroscopic images. J Endourol 2007;21(5):460–5; with permission.)

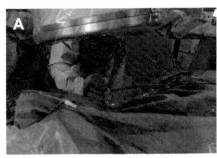
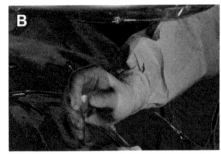

Fig. 15. Laser DARTT. (*A, B*) Using the laser guide, the surgeon can directly hold and insert the needle without concern for self-radiation. This technique allows tactile feedback when puncturing renal capsule and calyx.

the laser beam on the small conventional needle hub (**Fig. 15**). A specialized needle with a large hub containing a laser targeting feature is being developed to simplify this approach (**Fig. 16**). In a benchtop study, the laser DARRT reduced fluoroscopy time (63%) compared with the conventional bull's-eye technique and was easier to learn by novice surgeons.[38] However, the laser targeting does not work with the triangulation technique.

Ultrasonography combined with retrograde ureteroscopy and low-dose fluoroscopy

US renal access has been frequently reported, but tract dilation and other steps are more challenging.

Inserting the balloon too far into the system could tear the infundibulum, or push the stone extra-mural, so precision is important. Recently, Alsyouf and colleagues[39] reported a technique in which a retrograde ureteroscopic approach was combined with US and occasional fluoroscopy.

The patient is positioned prone, split-legged, and a fluoroless ureteroscopic technique[40] is used to hydrodistend the selected optimal calyx (**Fig. 17**). Ureteroscope deflection enhances US calyceal visualization (**Fig. 18**) (Video 5). Using US, the needle is inserted while avoiding the lung and viscera. Next, a ureteroscopic basket pulls the wire into the ureter. Dilation and sheath

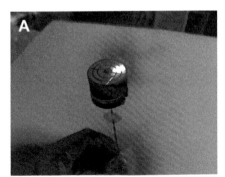
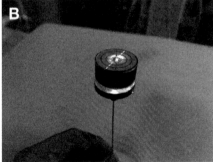
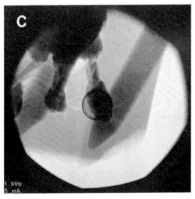

Fig. 16. Laser DARTT needle prototype. (*A*) Needle is misaligned and laser does not reach illumination chamber (improper alignment). (*B*) Laser reaches illumination chamber (properly aligned). (*C*) Fluoroscopic image of laser DARTT needle in benchtop model.

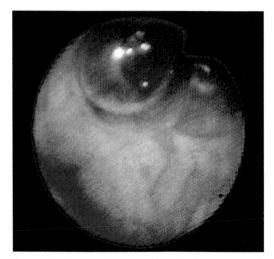

Fig. 17. Ureteroscopic view of posterior upper pole calyx.

placement are performed under ureteroscopic visualization. The mean fluoroscopy time for renal access was 3.5 seconds and the mean total PCNL fluoroscopy time was 8.8 seconds (n = 20). The direct ureteroscopic vision allows optimal calyx selection, facilitates guidewire passage, and allows precise dilation and sheath positioning. In addition, ureteroscopic access allows a second viewpoint for calyceal mapping.

Robotics

During conventional PCNL access, the surgeon uses two-dimensional images to precisely insert a needle in three-dimensional (3D) space. It is not surprising that a minority of urologist perform

this task. These highly cognitive and technical skills could be facilitated using robotics.[41,42]

Percutaneous renal access to the kidney

Cadeddu and colleagues[41] introduced the first robotic device for PCNL access (percutaneous renal access to the kidney [PAKY]) in 1998. Holding respiration, a robotic arm mounted on the operative table was used to insert the needle. The benchtop study (n = 70) was 100% successful. A subsequent clinical trial was successful but had a long access time (8.2 minutes) because of the setup time.[41] A second generation of this robot with a remote center of motion (RCM) device successfully inserted the needle robotically in 87% of patients (**Fig. 19**).[43] These designs were not adopted widely for clinical use, likely because of their high cost and setup complexity.

Automated needle targeting with x-ray

A recent robotic renal access device is the ANT-X (automated needle targeting with x-ray) described by Oo and colleagues[42] (**Fig. 20**). The ANT-X computer-assisted navigation system uses automatic robotic needle alignment with manual needle insertion. The ANT-X system uses fluoroscopy images to perform the bull's-eye technique for needle insertion and is able to compensate for respiratory motion, a limitation of prior robotic technology. The robotic needle holder is placed over the opacified target calyx. The device automatically aligns the needle by integrating real-time fluoroscopic images. This device showed a 26% radiation reduction in an animal model and has been successfully used clinically (Video 6).[42]

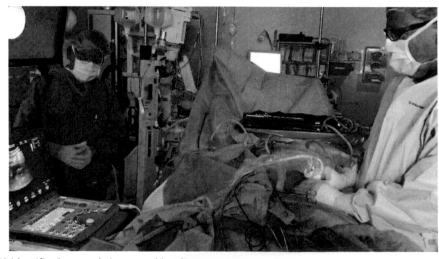

Fig. 18. US identifies lung and viscera and localizes ureteroscope tip.

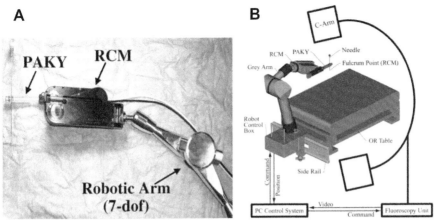

Fig. 19. (*A*) PAKY-RCM. (*B*) PAKY mounted on the side rail of the operating table. (*From* Su LM, Stoianovici D, Jarrett TW, et al. Robotic percutaneous access to the kidney: comparison with standard manual access. J Endourol 2002;16(7):471–5; with permission.)

The robotic PCNL needle insertion designs, although accurate and safe, are still costly, complex to set up, and dependent on fluoroscopy. The ideal robot would be inexpensive, portable, easy to set up, and require minimal use of fluoroscopy.

Other Technologies

Computed tomography–guided renal access

Jiao and colleagues[44] showed that C-arm CT was successful in obtaining renal access in 33 prior US failures. They used a 3D virtual syngo iGuide navigation system (Siemens Healthcare) to help create the needle trajectory, facilitating the real-time fluoroscopic puncture of the target calyx. CT allows clear localization of adjacent soft tissues while confirming needle placement. The associated high radiation exposure (4.8 mSv) should probably limit its application to patients with abnormal or complex anatomy.[45] Other limitations include high cost, failure to account for respiratory excursion, and long procedure times.[37]

Electromagnetic guidance

An electromagnetic tracking system has been developed to assist in PCNL needle placement. Using a chip on the needle and ureteric catheter tip as a homing beacon, computer software determines a 3D trajectory, which is displayed on a monitor. Both audio and visual cues assist in maintaining correct needle orientation. In a phase 1 study, Lima and colleagues[31] tested the Aurora Electromagnetic Tracking device (Northern Digital, Waterloo, Canada) for PCNL needle insertion. With the patient supine, ureteroscopy is

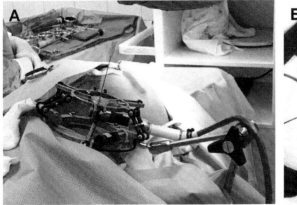
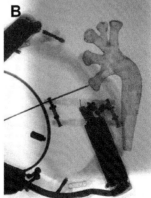

Fig. 20. ANT-X. (*A*) ANT-X set up at the bedside. (*B*) Fluoroscopic image of lower pole puncture of renal phantom model. Tan, Y. K and colleagues.)

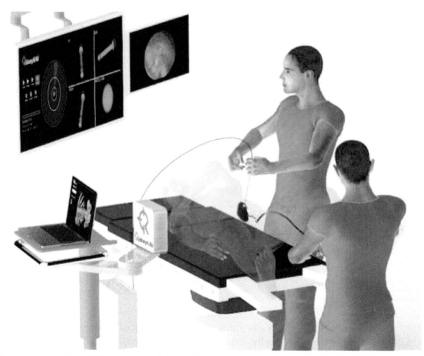

Fig. 21. Renal puncture before PCNL using real-time electromagnetic sensors in the tip of the needle and ureteric catheter. (*From* Lima E, Rodrigues PL, Mota P, et al. Ureteroscopy-assisted percutaneous kidney access made easy: first clinical experience with a novel navigation system using electromagnetic guidance (IDEAL stage 1). Eur Urol 2017;72(4):610–6; with permission.)

performed to place the catheter in the target calyx. The generator is placed near the patient (outside the surgical field) to create the electromagnetic field for tracking the position of the catheter and needle electromagnetic sensors (**Fig. 21**).[31] In addition, the 3D puncture software, integrating all inputs, directs needle placement (**Fig. 22**). Although this technology is promising, the device is complex, expensive, and has not seen wide adoption.[46]

iPAD

Rassweiler and colleagues[47] recently reported a technique using a high-resolution 3D reconstruction and marker-based tracking technology to guide renal access. It requires a preoperative dedicated prone CT with 5 colored metallic skin markers surrounding the access location. The CT images are segmented and all relevant anatomy is displayed on an iPad (Apple Inc, Cupertino, CA) (**Fig. 23**). The puncture site is determined by the relative location of the needle tip and the collecting system and is confirmed by intraoperative fluoroscopy. Although 3D iPad images are not real-time images, fusion with the metal markers minimizes risk for injury to surrounding structures.[47] The limitations of this technique are the need for additional CT and the

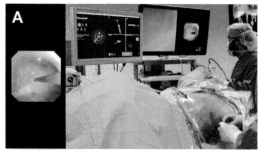

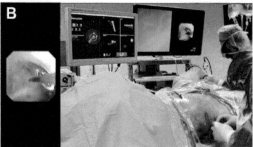

Fig. 22. Renal puncture using 3D navigation software. (*A*) Electromagnetic tracking system localizes the ureteric catheter and needle sensors. (*B*) Needle puncture into patient's lower calyx also confirmed with ureteroscope images. (*From* Lima E, Rodrigues PL, Mota P, et al. Ureteroscopy-assisted percutaneous kidney access made easy: first clinical experience with a novel navigation system using electromagnetic guidance (IDEAL stage 1). Eur Urol 2017;72(4):610–6; with permission.)

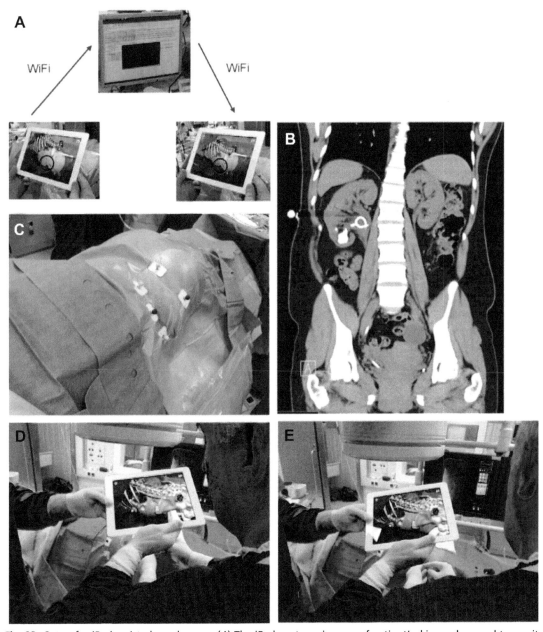

Fig. 23. Setup for iPad-assisted renal access. (*A*) The iPad captures images of patient's skin markers and transmits these to the server. (*B*) Coronal CT showing left renal stone and skin marker. (*C*) Patient prone at time of PCNL (identical position to CT). (*D*) Selecting puncture site using iPad and intraoperative fluoroscopy. (*E*) Inserting the needle into the target calyx. (*From* Rassweiler JJ, Muller M, Fangerau M, et al. iPad-assisted percutaneous access to the kidney using marker-based navigation: initial clinical experience. Eur Urol 2012;61(3):628–31; with permission.)

cumbersome nature of processing and setting up the images.

SUMMARY

PCNL advances have improved the safety, efficacy, and simplicity of obtaining renal access and decreased radiation exposure. It will also be important to ensure that the costs of these new technologies are balanced by improved outcomes. The integration of the best portions of these novel technologies shows promise for a better and safer renal access in the future.

SUPPLEMENTARY DATA

Supplementary data related to this article can be found online at https://doi.org/10.1016/j.ucl.2019.01.001.

REFERENCES

1. Fernström I, Johansson B. Percutaneous pyelolithotomy. A new extraction technique. Scand J Urol Nephrol 1976;10(3):257–9.
2. Lee CL, Anderson JK, Monga M. Residency training in percutaneous renal access: does it affect urological practice? J Urol 2004;171(2 Pt 1):592–5.
3. Antonelli JA, Pearle MS. Advances in percutaneous nephrolithotomy. Urol Clin North Am 2013;40(1):99–113.
4. Watterson JD, Soon S, Jana K. Access related complications during percutaneous nephrolithotomy: urology versus radiology at a single academic institution. J Urol 2006;176(1):142–5.
5. Aslam MZ, Thwaini A, Duggan B, et al. Urologists versus radiologists made PCNL tracts: the U.K. experience. Urol Res 2011;39(3):217–21.
6. Andonian S, Scoffone CM, Louie MK, et al. Does imaging modality used for percutaneous renal access make a difference? A matched case analysis. J Endourol 2013;27(1):24–8.
7. Mahesh M. Fluoroscopy: patient radiation exposure issues. Radiographics 2001;21(4):1033–45.
8. Linet MS, Freedman DM, Mohan AK, et al. Incidence of haematopoietic malignancies in US radiologic technologists. Occup Environ Med 2005;62(12):861–7.
9. US Food and Drug Administration. Initiative to reduce unnecessary radiation exposure from medical imaging. Silver Spring (MD): US Food and Drug Administration; 2010.
10. Miller NL, Matlaga BR, Lingeman JE. Techniques for fluoroscopic percutaneous renal access. J Urol 2007;178(1):15–23.
11. Smith DL, Heldt JP, Richards GD, et al. Radiation exposure during continuous and pulsed fluoroscopy. J Endourol 2013;27(3):384–8.
12. Hajiha M, Wilkinson M, Ewald J, et al. Bench-top comparison of conventional bulls-eye, the laser direct alignment radiation reduction technique and a novel low-radiation targeting needle to reduce fluoroscopy during percutaneous renal access. J Urol 2018;199(4):e476.
13. Lawson RK, Murphy JB, Taylor AJ, et al. Retrograde method for percutaneous access to kidney. Urology 1983;22(6):580–2.
14. Kawahara T, Ito H, Terao H, et al. Ureteroscopy assisted retrograde nephrostomy: a new technique for percutaneous nephrolithotomy (PCNL). BJU Int 2012;110(4):588–90.
15. Wynberg JB, Borin JF, Vicena JZ, et al. Flexible ureteroscopy-directed retrograde nephrostomy for percutaneous nephrolithotomy: description of a technique. J Endourol 2012;26(10):1268–74.
16. Khan F, Borin JF, Pearle MS, et al. Endoscopically guided percutaneous renal access: "seeing is believing". J Endourol 2006;20(7):451–5 [discussion: 455].
17. Grasso M, Lang G, Taylor FC. Flexible ureteroscopically assisted percutaneous renal access. Tech Urol 1995;1(1):39–43.
18. Isac W, Rizkala E, Liu X, et al. Endoscopic-guided versus fluoroscopic-guided renal access for percutaneous nephrolithotomy: a comparative analysis. Urology 2013;81(2):251–6.
19. Lojanapiwat B. The ideal puncture approach for PCNL: fluoroscopy, ultrasound or endoscopy? Indian J Urol 2013;29(3):208–13.
20. Li J, Xiao B, Hu W, et al. Complication and safety of ultrasound guided percutaneous nephrolithotomy in 8,025 cases in China. Chin Med J (Engl) 2014;127(24):4184–9.
21. Krueger PM, Coleman-Minahan K, Rooks RN. Race/ethnicity, nativity and trends in BMI among U.S. adults. Obesity (Silver Spring) 2014;22(7):1739–46.
22. Chu C, Masic S, Usawachintachit M, et al. Ultrasound-guided renal access for percutaneous nephrolithotomy: a description of three novel ultrasound-guided needle techniques. J Endourol 2016;30(2):153–8.
23. Usawachintachit M, Tzou DT, Hu W, et al. X-ray-free ultrasound-guided percutaneous nephrolithotomy: how to select the right patient? Urology 2017;100:38–44.
24. Thomas A, Ewald J, Kelly I, et al. Conventional vs computer-assisted stereoscopic ultrasound needle guidance for renal access: a randomized crossover bench-top trial. J Endourol 2018;32(5):424–30.
25. Basiri A, Kashi AH, Zeinali M, et al. Ultrasound-guided access during percutaneous nephrolithotomy: entering desired calyx with appropriate entry site and angle. Int Braz J Urol 2016;42(6):1160–7.
26. Chi Q, Wang Y, Lu J, et al. Ultrasonography combined with fluoroscopy for percutaneous nephrolithotomy: an analysis based on seven years single center experiences. Urol J 2014;11(1):1216–21.
27. Chi T, Masic S, Li J, et al. Ultrasound guidance for renal tract access and dilation reduces radiation exposure during percutaneous nephrolithotomy. Adv Urol 2016;2016:3840697.
28. Hosseini MM, Yousefi A, Rastegari M. Pure ultrasonography-guided radiation-free percutaneous nephrolithotomy: report of 357 cases. Springerplus 2015;4:313.
29. Taylor KJ, Riely CA, Hammers L, et al. Quantitative US attenuation in normal liver and in patients with diffuse liver disease: importance of fat. Radiology 1986;160(1):65–71.
30. Zhu W, Li J, Yuan J, et al. A prospective and randomised trial comparing fluoroscopic, total ultrasonographic, and combined guidance for renal access

in mini-percutaneous nephrolithotomy. BJU Int 2017; 119(4):612–8.

31. Lima E, Rodrigues PL, Mota P, et al. Ureteroscopy-assisted percutaneous kidney access made easy: first clinical experience with a novel navigation system using electromagnetic guidance (IDEAL Stage 1). Eur Urol 2017;72(4):610–6.

32. Li X, Long Q, Chen X, et al. Real-time ultrasound-guided PCNL using a novel SonixGPS needle tracking system. Urolithiasis 2015;29(2):158–61.

33. Hopkins RE, Bradley M. In-vitro visualization of biopsy needles with ultrasound: a comparative study of standard and echogenic needles using an ultrasound phantom. Clin Radiol 2001;56(6):499–502.

34. Usawachintachit M, Tzou DT, Mongan J, et al. Feasibility of retrograde ureteral contrast injection to guide ultrasonographic percutaneous renal access in the nondilated collecting system. J Endourol 2017;31(2):129–34.

35. Li R, Li T, Qian X, et al. Real-time ultrasonography-guided percutaneous nephrolithotomy using SonixGPS navigation: clinical experience and practice in a single center in China. J Endourol 2015;29(2): 158–61.

36. Bader MJ, Gratzke C, Seitz M, et al. The "all-seeing needle": initial results of an optical puncture system confirming access in percutaneous nephrolithotomy. Eur Urol 2011;59(6):1054–9.

37. Mozer P, Conort P, Leroy A, et al. Aid to percutaneous renal access by virtual projection of the ultrasound puncture tract onto fluoroscopic images. J Endourol 2007;21(5):460–5.

38. Khater N, Shen J, Arenas J, et al. Bench-top feasibility testing of a novel percutaneous renal access technique: the laser direct alignment radiation reduction technique (DARRT). J Endourol 2016; 30(11):1155–60.

39. Alsyouf M, Arenas JL, Smith JC, et al. Direct endoscopic visualization combined with ultrasound guided access during percutaneous nephrolithotomy: a feasibility study and comparison to a conventional cohort. J Urol 2016;196(1):227–33.

40. Olgin G, Smith D, Alsyouf M, et al. Ureteroscopy without fluoroscopy: a feasibility study and comparison with conventional ureteroscopy. J Endourol 2015;29(6):625–9.

41. Cadeddu JA, Stoianovici D, Chen RN, et al. Stereotactic mechanical percutaneous renal access. J Endourol 1998;12(2):121–5.

42. Oo MM, Gandhi HR, Chong KT, et al. Automated needle targeting with x-ray (ANT-X) - Robot-assisted device for percutaneous nephrolithotomy (PCNL) with its first successful use in human. J Endourol 2018. https://doi.org/10.1089/end.2018.0003.

43. Su LM, Stoianovici D, Jarrett TW, et al. Robotic percutaneous access to the kidney: comparison with standard manual access. J Endourol 2002; 16(7):471–5.

44. Jiao D, Zhang Z, Sun Z, et al. Percutaneous nephrolithotripsy: C-arm CT with 3D virtual navigation in non-dilated renal collecting systems. Diagn Interv Radiol 2018;24(1):17–22.

45. Munver R, Delvecchio FC, Newman GE, et al. Critical analysis of supracostal access for percutaneous renal surgery. J Urol 2001;166(4):1242–6.

46. Rodrigues PL, Rodrigues NF, Fonseca J, et al. Kidney targeting and puncturing during percutaneous nephrolithotomy: recent advances and future perspectives. J Endourol 2013;27(7): 826–34.

47. Rassweiler JJ, Muller M, Fangerau M, et al. iPad-assisted percutaneous access to the kidney using marker-based navigation: initial clinical experience. Eur Urol 2012;61(3):628–31.

Innovations in Ureteral Stent Technology

Connor Forbes, MD, Kymora B. Scotland, MD, PhD, Dirk Lange, PhD, Ben H. Chew, MD, MSC*

KEYWORDS

• Ureteral stent • Ureteric stent • Innovation

KEY POINTS

- Ureteral stents are indispensable in modern urology.
- Polymeric ureteral stents have undergone recent changes in design.
- Biodegradable/bioresorbable stents and a plethora of stent coatings have been developed to address stent-associated complications including infection, pain, and encrustation.

INTRODUCTION

The history of ureteral stents begins with Charles Thomas Stent, after whom the stent is named. Dr Stent was a dentist in London who developed a material in the 1850s that he used to take impressions of teeth.[1] This material consisted of gutta percha (a natural latex) mixed with tallow and talc.[1] His material ("Stent's compound") was used during the First World War and described shortly thereafter by surgeon J.F. Esser to fix skin grafts in place.[1] "Stenting" became the verb for this practice,[1] and the term eventually made its way to other fields, including urology to describe placing a tube in an organ.[2]

Ureteric stents were first described in 1949 by Herdman.[3] They were made from polyethylene, and projected from the kidney all the way to the exterior of the urethra.[2] Silicone and polyurethane eventually became the materials of choice because they reduced encrustation.[2] A urologist named R.P. Gibbons improved the shape of stents from a straight tube exiting the urethra to one with a distal bulb that could reside in the bladder and prevent proximal dislodgment.[2] Finally, the familiar single J and double J stents were developed in the 1970s by Thomas Hepperlen and Roy Finney.[2] A summary of these historical advances is found in **Fig. 1**.

Today, ureteric stent technology is changing to meet clinical demands. Used primarily for relief of obstruction or to promote ureteral healing, ureteral stents have drawbacks: indwelling stents are associated with infection; pain; encrustation; drainage failure; dislodgment; hematuria; and urinary symptoms, such as frequency and urgency. They may cause interference with normal ureteric physiology and if forgotten or patients are lost to follow-up, can result in kidney injury and even renal failure. There is no ideal ureteric stent currently available. The aim of most recent stent innovation has been to make steps toward properties of an ideal stent. These include prolonged dwell time without sequelae, ease of extraction, and lack of patient discomfort. In previous reviews we have addressed advances in the domain of ureteric stents.[4,5] Here, we expand further on innovations in the changing space of ureteric stent technology, focusing on recent progress.

STENT MATERIALS
Polymeric Ureteric Stents

Polymeric ureteric stents form the basis of today's most commonly used base material. Current-generation polymeric stents are composed of proprietary polymer blends that offer improved

Disclosure Statement: Dr. Chew is a consultant with Olympus Medical, Boston Scientific, Cook Medical, Adva-Tec, Auris Surgical, Coloplast. All other authors have nothing to disclose.
Department of Urologic Sciences, Level 6-2775 Laurel Street, Vancouver, British Columbia V5Z 1M9, Canada
* Corresponding author.
E-mail address: Ben.chew@ubc.ca

Urol Clin N Am 46 (2019) 245–255
https://doi.org/10.1016/j.ucl.2018.12.013

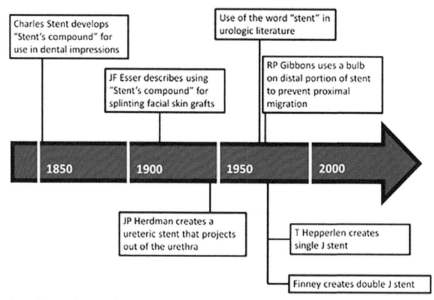

Fig. 1. Timeline of major historical innovations in ureteric stents.

stability and reduced friction.[6] Many of these include polyurethane, with or without an outer layer coating. Novel polymeric stents aim to improve biocompatibility, biodurability, ease of insertion and retrieval, duration of effective dwell time, and cost, all while remaining radiopaque.[7] Polymers tend to be inert, with a typical recommended dwell time of 3 months, although they are often approved for up to 12 months of dwell time. Numerous polymeric blends are available, each with its own reported advantages often shown *in vitro*. However, all materials suffer from some degree of encrustation while in the urine. At 10 weeks, polyurethane and polymeric blends showed 100% surface encrustation in an artificial urine solution.[8] A detailed description of the specific polymers available is found in a review by Venkatesan and colleagues.[6] Examples of frequently used polymers in ureteric stents are found in **Fig. 2**.

The standard shape of the polymeric ureteric stent is the double pigtail (double J) catheter, with a coil to secure the stent in the collecting system and the bladder. Variations on this theme aim to improve performance. A polymeric double J stent with two lumens has been shown *in vitro* to improve flow in a model of extrinsic compression.[9]

Novel shapes also aim to reduce pain. A small, nonrandomized study found a reduction in analgesic use postureteroscopy for patients who received a double J stent with a helical spiral stent (Percuflex Helical stent, Boston Scientific, Natick, MA) compared with the regular Percuflex stent.[10] The spiral shape is theorized to reduce pain by making the stent more flexible, thus conforming

to the ureter.[11] A second approach to pain focuses on reducing reflux along the stent, with the theoretic benefit of reducing pyelonephritis and scarring.[12] Recently, Park and colleagues[12] have produced three-dimensional printed stents with a small antirefluxing polymeric flap valve. This type of antirefluxing stent could improve on previous designs[13,14] by the unobtrusiveness of the valve. In a pig model, less frequent and lower grade reflux was seen on simulated voiding cystourethrogram with the flap valve stent.[15] Clinical trials are needed to confirm safety and effectiveness. An alternative approach to reducing reflux is to use a stent that does not pass through the ureteric orifice. This has been trialed in pigs with a stent that has a single polymeric coil in the renal pelvis and an anchoring tip that remains in the distal ureter.[16] The obvious drawback to this design is that retrieval requires ureteroscopy, and the long-term risk of stricture is not known. Furthermore, the benefits of reducing stent-related reflux in humans have not been convincingly demonstrated.

A variation in polymeric stent design has been seen with the release of the Polaris stent (Boston Scientific), which is a dual durometer stent that has a firmer coil material in the kidney portion and a softer polymer in the bladder coil. One randomized trial showed a decrease in certain domains of pain scores with this stent in limited circumstances, whereas in another study no significant improvement was found.[17,18] Further studies are needed to determine if the softness of the material affects patient comfort.

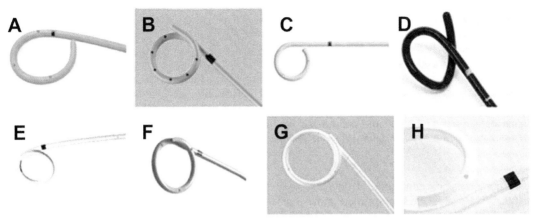

Fig. 2. Representative polymeric, commercially available ureteric stents. (*A*) Bardex double pigtail soft stent composed of polyurethane. (*B*) Sof-Flex double pigtail stent composed of polyurethane. (*C*) Yellow Star ureteral stent composed of polyurethane. (*D*) Fluoro-4 silicone ureteral stent composed of silicone/tantalum. (*E*) Percuflex ureteral stent composed of Percuflex. (*F*) Vortek double loop ureteral stent composed of Vortek. (*G*) C-Flex ureteral stent composed of C-Flex. (*H*) LithoStent composed of Tecoflex. (*Courtesy of* [*A, D*] Bard Medical, Covington, GA; [*B, G*] Cook Medical, Bloomington, IN; [*C*] Urotech/Medi-Globe Group, Achenmuhle, Germany; [*E*] Boston Scientific, Marlborough, MA; [*F*] Coloplast A/S, Humlebaek, Denmark; and [*H*] Olympus Corporation, Shinjuku, Japan with permission.)

There has been renewed interest in silicone ureteric stents. Silicone is an inert material, with reduced encrustation compared with polyurethane and other polymeric stents *in vitro*.[8] Bacteria are also less able to migrate along silicone stents.[19]

Silicone is less stiff compared with other commercially available ureteric stents, which is theorized to increase tolerability.[20] In a small study of patients stented after upper tract endoscopy or laparoscopic pyeloplasty, silicone stents resulted in less discomfort than Percuflex stents on univariate (but not multivariate) analysis.[21] However, this softness can decrease the force transmitted along the stent, reducing the ability of silicone stents to advance along tight ureters. Commercially available silicone stents include the Black Silicone Ureteric Stent (Cook Medical, Bloomington, IN) and the ImaJin Ureteral Stent (Coloplast A/S, Humlebaek, Denmark).

Metallic Ureteral Stents

Metallic stents have been investigated more commonly in recent years. Metal is attractive as a ureteric stent material because its increased rigidity lends itself to resistance to compression, which is often an issue in malignant ureteric obstruction. Some metallic stents are double pigtail in design, whereas others have a novel shape for prolonged dwell time. In addition to requiring data on effectiveness, the challenges for metallic stents include demonstrating

biocompatibility because metal is more prone to corrosion and is less inert compared with polymers.

Previously, the metallic stents used for ureteric obstruction were mostly off-label vascular metal-mesh stents.[22] A 10-year review of the palliative use of these vascular stents for malignant ureteric obstruction noted a 51.2% patency rate, with adverse sequelae including stent migration and hyperplastic ingrowth of ureteric tissues.[22] To help address tissue ingrowth, coated metal ureteric stents were developed. This included the Passager (Meadox, Boston Scientific Corporation, Oakland, NJ) stent, a self-expanding nitinol stent that is covered by a thin layer of polyester fabric. Comparison with the vascular metal-mesh Wallstent (Schneider, Zurich, Switzerland) was not favorable with severe ureteric reactions and frequent stent migration noted.[23,24] Further discussion of the benefits and drawbacks of these and other early metallic stents is found in a 2010 review by Sountoulides and colleagues.[25]

Metallic stents in the double J configuration were then developed. There are two double J type metallic ureteric stents now available: the Silhouette stent (Applied Medical, Rancho Santa Margarita, CA) and the Resonance stent (Cook Medical). The Silhouette is a double J stent constructed with nitinol wire reinforcing the walls of the stent and covered with a polymer (**Fig. 3**A). The nitinol is not visible and the polymer interfaces with tissue to maintain biocompatibility. *In vitro* studies have found superior resistance to kinking

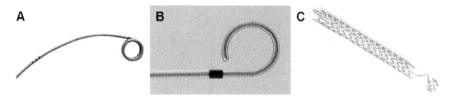

Fig. 3. Metallic ureteral stents. (*A*) The Silhouette polymeric stent incorporates nitinol. (*B*) Resonance double pigtail metallic stent. (*C*) Allium URS expandable ureteral stent with intravesical anchor. (*Courtesy of* [*A*] Applied Medical ancho Santa Margarita, CA; [*B*] Cook Medical, Bloomington, IN; [*C*] Allium Ltd, Caesarea, Israel.)

and compression compared with polymeric stents.[26,27] However, to our knowledge there are no published peer-reviewed *in vivo* studies clinically confirming these findings.

The Resonance stent has been examined in more detail in many studies (**Fig. 3**B). It is composed of a nickel-cobalt-chromium-molybdenum alloy, with a double J configuration and is approved for a maximum dwell time of 12 months.[28] The benefit of metallic stents, including the Resonance, is resistance to extrinsic compression. In a retrospective case series of 42 patients with malignant ureteric obstruction, the Resonance stent's dwell time was 4 months longer than the polymeric stent, which had been placed prior (5.3 vs 1.7 months; *P*<.0001).[28] Renal function was maintained in 90% of patients throughout the stent's dwell time, with no major complications.[28] Further research is needed to clarify indications for the Resonance stent. Reported patency rates and dwell time have been inconsistent for malignant and nonmalignant obstruction.[29,30] Similarly, reported risk factors for failure of Resonance ureteral stenting have been conflicting.[31,32] Reported risk factors include type of cancer, positive cancer response to treatment, and antegrade stent insertion.[31,32] Age and renal function were identified as risk factors in one study, but not in a separate study.[31,32] Encrustation remains an issue, with 22% of stents showing signs of encrustation on removal.[29]

The Resonance stent is a more expensive item compared with a standard polymer stent ($880 vs $109), but for patients requiring 12 months of stenting an average cost savings of $10,362 was observed in one study of 13 patients.[33] This cost savings relies on the assumption of a 12-month dwell time, which does not always occur.[28] However, a recent study reported a maximum dwell time of a single stent in malignant obstruction of 21.3 months without compromise.[34] Case series have also described Resonance stenting for rarer causes of urinary obstruction. The Resonance stent has been placed in the transplanted kidney ureter[35,36] and for stenting of obstructed ureterocutaneostomies.[37]

At present, Resonance stents may serve as a reasonable alternative in patients with anticipated prolonged stenting requirements and a desire to increase the interval between stent changes. These patients should have their renal function measured regularly to screen for stent dysfunction, with consideration of periodic imaging for the development of hydronephrosis and/or encrustation.

The remainder of the metallic stents available on the market are expandable stents that build on the previous technology of vascular metal-mesh stents. These are cylindrical, without coils, and anchor themselves into the ureter by expanding after deployment. The Allium URS (Allium LTD, Caesarea, Israel) is another current-generation metallic ureteric stent that is self-expanding. It is a nickel-titanium alloy covered by a polymer coating, and is wide in diameter (24F or 30F catheter) for increased intraluminal drainage.[38] This stent has a unique intravesical anchor that allows for complete unraveling of the stent for ease of extraction (**Fig. 3**C). A nonrandomized study of Allium URS stenting of 49 ureters (40 patients) with a mean follow-up of 21 months showed a 95% patency rate.[38] Stent dislodgment occurred in 14.2% of patients.[38] Encrustation was not noted clinically in this study,[38] although an *in vitro* study found the presence of some degree of encrustation on 100% of the surface area of Allium stents after 6 weeks.[39] Although results of a multicenter study were reported in Hebrew in 2015, there have been no subsequent peer-reviewed English-language clinical studies.

The Uventa stent (Taewoong Medical, Gyeonggi-do, South Korea) is a metal mesh stent that is deployed within a sheath. Once the sheath is removed, the stent expands and is left in place semipermanently. It is removed with laser treatment if required. The Uventa stent has a polymeric (polytetrafluoroethylene) coating to try to prevent the previous issue of hyperplastic reactions to metal-mesh stenting.[40] Initial studies showed promising results.[41] A 100% initial technical success rate was reported from a retrospective review of stenting of 40 ureters, with obstruction later occurring in nine ureters (22.5%).[42] However, a recent series of 44 patients who underwent segmental ureteric stenting with the Uventa stent had an overall long-term success rate of only 34%, and a major complication rate of 28%.[40] In two cases (4%), a major complication was the result of obstruction of the stent from encrustation.[40] The authors of that study attributed their decreased long-term success rate to longer duration of follow-up compared with previous studies.[40] Caution should be used with current-generation metal-mesh stents because their long-term consequences on ureteric physiology are not fully characterized. Changes reported to date include edema, fibrosis, and ureteric wall thickening.[42]

The Memokath 051 (PNN Medical, Kvistgaard, Denmark) is another expandable metallic stent designed specifically for the ureter. It is cylindrical with a funnel-shaped proximal end toward the renal pelvis. It is composed of nickel and titanium and is thermoexpandable.[43] After deploying, it is either flushed with warm saline or left to warm up to body temperature, which results in expansion of the stent in diameter. Cool saline is used to contract the stent for removal.[43] Like other metal stents, the goal is to have a longer dwell time than polymeric stents. The manufacturer does not recommend a specific time period for stent change. In a retrospective analysis of 125 patients with benign and malignant causes of obstruction who underwent Memokath 051 stenting of the ureter, the median dwell time was 355 days (range, 7–2125 days).[44] Predictors of longer dwell time included estimated glomerular filtration rate greater than 60 mL/min/1.73 m^2 and nonmalignant cause of ureteric obstruction.[44] A recent review included five studies where the Memokath 051 was used to stent malignant ureteric obstruction. Patency rates ranged from 19% to 100% with mean follow-up ranging from 10.6 to 22 months.[43] Complications included stent migration and encrustation, and small sample sizes (15–73 patients per study) limit generalizability.[43]

Advances have been made in metallic materials science in the last several years. Magnesium's antimicrobial properties have been studied in vitro on Escherichia coli using artificial urine media.[45] Magnesium discs were found to inhibit bacterial growth and were found to decrease bacterial viability compared with polymer or controls.[45] Magnesium also displayed biodegradability, which may be useful in next-generation stents.[45] This early in vitro study requires confirmation before clinical applications.

As with polymeric stents, complications with metallic ureteric stents have been reported in the literature. These include ureteroarterial fistulae, ureteroenteric fistulae, and ureterovaginal fistulae.[46,47] The incidence of this is too rare for accurate calculation, but fistula development can be life-threatening and highlights that metallic stenting can have serious sequelae.

Despite success in cardiology, there are no strong data supporting the use of drug-eluting metallic stents in urology to date. Further detailed information about metallic stents is found in a recent systematic review by Kallidonis and colleagues.[43]

An alternative to metallic stents for the conservative management of persistent ureteral strictures or extrinsic ureteral compression is the technique of placing two standard polymer ureteric stents in the same ureter, known as tandem ureteral stenting. The expected mechanism is increased resistance to compressive forces compared with a single stent, thus maintaining ureteral patency. In addition, intraluminal and extraluminal flow are improved with tandem ureteric stents compared with a single stent in an ex vivo model,[9] possibly because of increased space between the stents. A review by Elsamra and colleagues[48] summarized evidence for tandem ureteric stenting in malignant obstruction compared with other options. An approximately 0% to 47% failure rate for tandem ureteric stenting was found, compared with 15% to 44% for standard polymeric stenting.[48] Thus tandem stenting may prove useful in some patients with ureteral compression from external or internal etiologies.

Biodegradable/Bioresorbable Ureteric Stents

Recent advances have been made in biodegradable ureteric stents, although they are largely at the preclinical stage of development. These stents have been theorized to reduce morbidity associated with stent removal and serve as a vehicle for drug delivery. Major challenges include control over the timing of resorption, avoiding obstructive sequelae, and understanding effects on ureteric physiology. Previous generations of biodegradable stents, such as the temporary ureteral drainage stent, have suffered from incomplete degradation, in some cases requiring intervention for removal of fragments.[49] The temporary ureteral drainage stent is not commercially available as a result of these concerns.

Chitosan is a biodegradable material that has been studied in ureteric stents. It is a linear polysaccharide with antimicrobial properties and potential applications in drug-delivery.[50] Chitosan

Table 1
Stent coatings in development

Strategy	Short-Term Outcome	Long-Term Outcome
Antibiotic-impregnated catheters	Some in vitro, animal success	Concern for resistance
Silver alloy coating	Some in vitro success	Clinical trial: not effective
Hydrophilic coating (hydrogel)	Some in vitro success	Not clinically effective
Heparin	Little in vitro success	Not effective
Triclosan	Some in vitro, animal success	Clinical trials: not effective
Gendine	Some in vitro, animal success	No new data
Chitosan derivatives	Some in vitro success	No new data
Diamond-like carbon coatings	Some in vitro success	No new data
Hyaluronic acid	Some in vitro success	No new data
Salicylic acid–releasing polymers	Some in vitro success	No new data

alone does not have ideal mechanical characteristics for a ureteric stent. Its deformability and other mechanical properties are improved by blending with other polymers, such as polyethylene oxide (which is also biodegradable).[50] Although chitosan has not been used as the primary constituent of ureteral stents, it has been used as a coating in vitro (**Table 1**). Nanoparticles of chitosan with kanamycin were attached to the surface of polyurethane ureteral stents.[51] In an in vitro model of colonized urine, the stents coated with these nanoparticles had decreased viable bacterial adherence.[51] Drug delivery of kanamycin with chitosan continued for 7 days.[51] Clinical applicability remains to be seen with in vivo studies planned.

New materials and production methods have been proposed for biodegradable ureteric stents. Investigators have braided together combinations of polyglycolic acid (PGA) and poly-lactic-co-glycolic acid (PLGA), which are approved suture materials, and treated them thermally to create five different prototype stents.[52] When compared with the commercially available Percuflex (Boston Scientific) stent composed of modified polyurethane, these braided stents had a decreased compression recovery in vitro. Some of the PGA/PLGA blends also had improved tensile strength.[52] Computational models based on laboratory data reduce testing costs by determining the optimal ratio of PGA/PLGA.[53]

Previous stents made of polylactic acid in an animal model showed a longer than desirable degradation time of greater than 80 days.[54] More recently, PLGA/poly-caprolactone stents created using a specialized nanostructural technique called electrospinning showed complete degradation at 70 days in pigs, without evidence of fragments causing hydronephrosis.[55] The pathologic evaluation showed less urothelial inflammation caused by these stents compared with a polyurethane stent.[55] Other specialized techniques for PLGA stent production include repeated immersion to create a multilayered stent.[56]

Natural polysaccharides are also being developed into ureteric stents, using gellan gum, alginate, and gelatin.[57] These stents reabsorb quickly in artificial urine, between 14 and 60 days, and show reduced adherence of selected bacteria compared with a polymeric stent.[57] A subsequent trial of gelatin-based natural polysaccharide stents in seven pigs showed complete degradation of the stent in 10 days.[58] Histopathologic scoring showed increased tolerability of the natural polysaccharide stent compared with the commercial stent.[58] This preliminary equivalence study in animals demonstrated that natural polysaccharide stents may require increased biostability before longer clinical use.

Novel stent shapes are also being used for biodegradable stents. A recent study used a biodegradable antireflux stent in a pig model. This stent has no distal coil to reduce the chance of reflux.[16] The stents were composed of PGA and a biodegradable trademarked polymer named Glycomer-631. Degradation occurred between 3 and 6 weeks without obstructive fragments.[16] There were no complications, with no changes in serum creatinine in any group. There was less migration of the antirefluxing stent, with less edema around the ureteric orifice on pathology at 5 months.[16] These novel products are years away from generalized use in humans but present an interesting research avenue and hold promise for future ureteral stent designs.

STENT COATINGS

Research efforts aimed at addressing stent-associated complications, such as infection, encrustation, and stent pain, have focused on alterations of stent characteristics. In particular, the use of various coatings as a means of modification has been advocated by several groups. Initial efforts to address ureteral stent pain used a strategy of a nonsteroidal anti-inflammatory drug-eluting coating. A ketorolac-eluting stent was thought to be effective on *in vitro* and *in vivo* porcine studies,[59] but did not demonstrate significant efficacy in a subsequent clinical trial.[60] Indwelling ureteral stents are often associated with a variety of bothersome symptoms including generalized abdominal discomfort, flank pain, dysuria, frequency, and urgency. More than 80% of stented patients experience adverse symptoms, which can range from tiresome to debilitating.[61] Although there have been many theories postulated, the cause of these stent-associated symptoms has yet to be elucidated. As such, a variety of stent modifications have been devised to address possible causes including inflammation, bladder irritation, muscle spasm, and vesicoureteral reflux.[62]

There have been several attempts to produce so-called comfort stents where the stent durometer or firmness has been modulated to fabricate soft stents. This was based largely on the theory that stent rigidity affects patient tolerance. However, early studies found no significant difference in pain symptoms or patient quality of life with soft stents as compared with those crafted with firmer materials.[6]

One theory accounting for the urinary symptoms often associated with stent insertion is that of bladder and distal ureter irritation. In support of this theory, a recent study by Vernez and colleagues[63] demonstrated that ureteral nerve density was highest at the distal ureter. To combat this issue, several groups devised stents where the distal coil was replaced by loops of material or a tapered end.[64] However, there have been mixed results with few studies showing any significant difference in symptoms as compared with standard stents.[65] Moreover, concerns for these stents include suture migration caused by the loss of the distal pigtail coil, which serves to anchor the stent in the bladder. A new stent where the distal coil has been replaced by suture connected to a magnet attempts to address these issues. The magnet is proposed to prevent migration and allow for ease of removal while the tapered end decreases reflux. A clinical study investigating patient outcomes is underway (K.S. private communication).

The theories of bladder irritation and that of stent composition as reasons for stent-mediated discomfort have also led to the development of dual-durometer stents where the stent is composed of softer material at the distal end. It is unclear whether these stents result in subjectively improved patient pain. However, a recent study by this group showed decreased analgesic use with placement of a helical dual durometer stent as compared with the control dual durometer stent.[10]

Stents have also been designed to prevent vesicoureteral reflux with an antireflux membrane valve. A single clinical study showed significantly decreased pain as compared with typical stents.[66] However, no such stent is currently commercially available. Finally, an earlier school of thought held that stent size played a role in patient discomfort. However, Erturk and colleagues[67] demonstrated no difference in patient discomfort with 4.7F versus 7F stents.

The underlying rationale for the use of stent coatings in combating infection has been the need to prevent or reduce biofilm formation. Biofilms are complex communities of microorganisms and proteins that adhere onto the surface of an implant and incorporate extracellular polymers to form a near impenetrable matrix. As with the various attempts to mitigate stent colic, there have been numerous stent coatings developed to resist infection.[68] Preclinical data for many of these coatings have been promising. However, several of these devices have been insufficiently effective *in vivo* (see **Table 1**).[68,69] Some of the first models were antimicrobial-eluting ureteral stents. These proved problematic because of concerns for the development of bacterial resistance. Future prototypes need to demonstrate more controlled elution of antimicrobials incorporated into the device coatings. Efforts are now focused on drug-eluting stents in which combinations of antibiotics have been incorporated and broad-spectrum biomaterials, such as antimicrobial peptides, to avoid the development of antibiotic-resistant bacteria.[70]

In contrast to initial work that had largely centered on the prevention of biofilm formation, some more recent efforts have concentrated on bypassing the antimicrobial resistance of biofilm components. Our laboratory and collaborators have demonstrated a novel coating that uses polymer brushes to move antimicrobial peptides away from the surface of the implant, thus protecting them from being made ineffective by the deposition of biofilm components on the stent.[71] This coating was also effective at resisting biofilm formation in an *in vivo* model. However, peptide synthesis may prove prohibitively expensive for patient use. Other attempts at combating biofilm have gone beyond coatings to include such techniques as the use of sound waves to disrupt biofilm.[72] However, there have been no recent data on clinical utility of this strategy.

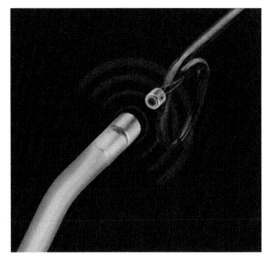

Fig. 4. The Blackstar magnetic ureteral stent uses a magnet for ease of extraction. (*Courtesy of* Urotech.)

Encrustation is another major complication of ureteral stent use. Previous work has shown demonstrated correlation between degree of encrustation and stent composition, leading to the use of such materials as silicone.[8] Attempts to inhibit stent encrustation have also involved the development of novel coatings. The rationale for devising these coatings has included the proposal that increased biocompatibility will lead to decreased encrustation.[73]

A recent report by Ron and colleagues[74] investigated the use of nanoparticles in repelling encrustation. These rhenium-doped fullerene-like molybdenum disulfide nanoparticles form a mosaic-like coating on the stent surface. The potential incorporation of nanoparticles into ureteral stents is a promising new avenue of investigation. The effort to devise successful stents with minimal complications needs to be multipronged, addressing stent-associated infection, encrustation, and pain using multiple synergistic strategies.

NOVEL TECHNIQUES DEVELOPED TO MANAGE INDWELLING STENTS

Several emerging techniques leverage existing technology in innovative ways. One attempt at decreasing the morbidity of stent removal has resulted in the development of the Blackstar stent (Urotech-Urovision, Medi-Glide Group, Rohrdorf, Germany) where the traditional double pigtail configuration has been modified by attaching a magnet to the distal coil (**Fig. 4**). A randomized trial of 40 patients who underwent magnetic stent placement compared with polymeric stent placement found that patients tolerated both stents well. Magnetic stents were retrieved successfully without cystoscopy 95% of the time, reducing cost and discomfort.[75]

"Forgotten" stents in patients who are lost to follow-up is a significant adverse event because stents left *in situ* over a prolonged period of time may cause serious sequelae. This includes renal failure from obstruction or sepsis, and may require multiple procedures for stent removal. A smartphone application (Ureteral Stent Tracker, Boston Scientific) allows providers to log placement of stents and receive periodic reminders regarding their placement.[76] A study that examined the usage of the stent tracking app demonstrated the ability to log ureteral stent insertion and dwell time conveniently in a patient population.[76] The study was unfortunately limited by lack of historical data. Ultimately the effectiveness of the app will depend on provider diligence, but it could represent a convenient tool for endourologists.

One means of protecting the ureter during pelvic or abdominal surgery where there is a significant concern for inadvertent injury is the use of ureteric catheters that emit light. These lighted catheters incorporate mounted lights that flash and allow for intraoperative identification of the ureter. Some authors advocate for their use, despite increased cost, as a method to reduce intraoperative ureteric injury, particularly in laparoscopic colorectal surgery.[77]

As smart devices gain in popularity, the use of sensors has been suggested for ureteral stents. Smart stents that use microelectromechanical systems to sense and communicate are in the early stages of development in cardiology.[78] Detection of flow of blood in a pig model with a vascular smart stent provides proof of principle.[78] To our knowledge, there are currently no published *in vivo* studies for smart ureteric stents. However, this likely represents the next frontier in stent innovation.

SUMMARY

Polymeric stents continue to dominate the market for ureteric stents. Their relative inertness makes for a satisfactory short-term solution. Incremental improvements in polymer blends and stent coatings have advanced this space. Biodegradable/bioresorbable stents and a plethora of stent coatings have been developed to address stent-associated complications including infection, pain, and encrustation. However, these innovations continue to be preclinical and, in several cases, have proven ineffective in clinical studies. Work continues on evolving stent designs. The development of metallic stents has had some utility for patients with chronic ureteral narrowing, particularly in cases of malignant obstruction. Finally, new frontiers of ureteric stent research may include smart stents with monitoring/communication capabilities. With continued design and innovation, it is hoped that stent morbidity will be decreased for all patients with ureteral stents.

REFERENCES

1. Morgenstern L. Stenting...where credit is due. Surg Endosc 2001;15(4):423.

2. Williams KG, Blacker AJ, Kumar P. Ureteric stents: the past, present and future. J Clin Urol 2018; 11(4):280–4.

3. Herdman JP. Polythene tubing in the experimental surgery of the ureter. Br J Surg 1949;37(145):105.

4. Chew BH, Lange D. Advances in ureteral stent development. Curr Opin Urol 2016;26(3):277–82.

5. Brotherhood H, Lange D, Chew BH. Advances in ureteral stents. Transl Androl Urol 2014;3(3):314–9.

6. Venkatesan N, Shroff S, Jayachandran K, et al. Polymers as ureteral stents. J Endourol 2010;24(2):191–8.

7. Mardis HK, Kroeger RM, Morton JJ, et al. Comparative evaluation of materials used for internal ureteral stents. J Endourol 1993;7(2):105–15.

8. Tunney MM, Keane PF, Jones DS, et al. Comparative assessment of ureteral stent biomaterial encrustation. Biomaterials 1996;17(15):1541–6.

9. Hafron J, Ost MC, Tan BJ, et al. Novel dual-lumen ureteral stents provide better ureteral flow than single ureteral stent in ex vivo porcine kidney model of extrinsic ureteral obstruction. Urology 2006; 68(4):911–5.

10. Chew BH, Rebullar KA, Harriman D, et al. Percuflex helical ureteral stents significantly reduce patient analgesic requirements compared to control stents. J Endourol 2017;31(12):1321–5.

11. Mucksavage P, Pick D, Haydel D, et al. An in vivo evaluation of a novel spiral cut flexible ureteral stent. Urology 2012;79(3):733–7.

12. Park CJ, Kim HW, Jeong S, et al. Anti-reflux ureteral stent with polymeric flap valve using three-dimensional printing: an in vitro study. J Endourol 2015;29(8):933–8.

13. Ritter M, Krombach P, Knoll T, et al. Initial experience with a newly developed antirefluxive ureter stent. Urol Res 2012;40(4):349–53.

14. Yamaguchi O, Yoshimura Y, Irisawa C, et al. Prototype of a reflux-preventing ureteral stent and its clinical use. Urology 1992;40(4):326–9.

15. Kim HW, Park CJ, Seo S, et al. Evaluation of a polymeric flap valve-attached ureteral stent for preventing vesicoureteral reflux in elevated intravesical pressure conditions: a pilot study using a porcine model. J Endourol 2016;30(4):428–32.

16. Soria F, Morcillo E, Serrano A, et al. Evaluation of a new design of antireflux-biodegradable ureteral stent in animal model. Urology 2018;115:59–64.

17. Park HK, Paick SH, Kim HG, et al. The impact of ureteral stent type on patient symptoms as determined by the ureteral stent symptom questionnaire: a prospective, randomized, controlled study. J Endourol 2015;29(3):367–71.

18. Lee JN, Kim BS. Comparison of efficacy and bladder irritation symptoms among three different ureteral stents: a double-blind, prospective, randomized controlled trial. Scand J Urol 2015;49(3): 237–41.

19. Watterson JD, Cadieux PA, Stickler D, et al. Swarming of Proteus mirabilis over ureteral stents: a comparative assessment. J Endourol 2003;17(7): 523–7.

20. Hendlin K, Dockendorf K, Horn C, et al. Ureteral stents: coil strength and durometer. Urology 2006; 68(1):42–5.

21. El-Nahas AR, El-Assmy AM, Shoma AM, et al. Self-retaining ureteral stents: analysis of factors responsible for patients' discomfort. J Endourol 2006; 20(1):33–7.

22. Liatsikos EN, Karnabatidis D, Katsanos K, et al. Ureteral metal stents: 10-year experience with malignant ureteral obstruction treatment. J Urol 2009; 182(6):2613–7.

23. Barbalias GA, Liatsikos EN, Kalogeropoulou C, et al. Externally coated ureteral metallic stents: an unfavorable clinical experience. Eur Urol 2002;42(3): 276–80.

24. Liatsikos EN, Siablis D, Kalogeropoulou C, et al. Coated v noncoated ureteral metal stents: an experimental model. J Endourol 2001;15(7):747–51.

25. Sountoulides P, Kaplan A, Kaufmann OG, et al. Current status of metal stents for managing malignant ureteric obstruction. BJU Int 2010;105(8):1066–72.

26. Christman MS, L'Esperance JO, Choe CH, et al. Analysis of ureteric stent kinking forces: the role of curvature in stent failure. BJU Int 2010;105(6): 866–9 [discussion: 868–9].

27. Miyaoka R, Hendlin K, Monga M. Resistance to extrinsic compression and maintenance of intraluminal flow in coil-reinforced stents (Silhouette Scaffold Device): an in vitro study. J Endourol 2010;24(4):595–8.

28. Chow PM, Chiang IN, Chen CY, et al. Malignant ureteral obstruction: functional duration of metallic versus polymeric ureteral stents. PLoS One 2015; 10(8):e0135566.

29. Liatsikos E, Kallidonis P, Kyriazis I, et al. Ureteral obstruction: is the full metallic double-pigtail stent the way to go? Eur Urol 2010;57(3):480–6.

30. Nagele U, Kuczyk MA, Horstmann M, et al. Initial clinical experience with full-length metal ureteral stents for obstructive ureteral stenosis. World J Urol 2008;26(3):257–62.

31. Hsu JS, Huang CY, Liu KL, et al. Risk factors for primary failure of metallic ureteral stents: experience from a tertiary center. J Endourol 2018. https://doi.org/10.1089/end.2017.0611.

32. Chow PM, Hsu JS, Wang SM, et al. Metallic ureteral stents in malignant ureteral obstruction: short-term results and radiological features predicting stent failure in patients with non-urological malignancies. World J Urol 2014;32(3):729–36.

33. Lopez-Huertas HL, Polcari AJ, Acosta-Miranda A, et al. Metallic ureteral stents: a cost-effective method of managing benign upper tract obstruction. J Endourol 2010;24(3):483–5.

34. Kang Q, Jiang F, Yu Y, et al. Application of resonance metallic stents for malignant ureteral obstruction. Minim Invasive Ther Allied Technol 2018;1–6. https://doi.org/10.1080/13645706.2018.1443944.

35. Abdulmajed MI, Jones VW, Shergill IS. The first use of Resonance((R)) metallic ureteric stent in a case of obstructed transplant kidney. Int J Surg Case Rep 2014;5(7):375–7.

36. Stainer V, Jones R, Agawal S, et al. The use of cook resonance metallic ureteral stent in cases of obstructive uropathy from persistent neoureteral stenosis, following kidney transplantation. J Endourol Case Rep 2017;3(1):39–41.

37. Proietti S, Sofer M, Giannantoni A, et al. Resonance((R)) metallic stent in patients with ureterocutaneostomies. Int Urol Nephrol 2016;48(2):207–12.

38. Moskovitz B, Halachmi S, Nativ O. A new self-expanding, large-caliber ureteral stent: results of a multicenter experience. J Endourol 2012;26(11):1523–7.

39. Shaheen T, Edirisinghe T, Gabriel M, et al. In vitro encrustation of a semi-permanent polymer-covered nitinol ureter stent: an artificial urine model. Urolithiasis 2014;42(3):203–7.

40. Kim M, Hong B, Park HK. Long-term outcomes of double-layered polytetrafluoroethylene membrane-covered self-expandable segmental metallic stents (Uventa) in patients with chronic ureteral obstructions: is it really safe? J Endourol 2016;30(12):1339–46.

41. Kim KS, Choi S, Choi YS, et al. Comparison of efficacy and safety between a segmental thermo-expandable metal alloy spiral stent (Memokath 051) and a self-expandable covered metallic stent (UVENTA) in the management of ureteral obstructions. J Laparoendosc Adv Surg Tech A 2014;24(8):550–5.

42. Kim KH, Cho KS, Ham WS, et al. Early application of permanent metallic mesh stent in substitution for temporary polymeric ureteral stent reduces unnecessary ureteral procedures in patients with malignant ureteral obstruction. Urology 2015;86(3):459–64.

43. Kallidonis P, Kotsiris D, Sanguedolce F, et al. The effectiveness of ureteric metal stents in malignant ureteric obstructions: a systematic review. Arab J Urol 2017;15(4):280–8.

44. Bier S, Amend B, Wagner E, et al. The thermoexpandable nitinol stent: a long-term alternative in patients without nephropathy or malignancy. Scand J Urol 2017;51(5):388–91.

45. Lock JY, Wyatt E, Upadhyayula S, et al. Degradation and antibacterial properties of magnesium alloys in artificial urine for potential resorbable ureteral stent applications. J Biomed Mater Res A 2014;102(3):781–92.

46. Song G, Lim B, Han KS, et al. Complications after polymeric and metallic ureteral stent placements including three types of fistula. J Endourol 2015;29(4):485–9.

47. Das K, Ordones F, Welikumbura S, et al. Ureteroiliac artery fistula caused by a metallic Memokath ureteral stent in a radiation-induced ureteral stricture. J Endourol Case Rep 2016;2(1):162–5.

48. Elsamra SE, Leavitt DA, Motato HA, et al. Stenting for malignant ureteral obstruction: tandem, metal or metal-mesh stents. Int J Urol 2015;22(7):629–36.

49. Lingeman JE, Preminger GM, Berger Y, et al. Use of a temporary ureteral drainage stent after uncomplicated ureteroscopy: results from a phase II clinical trial. J Urol 2003;169(5):1682–8.

50. Thierry B, Merhi Y, Silver J, et al. Biodegradable membrane-covered stent from chitosan-based polymers. J Biomed Mater Res A 2005;75(3):556–66.

51. Venkat Kumar G, Su CH, Velusamy P. Surface immobilization of kanamycin-chitosan nanoparticles on polyurethane ureteral stents to prevent bacterial adhesion. Biofouling 2016;32(8):861–70.

52. Zou T, Wang L, Li W, et al. A resorbable bicomponent braided ureteral stent with improved mechanical performance. J Mech Behav Biomed Mater 2014;38:17–25.

53. Liu X, Li F, Ding Y, et al. Intelligent optimization of the film-to-fiber ratio of a degradable braided bicomponent ureteral stent. Materials (Basel) 2015;8(11):7563–77.

54. Li G, Wang ZX, Fu WJ, et al. Introduction to biodegradable polylactic acid ureteral stent application for treatment of ureteral war injury. BJU Int 2011;108(6):901–6.

55. Wang X, Shan H, Wang J, et al. Characterization of nanostructured ureteral stent with gradient degradation in a porcine model. Int J Nanomedicine 2015;10:3055–64.

56. Yang G, Xie H, Huang Y, et al. Immersed multilayer biodegradable ureteral stent with reformed biodegradation: an in vitro experiment. J Biomater Appl 2017;31(8):1235–44.

57. Barros AA, Rita A, Duarte C, et al. Bioresorbable ureteral stents from natural origin polymers. J Biomed Mater Res B Appl Biomater 2015;103(3):608–17.

58. Barros AA, Oliveira C, Ribeiro AJ, et al. In vivo assessment of a novel biodegradable ureteral stent. World J Urol 2018;36(2):277–83.

59. Chew BH, Davoudi H, Li J, et al. An in vivo porcine evaluation of the safety, bioavailability, and tissue penetration of a ketorolac drug-eluting ureteral stent designed to improve comfort. J Endourol 2010; 24(6):1023–9.

60. Krambeck AE, Walsh RS, Denstedt JD, et al. A novel drug eluting ureteral stent: a prospective, randomized, multicenter clinical trial to evaluate the safety and effectiveness of a ketorolac loaded ureteral stent. J Urol 2010;183(3):1037–42.

61. Joshi HB, Okeke A, Newns N, et al. Characterization of urinary symptoms in patients with ureteral stents. Urology 2002;59(4):511–6.

62. Chew BH, Seitz C. Impact of ureteral stenting in ureteroscopy. Curr Opin Urol 2016;26(1):76–80.

63. Vernez SL, Okhunov Z, Wikenheiser J, et al. Precise characterization and 3-dimensional reconstruction of the autonomic nerve distribution of the human ureter. J Urol 2017;197(3 Pt 1):723–9.

64. Vogt B, Desgrippes A, Desfemmes FN. Changing the double-pigtail stent by a new suture stent to improve patient's quality of life: a prospective study. World J Urol 2015;33(8):1061–8.

65. Davenport K, Kumar V, Collins J, et al. New ureteral stent design does not improve patient quality of life: a randomized, controlled trial. J Urol 2011;185(1): 175–8.

66. Ecke TH, Bartel P, Hallmann S, et al. Evaluation of symptoms and patients' comfort for JJ-ureteral stents with and without antireflux-membrane valve. Urology 2010;75(1):212–6.

67. Erturk E, Sessions A, Joseph JV. Impact of ureteral stent diameter on symptoms and tolerability. J Endourol 2003;17(2):59–62.

68. Lo J, Lange D, Chew BH. Ureteral stents and foley catheters-associated urinary tract infections: the role of coatings and materials in infection prevention. Antibiotics (Basel) 2014;3(1):87–97.

69. El-Nahas AR, Lachine M, Elsawy E, et al. A randomized controlled trial comparing antimicrobial (silver sulfadiazine)-coated ureteral stents with non-coated stents. Scand J Urol 2018;52(1):76–80.

70. Glinel K, Thebault P, Humblot V, et al. Antibacterial surfaces developed from bio-inspired approaches. Acta Biomater 2012;8(5):1670–84.

71. Yu K, Lo JC, Mei Y, et al. Toward infection-resistant surfaces: achieving high antimicrobial peptide potency by modulating the functionality of polymer brush and peptide. ACS Appl Mater Interfaces 2015;7(51):28591–605.

72. Hazan Z, Zumeris J, Jacob H, et al. Effective prevention of microbial biofilm formation on medical devices by low-energy surface acoustic waves. Antimicrob Agents Chemother 2006;50(12): 4144–52.

73. Cauda F, Cauda V, Fiori C, et al. Heparin coating on ureteral double J stents prevents encrustations: an in vivo case study. J Endourol 2008;22(3):465–72.

74. Ron R, Zbaida D, Kafka IZ, et al. Attenuation of encrustation by self-assembled inorganic fullerene-like nanoparticles. Nanoscale 2014;6(10):5251–9.

75. Rassweiler MC, Michel MS, Ritter M, et al. Magnetic ureteral stent removal without cystoscopy: a randomized controlled trial. J Endourol 2017;31(8): 762–6.

76. Ziemba JB, Ludwig WW, Ruiz L, et al. Preventing the forgotten ureteral stent by using a mobile point-of-care application. J Endourol 2017;31(7):719–24.

77. Boyan WP Jr, Lavy D, Dinallo A, et al. Lighted ureteral stents in laparoscopic colorectal surgery; a five-year experience. Ann Transl Med 2017;5(3):44.

78. Chen X, Assadsangabi B, Hsiang Y, et al. Enabling angioplasty-ready "smart" stents to detect in-stent restenosis and occlusion. Adv Sci 2018;5(5): 1700560.

New Imaging Techniques in the Management of Stone Disease

Kevin Koo, MD, MPH, MPhil*, Brian R. Matlaga, MD, MPH

KEYWORDS

- Diagnostic imaging • Urinary calculi • Computed tomography • Ultrasonography
- Radiation exposure

KEY POINTS

- Advances in computed tomography, X-ray–based imaging, and ultrasonography have improved the accuracy of stone detection while minimizing radiation exposure.
- Dual-energy computed tomography uses 2 X-ray sources to differentiate the attenuation profile of calcium, uric acid, cystine, and other stone types.
- Digital tomosynthesis is an X-ray–based technology with superior diagnostic accuracy over conventional X-ray or intravenous pyelography and reduced radiation exposure compared with computed tomography.
- Electromagnetic tracking shows promise in enhancing the use of ultrasonography to achieve percutaneous renal access for nephrolithotomy.

INTRODUCTION

Urolithiasis is one of the most common urologic conditions among US adults,[1] and its prevalence and socioeconomic burden continue to increase.[2] The need for fast, accessible, inexpensive, and accurate radiographic imaging techniques to diagnose stone disease, predict responses to potential treatment options, and guide medical and surgical decision-making to optimize outcomes and minimize morbidity remains a clinical and economic priority.[3] X-ray (XR) and ultrasound, historically the mainstays of radiographic surveillance and detection, have yielded to computed tomography (CT), which is widely available, easily obtained, and superior in terms of diagnostic accuracy. However, concerns about cumulative exposure to ionizing radiation from lifelong stone recurrences have motivated attempts to reduce the effective dose and implement alternative modalities for first-line testing.[4] This article reviews recent advances in computed tomography, X-ray–based imaging, and ultrasonography in the contemporary management of stone disease.

COMPUTED TOMOGRAPHY

CT has become a routine modality for detecting and investigating stone disease. CT provides fast, accurate, cross-sectional identification of stones anywhere in the upper and lower urinary tract, which makes it particularly effective in the acute emergency setting in patients who present with flank pain and renal colic.[5–7] As CT scanners have become more commonplace and accessible in emergency departments, a parallel, up to 10-fold increase in the use of CT as a first-line diagnostic test for symptomatic stone disease has been observed,[8] with concomitant reductions in the use of radiographs and ultrasound.[8,9] CT also

Disclosure Statement: The authors have nothing to disclose.
Department of Urology, Johns Hopkins University School of Medicine, 600 North Wolfe Street, Baltimore, MD 21287, USA
* Corresponding author.
E-mail address: kkoo@jhmi.edu

Urol Clin N Am 46 (2019) 257–263
https://doi.org/10.1016/j.ucl.2018.12.007
0094-0143/19/© 2018 Elsevier Inc. All rights reserved.

has the advantage of being able to identify radiolucent stones, an important observation in the development and prioritization of this technology over conventional fluoroscopy.[10]

In addition to aiding the identification of stones, CT is useful during preoperative planning. The American Urologic Association and Endourological Society Guideline for the Surgical Management of Stones specifically recommends that clinicians should obtain a noncontrast CT before performing percutaneous nephrolithotomy (PCNL) in adults and children.[11] The guideline also advises that clinicians may use noncontrast CT to help decide between shockwave lithotripsy (SWL) and ureteroscopy (URS) for stone management,[11] although other imaging modalities may also be helpful to clinicians and patients choosing between different surgical options.[12]

There have recently been concerns about increased cumulative radiation exposure in patients with stone disease, in particular younger patients who may undergo numerous scans over decades of recurrence,[13] as well as obese patients whose increased body mass index may triple the effective radiation dose that is absorbed when compared with nonobese patients.[14] To minimize these risks while preserving the advantages of cross-sectional imaging, low-dose CT (LDCT) and ultra-LDCT (ULDCT) protocols have been introduced. These protocols are subject to the same limitations as conventional CT when performed in patients with higher body mass index,[15] but the overall effective doses delivered to the patient are considerably lower.

LDCT typically delivers between 1.4 and 2.0 mSv of radiation, compared with 11.2 mSv for a typical noncontrast scan[16] or up to 1.5 mSv and 3.5 mSv for abdominal radiograph and intravenous pyelogram, respectively.[17] A meta-analysis of studies assessing the sensitivity and specificity of LDCT protocols has demonstrated excellent efficacy of greater than 95%.[18] ULDCT protocols aim to deliver less than 1.0 mSv of radiation, rivaling the effective dose of a typical abdominal plain film.[4] However, the sensitivity and specificity of ULDCT have been found to decline, as reduced quality of the images can lead to missed stones, particularly smaller stones, due to poor granularity and image noise. Although ULDCT compares favorably with LDCT in the detection of stones larger than 4 mm, one trial noted a substantial difference in performance when detecting stones of all sizes, as modest as 72% sensitivity for ULDCT.[19]

Several other techniques to reduce ionizing radiation exposure from CT have been proposed.[20,21] One strategy is to individualize each scan to the body habitus and body mass index of the patient. Patients with smaller cross-sectional dimensions would require a decreased effective dose, while tailoring exposure for larger patients would reduce the risk of having to repeat the scan to achieve better-quality images. A second technique is to adjust the parameters of the scan based on the anticipated purpose and clinical indications for the scan. For instance, in a patient with a large staghorn calculus, the slice thickness and table speed may be able to be increased without compromising the ability to discern anatomic details for surgical planning. Finally, contemporary scanning software may be able to modulate the radiation dose delivered over the course of a scan, depending on designated regions of interest or findings on initial CT scout images.

Another important advantage of CT over traditional radiography and ultrasound in the management of stone disease is the ability to characterize stone composition, with implications for surgical treatment and nonsurgical management.[22–25] The quantification in Hounsfield units (HU) of a stone's CT attenuation has a mainstay role in predicting the response to SWL. Stones primarily composed of calcium oxalate monohydrate or cystine, for instance, may not respond as effectively to SWL.[26,27] However, there is contrary evidence suggesting that composition alone does not accurately predict SWL outcomes, and stones with similar composition may respond differently to shockwaves.[28] Furthermore, although some categories of pure stones are known to exhibit distinct CT attenuations,[29] in practice stones are frequently of mixed composition, leading to overlap in their attenuation values and making response to SWL less predictable.

More recent evidence also suggests that conventional CT may not distinguish different stone types as readily as previously thought. For example, studies of patients with pure calcium oxalate, uric acid, or cystine stones have showed that CT effectively predicted the calcium oxalate stones based on attenuation and can distinguish between calcium oxalate and uric acid stones,[30] but the radiographic profiles of uric acid and cystine stones may in many cases be similar, thus adversely affecting the accuracy of identifying stone composition based exclusively on CT.[31] The characteristics and attenuation of stone types also may vary among scanners made by different manufacturers,[32] potentially precluding interscan comparisons and generalizations regarding predictability.

Combining CT attenuation with other clinical or computed information has the potential to improve the accuracy of predicting stone composition from conventional CT data. In a study of uric acid stones, the combination of HU and patients' urinary pH in moderate-sized stones (larger than 4 mm) achieved 86% sensitivity and 99% specificity in predicting uric acid composition.[33] Alternatively, computer algorithms may be able to process CT images to develop predictive distributions of radiographic profiles corresponding to different stone types. A recent report used a pixel-mapping software to compute a stone's HU, morphologic eccentricity, and kurtosis characteristics, then mathematically modeled these data to predict uric acid composition with 89% sensitivity and 91% specificity.[34] Additional studies will be needed to improve the algorithms and determine their success in distinguishing among other stone types.

Dual-energy CT (DECT) is a newer technology that may help to overcome a significant limitation of CT. Conventional protocols use a single energy source to determine attenuation, so when scanned materials, whether biological tissue or inorganic stone, share attenuation characteristics due to composition similarities, the resulting scan may not reliably distinguish them.[35] Instead of a single XR source, DECT uses 2 XR sources that may be operated simultaneously and at different energy levels, typically 80 kV and 140 kV.[20] As a result, 2 sets of photon spectra data are acquired and then merged to generate the CT images.[36] The key underlying advantage of DECT is that the CT attenuation profiles of different stone types are energy-dependent, and thus compositional analysis may enhanced by combining the profiles produced at both low-energy and high-energy levels.[36–40]

Initial studies using DECT to assess stone composition demonstrated that DECT was able to distinguish between uric acid and non–uric acid stones more accurately than conventional CT. One in vitro study of uric acid stones showed classification accuracy improved from 40% for single-energy CT to as high as 93% for DECT,[41] whereas in vivo DECT was 90% accurate, with 100% sensitivity and 94% specificity.[42] Spectral attenuation evaluation has also confirmed successful in vivo differentiation between uric acid and non-uric acid stones, based on unique spectral attenuation curves generated for different stone types.[43] Using DECT to discriminate among several stone types, however, has proved more challenging, with multiple studies having mixed conclusions.[37,39,44,45] For example, in an in vitro assessment of calcium-based stones, DECT was not only able to discriminate between calcium and uric acid stones, but also between calcium oxalate and calcium phosphate stones.[37]

Further work involving increasingly complex stone types has suggested that DECT can accurately differentiate among cystine, struvite, calcium, and brushite stones.[35,44] DECT can generate a low-to-high energy ratio, which accounts for the attenuation using both XR sources of a specific material. Differences in the ratios of different stone types may be used to predict composition. For instance, a ratio of 1.13 to 1.24 predicts cystine, whereas a ratio of greater than 1.24 suggests a calcium salt.[46] Other subtypes and mixed-composition stones remain a challenge, but advances in DECT technology, such as modification of the specific dual-energy levels, show promise in further discrimination of non–uric acid stones.[47]

With regard to radiation exposure, the initial use of DECT with conventional CT resulted in higher effective doses.[36] Subsequent studies comparing DECT and single-energy CT, however, have suggested that the exposures may be comparable, between 2.6 and 2.7 mSv for both techniques.[48] When applied to compositional analysis of stones, DECT has been shown in recent in vivo studies to result in up to 40% lower radiation doses compared with single-energy CT and statistically equivalent doses compared with LDCT.[49] These dose-reduced DECT protocols were able to achieve lower radiation exposure by decreasing the tube current of the scanner. Continued interest in still lower radiation doses has led to proposed ultra–low-dose DECT protocols, which in one in vivo study yielded total doses between 1.2 and 2.5 mSv, depending on body mass index,[36] which were lower than the mean effective doses delivered by various low-dose DECT protocols, ranging from 2.66 to 4.95 mSv.[50–52] The lower doses were achieved by reducing the DECT tube current by up to 38% of the recommended settings and resulted in excellent differentiation between uric acid stones (100% sensitivity and specificity) and non–uric acid stones (100% sensitivity and 79% specificity).

X-RAY RADIOGRAPHY

Plain abdominal radiographs as a first-line modality to detect stones have gradually yielded to CT due to the latter's superior accuracy and sensitivity for not only stones but also other abdominopelvic pathology.[5,12,53] XR continues to demonstrate utility, however, for surgical planning, particularly for SWL, because XR provides useful information about radiopacity and localization under fluoroscopy. In select cases when the radiographic characteristics of a stone on radiographs are different from on initial CT, treatment considerations, such as the feasibility of SWL, may change.[54] Furthermore, CT scout images may not be a reliable surrogate for XR and may not detect a quarter of the stones visualized on radiographs,[55] which can have important implications for subsequent management.

XR also remains a common modality for postsurgical follow-up. A contemporary analysis of adult patients undergoing imaging following SWL or URS showed that 84% of patients undergoing SWL and 61% of patients undergoing URS had at least one imaging study within 12 months of surgery.[56] Abdominal radiography was the most commonly obtained follow-up imaging, accounting for 76% of patients undergoing SWL and 40% of patients undergoing URS. In contrast, the use of CT for follow-up declined over the 7-year study period, attributed to concerns about radiation exposure and cost. Whether the growing use of LDCT and ULDCT protocols will affect modality choice for follow-up imaging will require further study.

A newer innovation expanding the use of XR-based technology in stone disease is digital tomosynthesis (DT), which can improve the image quality of conventional radiographs by generating multiple high-resolution coronal images during an approximately 60-degree tomographic sweep and then combining them with a scout radiographs or intravenous pyelogram.[20,57,58] The desired number of sections does not influence and is not limited by the tomographic sweep, because the images are algorithmically reconstructed. The enhanced visualization of DT in the anterior-posterior axis is a particular advantage over conventional plain films.[59]

Originally pioneered in breast and thoracic imaging to improve the detection of pulmonary nodules and related pathology that may be challenging to identify on conventional radiographs,[60] DT has been demonstrated to be similarly effective in the management of urolithiasis. Initial studies of this technology have suggested that DT outperforms radiography or intravenous pyelography alone in diagnostic accuracy.[61,62] Other strengths include decreased radiation exposure, with the effective dose of DT similar to XR and significantly lower than even LDCT[59]; preserved image quality regardless of body mass index[15]; and potential cost-savings compared with conventional CT.[63]

Emerging evidence suggests that DT may have a role in identifying specific stone types. A recent comparative study of radiography, DT, and conventional CT assessing stones implanted in fresh tissue cadavers found that the diagnostic accuracy of DT and CT were similar and also superior to radiography in the detection of renal stones

(DT 81% accurate, CT 81%, XR 48%) and uric acid stones (CT 56% accurate, DT 41%, XR 22%).[57] Detection of ureteral stones was lower (CT 38% accurate, DT 24%, XR 13%). Poorer accuracy across modalities overall was attributed to the cadaver model.

ULTRASOUND

The advantages of ultrasound in the detection and surveillance of stone disease are several-fold: the technique is noninvasive, may be performed efficiently at the bedside, and confers no ionizing radiation to the operator or the patient.[4,20] In contrast to XR and CT, ultrasound also allows for dynamic, real-time visualization of intrarenal and surrounding anatomy. In the setting of trial evidence demonstrating that ultrasound significantly reduced radiation exposure without increasing complication or hospital admission rates in patients with suspected symptomatic stones,[64] these features have led to the prioritization of ultrasound in acute emergency settings for the initial diagnostic evaluation of urolithiasis.

Ultrasonography, however, also has notable limitations. The pooled sensitivity and specificity of ultrasound in detecting renal stones has been reported to be as low as 45% and 88%, respectively, versus more than 95% for conventional CT.[65] Ultrasound measurements may be significantly dependent on operator experience and technique, potentially leading to interoperator and interstudy variation. Increased body habitus and body mass index also reduce the accuracy and imaging quality of ultrasound.[65] As a result, overestimation of stone size is a documented limitation of ultrasound, up to 1 mm in stones smaller than 5 mm.[66]

Use of color Doppler may help attenuate some of these limitations. When ultrasound echoes are reflected by a stone, the resulting "twinkle artifact" appears as alternating colors behind the stone and can increase diagnostic accuracy to 97% of stones seen by CT.[67] Conventional grayscale ultrasound, on the other hand, has been reported to miss one-third of these stones. Notably, color Doppler is subject to the same operator dependence as ultrasound in general. Consequently, the false-positive rate of the twinkle artifact may be as high as 50%,[68] which in acute settings in which diagnostic accuracy is paramount may result in patients having to undergo confirmatory CT.

Aside from its use in the detection of stones, another important application of ultrasound in stone management is sonographic guidance in percutaneous access for nephrolithotomy. When performed by an experienced operator, ultrasound-guided percutaneous access can have success rates as high as 88% to 99%, and has been reliably performed in a large series of percutaneous procedures.[69,70] Sonographic guidance reduces radiation exposure in obese patients, who might otherwise require higher effective doses under fluoroscopic guidance to achieve comparable image quality.[71,72]

To overcome the spatial limitations of 2-dimensional ultrasound images during a 3-dimensional access procedure, a promising area of innovation is the use of electromagnetic tracking to provide continuous, real-time guidance during needle puncture. Electromagnetic sensors allow the needle to be navigated to a selected target, avoiding surrounding anatomic obstacles and providing visual feedback to the surgeon regarding alignment and orientation.[69] Early demonstration of this technology in a porcine model confirmed technical feasibility of both renal and ureteral punctures with an average time of less than 1 minute.[73] A recent small patient series incorporated electromagnetic sensors into ureteroscopy-assisted percutaneous access, resulting in successful puncture with one attempt in each of the 10 patients and a median time to acceptable placement of 20 seconds.[74] In addition to technical feasibility, a potential advantage of electromagnetic tracking is the modest learning curve compared with conventional techniques for performing percutaneous access. Using porcine models, surgeons were able to achieve technical expertise after performing only 12 cases[73]; these findings will need to be further validated through in vivo patient trials.

SUMMARY

Notable advances in CT, XR-based imaging, and ultrasonography have helped to improve diagnostic accuracy, predict stone composition, and minimize patients' exposure to ionizing radiation. Ongoing investigations of dual-energy CT, digital tomosynthesis, and electromagnetic tracking may yield novel applications of these technologies to guide decision-making across the disease spectrum, from diagnosis to treatment. These innovations are urgently needed as the prevalence and economic consequences of stone disease continue to rise.

REFERENCES

1. Scales CD Jr, Smith AC, Hanley JM, et al, Urologic Diseases in America Project. Prevalence of kidney stones in the United States. Eur Urol 2012;62(1):160–5.
2. Ziemba JB, Matlaga BR. Epidemiology and economics of nephrolithiasis. Investig Clin Urol 2017; 58(5):299–306.
3. Matlaga BR. The need for better decision tools in managing stone disease. J Urol 2012;188(3):698–9.
4. Yecies T, Averch TD, Semins MJ. Identifying and managing the risks of medical ionizing radiation in endourology. Can J Urol 2018;25(1):9154–60.
5. Worster A, Preyra I, Weaver B, et al. The accuracy of noncontrast helical computed tomography versus intravenous pyelography in the diagnosis of suspected acute urolithiasis: a meta-analysis. Ann Emerg Med 2002;40(3):280–6.
6. Fowler KA, Locken JA, Duchesne JH, et al. US for detecting renal calculi with nonenhanced CT as a reference standard. Radiology 2002;222(1):109–13.
7. Rekant EM, Gibert CL, Counselman FL. Emergency department time for evaluation of patients discharged with a diagnosis of renal colic: unenhanced helical computed tomography versus intravenous urography. J Emerg Med 2001;21(4):371–4.
8. Westphalen AC, Hsia RY, Maselli JH, et al. Radiological imaging of patients with suspected urinary tract stones: national trends, diagnoses, and predictors. Acad Emerg Med 2011;18(7):699–707.
9. Fwu CW, Eggers PW, Kimmel PL, et al. Emergency department visits, use of imaging, and drugs for urolithiasis have increased in the United States. Kidney Int 2013;83(3):479–86.
10. Segal AJ, Spataro RF, Linke CA, et al. Diagnosis of nonopaque calculi by computed tomography. Radiology 1978;129(2):447–50.
11. Assimos D, Krambeck A, Miller NL, et al. Surgical management of stones: American Urological Association/Endourological Society Guideline, PART I. J Urol 2016;196(4):1153–60.
12. Fulgham PF, Assimos DG, Pearle MS, et al. Clinical effectiveness protocols for imaging in the management of ureteral calculous disease: AUA technology assessment. J Urol 2013;189(4):1203–13.
13. Katz SI, Saluja S, Brink JA, et al. Radiation dose associated with unenhanced CT for suspected renal colic: impact of repetitive studies. AJR Am J Roentgenol 2006;186(4):1120–4.
14. Wang AJ, Goldsmith ZG, Wang C, et al. Obesity triples the radiation dose of stone protocol computerized tomography. J Urol 2013;189(6):2142–6.
15. Poletti PA, Platon A, Rutschmann OT, et al. Low-dose versus standard-dose CT protocol in patients with clinically suspected renal colic. AJR Am J Roentgenol 2007;188(4):927–33.
16. Lukasiewicz A, Bhargavan-Chatfield M, Coombs L, et al. Radiation dose index of renal colic protocol CT studies in the United States: a report from the American College of Radiology National Radiology Data Registry. Radiology 2014;271(2):445–51.
17. Kluner C, Hein PA, Gralla O, et al. Does ultra-low-dose CT with a radiation dose equivalent to that of KUB suffice to detect renal and ureteral calculi? J Comput Assist Tomogr 2006;30(1):44–50.

18. Niemann T, Kollmann T, Bongartz G. Diagnostic performance of low-dose CT for the detection of urolithiasis: a meta-analysis. AJR Am J Roentgenol 2008; 191(2):396–401.

19. Pooler BD, Lubner MG, Kim DH, et al. Prospective trial of the detection of urolithiasis on ultralow dose (sub mSv) noncontrast computerized tomography: direct comparison against routine low dose reference standard. J Urol 2014;192(5):1433–9.

20. Villa L, Giusti G, Knoll T, et al. Imaging for urinary stones: update in 2015. Eur Urol Focus 2016;2(2): 122–9.

21. Zagoria RJ, Dixon RL. Radiology of urolithiasis: implications of radiation exposure and new imaging modalities. Adv Chronic Kidney Dis 2009;16(1): 48–51.

22. Marchini GS, Gebreselassie S, Liu X, et al. Absolute Hounsfield unit measurement on noncontrast computed tomography cannot accurately predict struvite stone composition. J Endourol 2013;27(2):162–7.

23. Nakada SY, Hoff DG, Attai S, et al. Determination of stone composition by noncontrast spiral computed tomography in the clinical setting. Urology 2000; 55(6):816–9.

24. Deveci S, Coskun M, Tekin MI, et al. Spiral computed tomography: role in determination of chemical compositions of pure and mixed urinary stones–an in vitro study. Urology 2004;64(2):237–40.

25. el-Assmy A, Abou-el-Ghar ME, el-Nahas AR, et al. Multidetector computed tomography: role in determination of urinary stones composition and disintegration with extracorporeal shock wave lithotripsy–an in vitro study. Urology 2011;77(2):286–90.

26. Perks AE, Schuler TD, Lee J, et al. Stone attenuation and skin-to-stone distance on computed tomography predicts for stone fragmentation by shock wave lithotripsy. Urology 2008;72(4):765–9.

27. Shah K, Kurien A, Mishra S, et al. Predicting effectiveness of extracorporeal shockwave lithotripsy by stone attenuation value. J Endourol 2010;24(7): 1169–73.

28. Williams JC Jr, Saw KC, Paterson RF, et al. Variability of renal stone fragility in shock wave lithotripsy. Urology 2003;61(6):1092–6 [discussion: 1097].

29. Grosjean R, Sauer B, Guerra RM, et al. Characterization of human renal stones with MDCT: advantage of dual energy and limitations due to respiratory motion. AJR Am J Roentgenol 2008;190(3):720–8.

30. Marchini GS, Remer EM, Gebreselassie S, et al. Stone characteristics on noncontrast computed tomography: establishing definitive patterns to discriminate calcium and uric acid compositions. Urology 2013;82(3):539–46.

31. Torricelli FC, Marchini GS, De S, et al. Predicting urinary stone composition based on single-energy noncontrast computed tomography: the challenge of cystine. Urology 2014;83(6):1258–63.

32. Grosjean R, Daudon M, Chammas MF Jr, et al. Pitfalls in urinary stone identification using CT attenuation values: are we getting the same information on different scanner models? Eur J Radiol 2013;82(8): 1201–6.

33. Spettel S, Shah P, Sekhar K, et al. Using Hounsfield unit measurement and urine parameters to predict uric acid stones. Urology 2013;82(1):22–6.

34. Ganesan V, De S, Shkumat N, et al. Accurately diagnosing uric acid stones from conventional computerized tomography imaging: development and preliminary assessment of a pixel mapping software. J Urol 2018;199(2):487–94.

35. Vernuccio F, Meyer M, Mileto A, et al. Use of dual-energy computed tomography for evaluation of genitourinary diseases. Urol Clin North Am 2018; 45(3):297–310.

36. Wilhelm K, Schoenthaler M, Hein S, et al. Focused dual-energy CT maintains diagnostic and compositional accuracy for urolithiasis using ultralow-dose noncontrast CT. Urology 2015;86(6):1097–102.

37. Matlaga BR, Kawamoto S, Fishman E. Dual source computed tomography: a novel technique to determine stone composition. Urology 2008;72(5): 1164–8.

38. Flohr TG, McCollough CH, Bruder H, et al. First performance evaluation of a dual-source CT (DSCT) system. Eur Radiol 2006;16(2):256–68.

39. Sheir KZ, Mansour O, Madbouly K, et al. Determination of the chemical composition of urinary calculi by noncontrast spiral computerized tomography. Urol Res 2005;33(2):99–104.

40. Johnson TR, Krauss B, Sedlmair M, et al. Material differentiation by dual energy CT: initial experience. Eur Radiol 2007;17(6):1510–7.

41. Wisenbaugh ES, Paden RG, Silva AC, et al. Dual-energy vs conventional computed tomography in determining stone composition. Urology 2014; 83(6):1243–7.

42. Bonatti M, Lombardo F, Zamboni GA, et al. Renal stones composition in vivo determination: comparison between 100/Sn140 kV dual-energy CT and 120 kV single-energy CT. Urolithiasis 2017;45(3): 255–61.

43. Lombardo F, Bonatti M, Zamboni GA, et al. Uric acid versus non-uric acid renal stones: in vivo differentiation with spectral CT. Clin Radiol 2017;72(6):490–6.

44. Graser A, Johnson TR, Bader M, et al. Dual energy CT characterization of urinary calculi: initial in vitro and clinical experience. Invest Radiol 2008;43(2): 112–9.

45. Li X, Zhao R, Liu B, et al. Gemstone spectral imaging dual-energy computed tomography: a novel technique to determine urinary stone composition. Urology 2013;81(4):727–30.

46. Hidas G, Eliahou R, Duvdevani M, et al. Determination of renal stone composition with dual-energy CT:

in vivo analysis and comparison with x-ray diffraction. Radiology 2010;257(2):394–401.

47. Duan X, Li Z, Yu L, et al. Characterization of urinary stone composition by use of third-generation dual-source dual-energy CT with increased spectral separation. AJR Am J Roentgenol 2015;205(6):1203–7.

48. Schenzle JC, Sommer WH, Neumaier K, et al. Dual energy CT of the chest: how about the dose? Invest Radiol 2010;45(6):347–53.

49. Jepperson MA, Cernigliaro JG, Ibrahim el SH, et al. In vivo comparison of radiation exposure of dual-energy CT versus low-dose CT versus standard CT for imaging urinary calculi. J Endourol 2015;29(2):141–6.

50. Eiber M, Holzapfel K, Frimberger M, et al. Targeted dual-energy single-source CT for characterisation of urinary calculi: experimental and clinical experience. Eur Radiol 2012;22(1):251–8.

51. Ascenti G, Siragusa C, Racchiusa S, et al. Stone-targeted dual-energy CT: a new diagnostic approach to urinary calculosis. AJR Am J Roentgenol 2010; 195(4):953–8.

52. Thomas C, Heuschmid M, Schilling D, et al. Urinary calculi composed of uric acid, cystine, and mineral salts: differentiation with dual-energy CT at a radiation dose comparable to that of intravenous pyelography. Radiology 2010;257(2):402–9.

53. Heidenreich A, Desgrandschamps F, Terrier F. Modern approach of diagnosis and management of acute flank pain: review of all imaging modalities. Eur Urol 2002;41(4):351–62.

54. Lamb AD, Wines MD, Mousa S, et al. Plain radiography still is required in the planning of treatment for urolithiasis. J Endourol 2008;22(10):2201–5.

55. Johnston R, Lin A, Du J, et al. Comparison of kidney-ureter-bladder abdominal radiography and computed tomography scout films for identifying renal calculi. BJU Int 2009;104(5):670–3.

56. Ahn JS, Holt SK, May PC, et al. National imaging trends after ureteroscopic or shock wave lithotripsy for nephrolithiasis. J Urol 2018;199(2):500–7.

57. Wollin DA, Gupta RT, Young B, et al. Abdominal radiography with digital tomosynthesis: an alternative to computed tomography for identification of urinary calculi? Urology 2018;120:56–61.

58. Lipkin ME, Preminger GM. Imaging techniques for stone disease and methods for reducing radiation exposure. Urol Clin North Am 2013;40(1):47–57.

59. Neisius A, Astroza GM, Wang C, et al. Digital tomosynthesis: a new technique for imaging nephrolithiasis. Specific organ doses and effective doses compared with renal stone protocol noncontrast computed tomography. Urology 2014;83(2):282–7.

60. Johnsson AA, Vikgren J, Bath M. Chest tomosynthesis: technical and clinical perspectives. Semin Respir Crit Care Med 2014;35(1):17–26.

61. Mermuys K, De Geeter F, Bacher K, et al. Digital tomosynthesis in the detection of urolithiasis: diagnostic performance and dosimetry compared with digital radiography with MDCT as the reference standard. AJR Am J Roentgenol 2010;195(1):161–7.

62. Wells IT, Raju VM, Rowberry BK, et al. Digital tomosynthesis–a new lease of life for the intravenous urogram? Br J Radiol 2011;84(1001):464–8.

63. Quaia E, Grisi G, Baratella E, et al. Diagnostic imaging costs before and after digital tomosynthesis implementation in patient management after detection of suspected thoracic lesions on chest radiography. Insights Imaging 2014;5(1):147–55.

64. Smith-Bindman R, Aubin C, Bailitz J, et al. Ultrasonography versus computed tomography for suspected nephrolithiasis. N Engl J Med 2014; 371(12):1100–10.

65. Ray AA, Ghiculete D, Pace KT, et al. Limitations to ultrasound in the detection and measurement of urinary tract calculi. Urology 2010;76(2):295–300.

66. Viprakasit DP, Sawyer MD, Herrell SD, et al. Limitations of ultrasonography in the evaluation of urolithiasis: a correlation with computed tomography. J Endourol 2012;26(3):209–13.

67. Mitterberger M, Aigner F, Pallwein L, et al. Sonographic detection of renal and ureteral stones. Value of the twinkling sign. Int Braz J Urol 2009;35(5): 532–9 [discussion: 540–1].

68. Dillman JR, Kappil M, Weadock WJ, et al. Sonographic twinkling artifact for renal calculus detection: correlation with CT. Radiology 2011;259(3): 911–6.

69. Slater RC, Ost M. Percutaneous stone removal: new approaches to access and imaging. Curr Urol Rep 2015;16(5):29.

70. Yan S, Xiang F, Yongsheng S. Percutaneous nephrolithotomy guided solely by ultrasonography: a 5-year study of >700 cases. BJU Int 2013;112(7):965–71.

71. Usawachintachit M, Masic S, Chang HC, et al. Ultrasound guidance to assist percutaneous nephrolithotomy reduces radiation exposure in obese patients. Urology 2016;98:32–8.

72. Chi T, Masic S, Li J, et al. Ultrasound guidance for renal tract access and dilation reduces radiation exposure during percutaneous nephrolithotomy. Adv Urol 2016;2016:3840697.

73. Rodrigues PL, Vilaca JL, Oliveira C, et al. Collecting system percutaneous access using real-time tracking sensors: first pig model in vivo experience. J Urol 2013;190(5):1932–7.

74. Lima E, Rodrigues PL, Mota P, et al. Ureteroscopy-assisted percutaneous kidney access made easy: first clinical experience with a novel navigation system using electromagnetic guidance (IDEAL stage 1). Eur Urol 2017;72(4):610–6.

Radiation Mitigation Techniques in Kidney Stone Management

Todd Samuel Yecies, MD[a], Michelle Jo Semins, MD[b],*

KEYWORDS

- Radiation safety • ALARA • Fluoroscopy • Nephrolithiasis

KEY POINTS

- Patients with nephrolithiasis are exposed to significant quantities of ionizing radiation with the potential to cause secondary malignancy.
- Appropriate radiation stewardship can significantly reduce the radiation dose associated with a nephrolithiasis episode.
- Principle avenues for radiation reduction consist of appropriate selection of preoperative and postoperative imaging modalities and alterations in fluoroscopy settings and usage patterns intraoperatively.

INTRODUCTION: THE SCOPE OF THE PROBLEM

The risks of exposure to medical ionizing radiation are of increasing concern both among medical professionals and the general public. Herein we aim to summarize the current evidence regarding the risks of medical ionizing radiation to patients with nephrolithiasis. We then identify techniques through which patient radiation exposure can be reduced in the preoperative, intraoperative, and postoperative settings.

To discuss techniques for radiation dose mitigation, one must first understand the underlying terminology used. Radiation quantities are discussed via 2 standard approaches. The first are the units rad or the SI equivalent of gray (Gy), which express the absolute amount of ionizing radiation delivered to a specific point or target tissue. The second is by expressing the effective dose, defined as the relative effect of a specified amount of radiation on the target tissue or individual. Effective dose is measured in either joules/kg or the SI equivalent of sievert (Sv), which is a calculated value using the equation effective dose (Sv) = absorbed dose (Gy) × tissue weighting factor. Effective dose accounts for the absorbed dose and the target tissue radiation sensitivity. The target tissue sensitivity to radiation injury is described by the tissue weighting factor. In the United States, estimated average annual background radiation exposure is 3 mSv.[1] This can provide context to future numbers discussed in this review.

There are 2 principal classifications of radiation-induced injury: deterministic and stochastic effects. Deterministic effects are defined by having a threshold dose below which there is no measurable effect, as occurs in cataract formation, dermal injury, and hair loss, estimated to occur above doses of 0.5 Gy, 2 Gy, and 3 Gy, respectively. These represent radiation doses rarely encountered during urologic intervention or imaging.[2] There is no threshold dose for injury for stochastic effects.

Disclosure Statement: Dr M.J. Semins is a consultant for Boston Scientific. Dr T.S. Yecies has nothing to disclose.
a Department of Urology, University of Pittsburgh Medical Center, 200 Lothrop Street, Kaufman Building, 701, Pittsburgh, PA 15213, USA; b Department of Urology, University of Pittsburgh Medical Center, Pittsburgh, PA, USA
* Corresponding author. 1350 Locust Street Suite G100A Building C, Pittsburgh, PA 15219.
E-mail address: seminsmj@upmc.edu

Urol Clin N Am 46 (2019) 265–272
https://doi.org/10.1016/j.ucl.2018.12.008
0094-0143/19/© 2018 Elsevier Inc. All rights reserved.

The risk of radiation-induced malignancy is believed to be a stochastic effect, and more specifically to follow a linear, no-threshold model. The evidence for this is based on 3 primary sources: identification of excess relative risk of malignancy in the survivors of nuclear explosions,[3] identification of excess relative risk of malignancy in nuclear power workers,[4] and epidemiologic assessments of the national health systems in England and Australia in which patients undergoing computed tomography (CT) scans were found to have an increased risk of future malignancy.[5,6] Although each approach has methodologic limitations and the validity of the linear no-threshold model is not above reproach,[7] the preponderance of evidence from these studies suggests a dose, age, and gender-dependent risk of radiation-induced malignancy. Based on these data, the Biological Effects of Ionizing Radiation (BEIR) VII Phase 2 report commissioned by the National Academy of Sciences provides a framework for estimating the lifetime attributable risk of cancer incidence associated with radiation exposure.[8]

Both diagnostic imaging and fluoroscopy-guided interventions expose patients with kidney stones to ionizing radiation. Ferrandino and colleagues[9] identified that patients with a kidney stone episode underwent an average of 1.7 CT scans, 1 abdominal radiograph, and 1 excretory urogram over a 1-year period, with a median patient dose of 29.7 mSv for diagnostic modalities alone. Fahmy and colleagues[10] had similar findings, with a median 1-year and 2-year dose of 29.3 mSv and 37.3 mSv, respectively; again not including radiation from fluoroscopy-guided interventions. Recurrence rates of nephrolithiasis are high, estimated to be up to 50% at 5 years. This translates to great potential for repeated high levels of radiation exposure in this patient population. In addition, the vast majority of treatments for nephrolithiasis are fluoroscopy-guided interventions, including percutaneous nephrolithotomy (PCNL), extracorporeal shock wave lithotripsy (SWL), and ureteroscopy (URS). Using patient dosimeters, PCNL has been estimated to carry a mean effective dose of 8.66 mSv, whereas URS and SWL have been estimated to carry median effective doses of 1.13 mSv and 1.63 mSv, respectively.[11–13]

The risk to an individual patient from this radiation exposure can be estimated using the models provided in the BEIR report. A dose of 37.3 mSv carries a lifetime attributable risk of secondary malignancy ranging from 0.40% in women aged 20 to 30 years old to 0.065% in men older than 70 years. Using a conservative estimate of 1.5 stone episodes per stone former, radiation usage in the

management of nephrolithiasis has been estimated to cause an additional 863 cases of malignancy annually in the United States.[14] As physicians, it is imperative that we avoid inflicting this potential harm on our patients, especially when avenues exist to drastically reduce radiation exposure in nephrolithiasis management, as is described in the following sections.

RADIATION REDUCTION IN THE DIAGNOSIS AND PREOPERATIVE EVALUATION OF NEPHROLITHIASIS

The single largest source of radiation exposure for patients with nephrolithiasis, and thus the largest target for radiation dose reduction, is the use of CT imaging. A standard single-phase CT scan carries an average radiation dose of 11.3 mSv, and many nephrolithiasis patients receive multiphasic CT scans with a corresponding increased dose.[15] The increase in utilization of CT scanning in evaluation and management of nephrolithiasis has significantly increased the ionizing radiation dose associated with a stone episode; however, there is no evidence demonstrating that this improves clinical outcomes. In fact, multiple studies have demonstrated that in patients with suspected renal colic, increasing CT utilization is not associated with any change in hospital admissions, diagnosis of nephrolithiasis, or diagnosis of significant alternative pathology.[16,17]

Therefore, a key intervention to reduce patient radiation exposure is to substitute diagnostic imaging with studies associated with lower radiation doses, such as kidney-ureter-bladder (KUB) radiographs or ultrasound. In addition to being less expensive than CT or ultrasound, the effective radiation dose of KUB is 0.6 to 1.1 mSv.[18] However, there are some limitations to using alternative imaging. A meta-analysis demonstrated KUB has a poor sensitivity (45%–59%) and specificity (71%–77%) for the detection of kidney stones.[19] Ultrasound too shows an inferior sensitivity (45%) and specificity (88%) for kidney stone diagnosis, compared with noncontrast CT scan (95% and 98%, respectively).[20] Ultrasound also frequently overestimates stone size, with a mean discordance of 1 mm for stones <5 mm in size, and may misdiagnose renal parenchymal plaques as discrete stones.[21] Nonetheless, the use of ultrasound carries many benefits, including that it is radiation-free, is noninvasive, and is less expensive than CT. The *New England Journal of Medicine* recently published a randomized controlled trial showing that use of ultrasound initially instead of CT for suspected kidney stones was associated with significantly less radiation exposure over a

6-month period.[22] Although there was no differ-ence in complication or readmission rate, subse-quent CT scan was required in up to 40% of patients during the same emergency room visit. Overall, patients assigned to initial ultrasound received an average radiation dose of 9.3 mSv compared with 17.2 mSv for patients assigned to initial CT scan. Based on these findings, many now advocate for ultrasound being the initial test of choice for suspected nephrolithiasis. It should be noted that the most current American Urological Association (AUA) recommendations on the sub-ject, a white paper published in 2012, advocate for use of CT scanning, either standard or low dose, in patients with suspected renal colic.[23] In the opinion of the authors, this guideline should be revised in light of more recent evidence. In addi-tion, if a CT scan is performed on initial evaluation, and a patient re-presents to the emergency room, KUB and ultrasound should be strongly considered if repeat imaging is deemed necessary.

Despite the demonstrated benefits of initial ultra-sound for evaluation of nephrolithiasis, many urolo-gists find the anatomic information provided by CT scan to be necessary for preoperative planning when treatment is necessary. Thus, another essen-tial component of reducing nephrolithiasis patient radiation exposure is increasing the use of low-dose CT (LDCT) and ultra-LDCT (ULDCT) scan technology. The accuracy of LDCT for diagnosis of nephrolithiasis is well established, with pooled sensitivity and specificity of 96% and 95%, respec-tively, on meta-analysis.[24] LDCT estimated radia-tion dose is 1.4 to 2.0 mSv versus 11.2 mSv for standard single-phase CT.[15] A CT protocol that emits an effective dose less than 1 mSv, compara-ble to a KUB, is considered a ULDCT. For stones larger than 4 mm, sensitivity and specificity have been shown to be high for ULDCT, 92% and 96%, respectively; however, sensitivity decreases to 72% for stones of all sizes.[25] Unfortunately, one potential drawback for both LDCT and ULDCT is that patient body mass index (BMI) significantly af-fects study sensitivity.[26]

Based on these data, a patient with a new symp-tomatic kidney stone could easily receive an ultra-sound as initial evaluation followed by an LDCT if necessary for diagnostic clarification or surgical planning. This would conceivably reduce the pre-operative radiation dose for a presentation of renal colic from 17.2 mSv to 1.4 to 2.0 mSv.[22]

TECHNIQUES TO REDUCE INTRAOPERATIVE RADIATION USE

Besides focusing on diagnostic imaging, another target for reducing radiation exposure to the

patient with a kidney stone is reducing the dose delivered in the operating room. As previously discussed, the average radiation doses associ-ated with PCNL, URS, and SWL are 8.66 mSv, 1.13 mSv, and 1.63 mSv, respectively.[11–13] This likely represents an underestimate, however, as these were nonblinded studies, and the act of measuring radiation dose has been demonstrated to reduce radiation utilization.[27] Although intrao-perative fluoroscopy represents a relatively small portion of the total radiation received by patients with nephrolithiasis, given that many patients will undergo multiple lifetime interventions, radiation reduction techniques can still offer a significant dose reduction.

The most readily available intervention to reduce fluoroscopy usage during endourologic proced-ures is education and visual cues to reduce unnec-essary image acquisition. Fluoroscopy usage can be reduced by more than 50% by implementing a curriculum for radiation safety training for physi-cians.[27] Fluoroscopy time also can be reduced by 24% just by reporting personal times to the oper-ating surgeon.[28] Formal radiation-reduction proto-cols also reduce fluoroscopy use, such as using C-arm lasers to target the location without image exposure, using markings on the drape to target the laser to the organ of interest, and using last im-age hold technology to avoid duplicate pictures.[29] In addition, using radiation technologists familiar with urologic procedures can reduce fluoroscopy usage due to increased familiarity with endouro-logic needs.[30] To minimize miscommunication, we advocate establishing a terminology ahead of time with the technologist to guide their machine movements, and we also encourage foot pedal control by the surgeon. To minimize fluoroscopy usage in transition from kidney to bladder images, the floor can be marked with tape to demonstrate the appropriate C-arm position, which increases in importance when the technologists turnover mid-case.

The next key method to reduce patient radia-tion exposure is through adjustment of C-arm set-tings. The low-dose setting can be used and the fluoroscopy pulse rate can be manipulated. The low-dose setting can reduce the absorbed radia-tion dose by 57%.[31] The importance of this sim-ple intervention is difficult to overstate, as through the press of a button at the beginning of an intervention, a drastic dose reduction can be performed. It is important to note that the use of fluoroscopy time as a proxy measurement of radiation exposure does not account for the use of low-dose fluoroscopy, meaning that fluo-roscopy time will not change even as the radiation dose is significantly reduced.

The standard pulse rate of most C-arms, also known as "continuous" fluoroscopy, is 30 pulses per second (pps); however, this can be set to as low as a single pps. Fluoroscopy time during URS has been shown to decrease by 34%, 55%, and 79% using settings of 12, 4, and 1 pps, respectively, with no difference in perioperative outcomes.[26,32,33] Similarly, fluoroscopy time decreased during PCNL, when using a multimodal radiation reduction protocol including the use of a dedicated fluoroscopy technician, low-dose setting and pulsed fluoroscopy at 1 pps.[30] Importantly, for a diverse range of interventional procedures, both surgeons and radiologists have found pulsed and continuous fluoroscopy images to be clinically equivalent.[34] Selection of pulsed fluoroscopy and the low-dose setting can occur in a matter of seconds, and can simply be installed as standard procedure within an operating room environment. In our experience, the use of both the low-dose setting and reduced fluoroscopy pulse rates results in completely adequate image quality and is a simple maneuver that allows for drastic reduction in radiation dose.

In addition to modifying fluoroscopy settings, surgical techniques have been established to significantly decrease or eliminate fluoroscopy usage during URS, SWL, and PCNL. Using direct visualization, tactile feedback, and external visual cues, URS without image guidance has been shown to be safe and feasible.[35,36] Alternatively, URS can be performed using ultrasound rather than fluoroscopic guidance and this has been found to be safe and technically feasible in multiple small randomized trials comparing the 2 imaging techniques in noncomplex cases.[37,38] Since the advent of second-generation extracorporeal lithotripter units in the 1990s, ultrasound-guided SWL has also been an available treatment option. Ultrasound guidance for SWL carries the potential benefit of improved visualization of radiolucent stones, while carrying the potential drawback of increased difficulty with stone localization. Although ultrasound and fluoroscopy-guided SWL have never been directly compared, the largest identified series of ultrasound-guided SWL was comparable to fluoroscopy-guided SWL with a success rate of 86%.[39] Other studies, however, have noted reduced success due to the challenge described previously with stone localization.[40] The use of ultrasound guidance during both URS and SWL has to date been limited to noncomplex cases and studies have not been powered to show differences in complications because rates are so low. Nonetheless, these results are promising.

Of all stone interventions, PCNL carries the highest radiation dose, of which the largest individual component comes from percutaneous renal access. Various alternative percutaneous renal access methods have been demonstrated to reduce this radiation exposure. Ureteroscopic-guided percutaneous access is associated with fewer puncture attempts and thus fluoroscopy exposure.[41] Because reduced photon energy is needed to penetrate air, use of an air pyelogram can reduce effective dose with the same fluoroscopy time compared with a contrast pyelogram to guide needle puncture.[42] More recently, percutaneous access under ultrasound guidance has been performed successfully with no difference in complications, and significantly lessens radiation exposure.[43,44] Finally, a technique entitled the "laser direct alignment radiation reduction technique" (DARRT) has been published in which a laser-aiming beam mounted on the C-arm is used to guide the trajectory of needle puncture rather than continuous fluoroscopy, which reduced fluoroscopy utilization to levels comparable with ultrasound-guided percutaneous access.[45,46]

Although the purpose of this review was to describe techniques to mitigate patient radiation exposure, it should be noted that measures to reduce patient radiation exposure intraoperatively also carry the additional benefit of reducing exposure to the urologist and operating room staff. For example, dosimetry measurements demonstrated that transitioning from continuous to single pulse per second fluoroscopy reduced surgeon effective dose by 60%.[32] There is currently no evidence demonstrating increased risk of radiation-induced malignancy in urologists. However, given that a busy urologist may perform thousands of fluoroscopy-guided interventions over the course of a career and the efficacy of lead aprons in preventing scatter radiation exposure may be limited, prudence dictates that urologists should act on readily available interventions to minimize radiation exposure as described in this section.[47,48]

RADIATION REDUCTION IN POSTOPERATIVE FOLLOW-UP OF PATIENTS WITH NEPHROLITHIASIS

Radiation reduction techniques in the postoperative setting can be achieved through 3 primary techniques: increased utilization of non-CT modalities in follow-up, reducing the rate of recurrent stone formation through metabolic therapy, and promoting patient-specific care pathways for recurrent stone formers to reduce the radiation dose associated with future stone episodes.

The need for routine postoperative imaging after ureteroscopy is controversial[49]; however, some argue that it is necessary due to the small but significant rate of silent obstruction after ureteroscopy, estimated at 1% to 5%.[50] Routine post-ureteroscopy renal ultrasound has been proven to be effective in detecting silent hydronephrosis and is cost-effective with an estimated cost per kidney saved of $6262.[51,52] The routine usage of renal ultrasound in asymptomatic patients after ureteroscopy is currently recommended by AUA guidelines, with CT imaging reserved for persistently symptomatic patients, those with hydronephrosis, or residual fragments identified on ultrasound at the discretion of the provider.[23] It is the opinion of the authors that even in the case when residual fragments are identified, CT scan should be used only if the additional information offered will immediately impact patient care; for example, the decision to perform a second stage ureteroscopy, and in this setting a low-dose CT scan can be performed.

Similar debate has occurred regarding the role of routine CT scanning after PCNL. CT scan is significantly more sensitive for detection of residual fragments after PCNL than ultrasound or KUB.[53] Furthermore, an estimated 20% of patients with residual stone fragments >2 mm will ultimately require additional surgical intervention.[54] LDCT has been demonstrated to be effective in this setting in detection of clinically significant residual fragments.[51] What has not been demonstrated is whether timely identification of these residual fragments alters surgical planning and patient outcomes. A reasonable course of action may be to perform LDCT in settings in which a "second-look" procedure would be considered in the setting of residual fragments, while otherwise following patients with renal ultrasound and additional imaging as indicated by clinical status.

Although the risk of a radiation-induced malignancy from the radiation exposure associated with a single stone episode is low, the high recurrence rate of nephrolithiasis means that patients may be exposed to higher doses of radiation over the course of multiple stone episodes. Thus, a key step to reduce radiation exposure in patients with stones is through reduction of recurrent stone episodes. Multiple prospective, randomized controlled trials have demonstrated the efficacy of various metabolic interventions for stone prevention, including modulating fluid, protein, and sodium intake; potassium citrate; thiazides; and allopurinol.[55–58] Stone recurrence rates were reduced from 50% to 90%, depending on the intervention studied. Furthermore, enrollment in a multidisciplinary stone clinic has been demonstrated to

reduce long-term stone recurrence, with data demonstrating significant improvement in metabolic parameters and reduction in stone episodes with follow-up as long as 20 years.[59] What remains controversial within the urologic literature, however, is the role of metabolic evaluation for first-time stone formers, with many arguing that comprehensive metabolic evaluation is not cost-effective compared with empiric management. Current AUA and European Association of Urology guidelines recommend that patients undergo comprehensive metabolic evaluation only if they are considered "high risk" for stone recurrence or express interest in metabolic evaluation, in the case of the AUA guidelines.[60,61] It is worth noting that the potential benefit of radiation dose reduction was not significantly considered in the formulation of the aforementioned guidelines and cost-effectiveness studies, and may alter the risk-benefit calculus when considering initial metabolic stone evaluation.

Despite stone prevention efforts, it is known that many patients will continue to have recurrent stone episodes and receive frequent CT imaging. Limited evidence exists in the urologic literature regarding radiation management strategies in these patients; however, lessons can be learned from the implementation of patient-specific care pathways in other disciplines. Multiple institutions have identified that creating patient-specific care plans, often automatically triggered through the electronic medical record, for frequent utilizers of health care services can reduce emergency room visits,[62] inpatient hospitalizations,[63] and reduce health care costs.[64] Similarly, care-plans could be created that direct physicians to order ultrasound or low-dose imaging studies for repeat stone formers to reduce radiation exposure in this high-risk patient population.

Another key point in reducing the radiation dose to recurrent stone formers is in the setting of monitoring known preexisting stones. Current AUA recommendations are to follow existing radiopaque stones with a combination of KUB and ultrasound, whereas radiolucent stones can be observed with LDCT.[23] Radiolucent stones also can be followed with ultrasound. In keeping with ALARA (as low as reasonably achievable) principles, follow-up imaging should be obtained only if the results, such as an increase in stone size, change in location, or absence of passage would alter patient management, such as affecting the decision to proceed with surgical intervention.

SUMMARY

Radiation exposure is an unfortunate and under-recognized consequence of nephrolithiasis management in the current era. A wide variety of evidence-based radiation mitigation techniques were herein described using current and widely available technology. It is thus incumbent on urologists to apply these techniques to reduce radiation exposure in this high-risk population.

REFERENCES

1. Radiation exposure from x-ray examinations. Web site. Available at: RadiologyInfo.org http://www.radiologyinfo.org/en/safety/index.cfm?pg=sfty_xray. Accessed August 26, 2010.

2. Authors on behalf of ICRP, Stewart FA, Akleyev AV, Hauer-Jensen M, et al. ICRP publication 118: ICRP statement on tissue reactions and early and late effects of radiation in normal tissues and organs, threshold doses for tissue reactions in a radiation protection context. Ann ICRP 2012; 41(1–2):1–322.

3. Pierce DA, Preston DL. Radiation-related cancer risks at low doses among atomic bomb survivors. Radiat Res 2000;154(2):178–86.

4. Cardis E, Vrijheid M, Blettner M, et al. The 15-country collaborative study of cancer risk among radiation workers in the nuclear industry: estimates of radiation-related cancer risks. Radiat Res 2007; 167:396–416.

5. Pearce M, Salotti J, Little M, et al. Radiation exposure from CT scans in childhood and subsequent risk of leukaemia and brain tumours: a retrospective cohort study. Lancet 2012;380(9840):499–505.

6. Mathews J, Forsythe A, Brady Z, et al. Cancer risk in 680 000 people exposed to computed tomography scans in childhood or adolescence: data linkage study of 11 million Australians. BMJ 2013;346:f2360.

7. Calabrese EJ, O'Connor MK. Estimating risk of low radiation doses - a critical review of the BEIR VII report and its use of the linear no-threshold (LNT) hypothesis. Radiat Res 2014;182(5):463–74.

8. National Research Council. Health risks from exposure to low levels of ionizing radiation: BEIR VII phase 2. Washington, DC: The National Academies Press; 2006. Available at: https://doi.org/10.17226/11340.

9. Ferrandino MN, Bagrodia A, Pierre SA, et al. Radiation exposure in the acute and short-term management of urolithiasis at 2 academic centers. J Urol 2009;181(2):668–72 [discussion: 673].

10. Fahmy NM, Elkoushy MA, Andonian S. Effective radiation exposure in evaluation and follow-up of patients with urolithiasis. Urology 2012;79(1):43–7.

11. Mancini JG, Raymundo EM, Lipkin M, et al. Factors affecting patient radiation exposure during percutaneous nephrolithotomy. J Urol 2010;184(6):2373–7.

12. Lipkin ME, Wang AJ, Toncheva G, et al. Determination of patient radiation dose during ureteroscopic treatment of urolithiasis using a validated model. J Urol 2012;187(3):920–4.

13. Sandilos P, Tsalafoutas I, Koutsokalis G, et al. Radiation doses to patients from extracorporeal shock wave lithotripsy. Health Phys 2006;90(6):583–7.

14. Yecies T, Semins M. Modeling the incidence of secondary malignancy and subsequent mortality related to ionizing radiation use in the evaluation and management of nephrolithiasis. MP50-19, presented at American Urological Association Annual Meeting. San Francisco, May 17–20, 2018.

15. Lukasiewicz A, Bhargavan-Chatfield M, Coombs L, et al. Radiation dose index of renal colic protocol CT studies in the United States: a report from the American College Radiology National Radiology Data Registry. Radiology 2014;271:445.

16. Westphalen AC, Hsia RY, Maselli JH, et al. Radiological imaging of patients with suspected urinary tract stones: national trends, diagnoses, and predictors. Acad Emerg Med 2011;18(7):699–707.

17. Kirpalani A, Khalili K, Lee S, et al. Renal colic: comparison of use and outcomes of unenhanced helical CT for emergency investigation in 1998 and 2002. Radiology 2005;236(2):554–8.

18. Astroza GM, Neisius A, Wang AJ, et al. Radiation exposure in the follow-up of patients with urolithiasis comparing digital tomosynthesis, non-contrast CT, standard KUB, and IVU. J Endourol 2013;27:1187.

19. Brisbane W, Bailey MR, Sorensen MD. An overview of kidney stone imaging techniques. Nat Rev Urol 2016;13(11):654–62.

20. Ray AA, Ghiculete D, Pace KT, et al. Limitations to ultrasound in the detection and measurement of urinary tract calculi. Urology 2010;76:295.

21. Viprakasit DP, Sawyer MD, Herrell SD, et al. Limitations of ultrasonography in the evaluation of urolithiasis: a correlation with computed tomography. J Endourol 2012;26:209.

22. Smith R, Aubin C, Bailitz J, et al. Ultrasonography versus computed tomography for suspected nephrolithiasis. N Engl J Med 2014;371(12):1100–10.

23. Fulgham PF, Assimos DG, Pearle MS. Clinical effectiveness protocols for imaging in the management of ureteral calculous disease: AUA technology assessment. J Urol 2013;189(4):1203–13.

24. Niemann T, Kollmann T, Bongartz G. Diagnostic performance of low-dose CT for the detection of urolithiasis: a meta-analysis AJR. Am J Roentgenol 2008; 191:396.

25. Pooler BD, Lubner MG, Kim DH, et al. Prospective trial of the detection of urolithiasis on ultralow dose (sub mSv) noncontrast computerized tomography: direct comparison against routine low dose reference standard. J Urol 2014;192:1433.

26. Poletti PA, Platon A, Rutschmann OT, et al. Low-dose versus standard-dose CT protocol in patients with

clinically suspected renal colic. AJR Am J Roentgenol 2007;188:927.

27. Weld LR, Nwoye UO, Knight RB, et al. Safety, minimization, and awareness radiation training reduces fluoroscopy time during unilateral ureteroscopy. Urology 2014;84(3):520–5.

28. Ngo TC, Macleod LC, Rosenstein DI, et al. Tracking intraoperative fluoroscopy utilization reduces radiation exposure during ureteroscopy. J Endourol 2011;25(5):763–7.

29. Chen TT, Wang C, Ferrandino MN, et al. Radiation exposure during the evaluation and management of nephrolithiasis. J Urol 2015;194(4):878–85.

30. Blair B, Huang G, Arnold D, et al. Reduced fluoroscopy protocol for percutaneous nephrostolithotomy: feasibility, outcomes and effects on fluoroscopy time. J Urol 2013;190(6):2112–6.

31. Mahesh M. Fluoroscopy: patient radiation exposure issues. Radiographics 2001;21(4):1033–45.

32. Canales BK, Sinclair L, Kang D. Changing default fluoroscopy equipment settings decreases entrance skin dose in patients. J Urol 2016;195(4 Pt 1):992–7.

33. Elkoushy MA, Shahrour W, Andonian S. Pulsed fluoroscopy in ureteroscopy and percutaneous nephrolithotomy. Urology 2012;79(6):1230–5.

34. Boland GW, Murphy B, Arellano R, et al. Dose reduction in gastrointestinal and genitourinary fluoroscopy: use of grid-controlled pulsed fluoroscopy. AJR Am J Roentgenol 2000;175(5):1453–7.

35. Olgin G, Smith D, Alsyouf M, et al. Ureteroscopy without fluoroscopy: a feasibility study and comparison with conventional ureteroscopy. J Endourol 2015;29(6):625–9.

36. Hein S, Schoenthaler M, Wilhelm K. Ultra-low radiation exposure during flexible ureteroscopy in nephrolithiasis patients - how far can we go? Urology 2017. https://doi.org/10.1016/j.urology.2017.06.016.

37. Deters LA, Dagrosa LM, Herrick BW, et al. Ultrasound guided ureteroscopy for the definitive management of ureteral stones: a randomized, controlled trial. J Urol 2014;192(6):1710–3.

38. Singh V, Purkait B, Sinha RJ. Prospective randomized comparison between fluoroscopy-guided ureteroscopy versus ureteroscopy with real-time ultrasonography for the management of ureteral stones. Urol Ann 2016;8(4):418–22.

39. Karlin G, Marino C, Badlani G, et al. Benefits of an ultrasound-guided SWL unit. Arch Esp Urol 1990; 43(5):579–81.

40. Goren MR, Goren V, Ozer C. Ultrasound-guided shockwave lithotripsy reduces radiation exposure and has better outcomes for pediatric cystine stones. Urol Int 2017;98(4):429–35.

41. Lantz A, O'Malley P, Ordon M, et al. Assessing radiation exposure during endoscopic-guided percutaneous nephrolithotomy. Can Urol Assoc J 2014; 8(9–10):347–51.

42. Lipkin ME, Mancini JG, Zilberman DE, et al. Reduced radiation exposure with the use of an air retrograde pyelogram during fluoroscopic access for percutaneous nephrolithotomy. J Endourol 2011;25(4):563–7.

43. Usawachintachit M, Masic S, Chang HC, et al. Ultrasound guidance to assist percutaneous nephrolithotomy reduces radiation exposure in obese patients. Urology 2016;98:32–8.

44. AChi T, Masic S, Li J, et al. Ultrasound guidance for renal tract access and dilation reduces radiation exposure during percutaneous nephrolithotomy. Adv Urol 2016;2016:3840697.

45. Khater N, Shen J, Arenas J, et al. Bench-top feasibility testing of a novel percutaneous renal access technique: the laser direct alignment radiation reduction technique (DARRT). J Endourol 2016; 30(11):1155–60.

46. Abourbih S, Keheila M, Yang P, et al. Comparison of ultrasound-guided, conventional fluoroscopic, and a novel laser direct alignment radiation reduction technique for percutaneous nephrolithotomy. Podium Presentation 21-04. Presented at the AUA annual meeting. Boston, MA, May 17–20, 2018.

47. Seung-ae H, Ki-Jeong K, Tae-Ahn J. Efficiency of lead aprons in blocking radiation – how protective are they? Heliyon 2016;2(5):e00117.

48. Bahreyni Toossi MT, Zare H, Bayani Sh, et al. Evaluation of the effectiveness of the lead aprons and thyroid shields worn by cardiologists in angiography departments of two main general hospitals in Mashhad, Iran. J Nucl Sci Tech 2008;45(sup 5):159–62.

49. Bugg CE Jr, El-Galley R, Kenney PJ. Follow-up functional radiographic studies are not mandatory for all patients after ureteroscopy. Urology 2002;59(5): 662–7.

50. Weizer AZ, Auge BK, Silverstein AD. Routine postoperative imaging is important after ureteroscopic stone manipulation. J Urol 2002;168(1):46–50.

51. Manger JP, Mendoza PJ, Babayan RK, et al. Use of renal ultrasound to detect hydronephrosis after ureteroscopy. J Endourol 2009;23(9):1399–402.

52. Sutherland TN, Pearle MS, Lotan Y, et al. How much is a kidney worth? Cost-effectiveness of routine imaging after ureteroscopy to prevent silent obstruction. J Urol 2013;189(6):2136–41.

53. Osman Y, El-Tabey N, Refai H, et al. Detection of residual stones after percutaneous nephrolithotomy: role of nonenhanced spiral computerized tomography. J Urol 2008;179:198–200.

54. Sountoulides P, Metaxa L, Cindolo L. Is computed tomography mandatory for the detection of residual stone fragments after percutaneous nephrolithotomy? J Endourol 2013;27(11):1341–8.

55. Ettinger B, Citron JT, Livermore B, et al. Chlorthalidone reduces calcium oxalate calculous recurrence

but magnesium hydroxide does not. J Urol 1988; 139:679–84.

56. Ettinger B, Pak CY, Citron JT, et al. Potassium-magnesium citrate is an effective prophylaxis against recurrent calcium oxalate nephrolithiasis. J Urol 1997;158:2069–73.

57. Ettinger B, Tang A, Citron JT, et al. Randomized trial of allopurinol in the prevention of calcium oxalate calculi. N Engl J Med 1986;315:1386–9.

58. Borghi L, Schianchi T, Meschi T, et al. Comparison of two diets for the prevention of recurrent stones in idiopathic hypercalciuria. N Engl J Med 2002;346:77–84.

59. Parks JH, Coe FL. Evidence for durable kidney stone prevention over several decades. BJU Int 2009;103(9):1238–46.

60. Skolarikos A, Straub M, Knoll T, et al. Metabolic evaluation and recurrence prevention for urinary stone patients: EAU guidelines. Eur Urol 2015;67(4): 750–63.

61. Pearle MS, Goldfarb DS, Assimos DG. Medical management of kidney stones: AUA guideline. J Urol 2014;192(2):316–24.

62. Olsen JC, Ogarek JL, Goldenberg EJ, et al. Impact of a chronic pain protocol on emergency department utilization. Acad Emerg Med 2016;23(4): 424–32.

63. Krishnamurti L, Smith-Packard B, Gupta A. Impact of individualized pain plan on the emergency management of children with sickle cell disease. Pediatr Blood Cancer 2014;61(10):1747–53.

64. Mercer T, Bae J, Kipnes J. The highest utilizers of care: individualized care plans to coordinate care, improve healthcare service utilization, and reduce costs at an academic tertiary care center. J Hosp Med 2015;10(7):419–24.

Innovations in Ultrasound Technology in the Management of Kidney Stones

Jessica C. Dai, MD[a],*, Michael R. Bailey, PhD, MS[a,b,c],
Mathew D. Sorensen, MD, MS, FACS[a,d],
Jonathan D. Harper, MD[a]

KEYWORDS

- Ultrasound • Nephrolithiasis • Twinkling • Acoustic shadow • Ultrasonic propulsion
- Burst wave lithotripsy

KEY POINTS

- Twinkling signal improves the detection of kidney stones on ultrasound examination.
- Posterior acoustic shadow measurements improve the accuracy of stone sizing on ultrasound examination.
- Ultrasonic propulsion allows noninvasive movement of stones in awake patients. This has many potential applications, including dislodging obstructing stones and mobilizing residual stone fragments after surgery.
- Burst wave lithotripsy is a promising ultrasound-based technology for transcutaneous stone fragmentation. Effectiveness and safety have been shown in animals.
- Ultrasonic propulsion and burst wave lithotripsy may be integrated and combined or used separately.

INTRODUCTION

The use of ultrasound (US) technology in the management of nephrolithiasis can be traced back to 1961, when Schlegel and colleagues[1] first published on amplitude (A)-mode sonography for the intraoperative localization of renal stones. Although US has continued to play a role in the management of stone disease, computed tomography (CT) scanning has become the imaging study of choice owing to its high sensitivity and specificity for stone detection.[2,3] Recent concern about the long-term effects of ionizing radiation exposure has given rise to renewed interest in US technology, which is already the preferred imaging study for children and pregnant patients with suspected nephrolithiasis.[2] Some even have suggested that US examination should be the initial imaging modality for patients presenting with acute renal colic.[4]

Continued refinement of US technology has expanded its use in diagnosis and follow-up, percutaneous access, minimally invasive renal surgery, and shockwave lithotripsy (SWL).[5] Recent research in diagnostic US technology for stone detection and sizing may further enhance its role

Disclosure Statement: Dr M.R. Bailey, and Dr M.D. Sorensen have equity in and consult for SonoMotion, Inc. Drs J.C. Dai and J.D. Harper have nothing to disclose.

[a] Department of Urology, University of Washington School of Medicine, University of Washington, 1959 Northeast Pacific Street, Box 356510, Seattle, WA 98195, USA; [b] Center for Industrial and Medical Ultrasound, University of Washington, 1014 NorthEast 40th Street, Seattle, WA 98105, USA; [c] Department of Mechanical Engineering, University of Washington, Stevens Way, Box 352600, Seattle, WA 98195, USA; [d] Puget Sound Veterans Affairs Hospital, 1660 S. Columbian Way, Seattle, WA 98108, USA

* Corresponding author.
E-mail address: jcdai@uw.edu

in the management of stone disease. US technology is also being applied to noninvasively move and break up kidney stones. Such innovative developments have the potential to generate a future paradigm shift in the management of kidney stones.

DEVELOPMENTS IN ULTRASOUND-BASED STONE IMAGING

Compared with CT scans, US examination has a low sensitivity and limited specificity for stone detection (24%–70% and 88%–94.4%, respectively).[6–8] Moreover, stone sizing on US imaging has poor accuracy, with average overestimation of 3.3 mm for stones 5 mm or smaller.[9] Because stone size has implications on the likelihood of spontaneous passage as well as optimal surgical treatment options, clinical decision making is predicated on this information. Management decisions made on US stone size alone result in miscounseling in up to 22% of cases.[10] Adequate stone detection and sizing accuracy therefore remain 2 of the primary challenges to more widespread use of US imaging.

Improving Stone Detection

Renal stones have been traditionally identified on grayscale brightness (B)-mode US imaging as echogenic foci that may be accompanied by a posterior acoustic shadow. However, some stones do not have this classic appearance, and elude detection. Twinkling artifact was first described in 1996 and refers to a rapidly changing, heterogeneous distribution of colors around a stone on color-flow Doppler mode (**Fig. 1**).[11] Twinkling is present for 43% to 96% of stones on US examination, and has been proposed as a useful adjunct for stone detection.[12–14] This artifact may highlight the presence of a stone not immediately evident on B-mode imaging.

The prevailing explanation for twinkling is that small bubbles trapped in stone surface crevices oscillate and generate random backscatter when struck by incident Doppler pulses. These signals are interpreted and displayed as noise. Lu and colleagues[15] provided evidence for this theory by demonstrating that twinkling could be extinguished with hyperbaric pressures and reinstated with reduced static pressure. Wetting stones with ethanol also decreased twinkling, presumably by influencing surface tension and bubble stabilization on the stone surface. Simon and colleagues[16] captured the presence of microbubbles by exposing stones to lithotripter pulses and varying static pressures. Stones demonstrated reproducible twinkling signals, and bubble activity was directly visualized on the stone with lithotripter pulses.

Preclinical studies have assessed the potential usefulness of twinkling for stone detection. In phantom and sheep kidneys, twinkling was found to have greater contrast (with respect to background) than acoustic shadowing, suggesting that this may be more readily identifiable on US examination.[17] In human studies, 85% of nonshadowing stones twinkled.[18] Moreover, twinkling contrast was 37 times greater than the hyperechoic stone signal on grayscale US images.[19] Although the strength of the twinkling signal varies by stone composition, in vitro studies suggest that this may be more related to the stone's structure.[20,21] Twinkling strength may also be related to the location of the focal zone during an ultrasound examination, likely because higher pressures at the focal zone cause greater microbubble oscillation.[18]

Clinical studies have evaluated the effect of twinkling on stone detection. Among patients with acute renal colic, twinkling signal demonstrated a sensitivity of 83% and a positive predictive value of 94%, compared with sensitivity of 80% and positive predictive value of 65% for grayscale sonography alone. Considered together, detection sensitivity increased to 88% and the positive predictive value to 96%.[22] In a clinic-based study of patients with CT scan-confirmed stones, twinkling alone had higher specificity than the hyperechoic stone signal on B-mode imaging (74% vs 48%).[12] In the acute setting, twinkling was seen in 97.1% of patients with renal colic and nephrolithiasis, with a sensitivity of 97.2% and specificity of 99%.[13]

Others have found that twinkling is less reliable among patients without known nephrolithiasis. In this population, twinkling alone was 78% sensitive and 40% specific for stones. When additional US features were considered (echogenic focus, posterior acoustic shadow, or both), sensitivity decreased to as low as 31%, but specificity increased to as high as 95%.[14] Thus, twinkling may be one of several US features to indicate stone presence on US imaging, but may be most useful among patients with a history of nephrolithiasis.

Twinkling has also been correlated with the duration of renal colic symptoms, pain, and difficulty with guidewire passage at time of endoscopic intervention.[23] Although this finding may have potential clinical implications by providing prognostic information at the time of stone diagnosis, further research validating these findings is warranted. Current understanding of the twinkling signal remains limited by single-institution studies

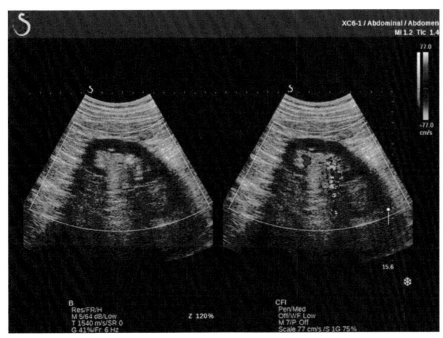

Fig. 1. Example of stone twinkling (*arrow*). The same stone is imaged on grayscale sonography alone (*left*) and on color flow Doppler (*right*). The flickering mosaic of color on color flow Doppler is called twinkling. Normal blood flow is also detected by Doppler (*solid red*) and can be readily distinguished from twinkling.

and variability in imaging techniques. Optimization and standardization of twinkling, which was once perceived an artifact, might provide greater usefulness in improving the identification of renal stones.

Optimizing Stone Sizing Accuracy

Improving stone sizing on US imaging has been another area of active research. The degree and wide variability of size overestimation limits the use of US imaging for clinical decision making, particularly in the acute setting where it has been promoted as first-line imaging modality for suspected nephrolithiasis.[4,24,25] Techniques to optimize the accuracy of stone sizing are therefore paramount.

Several US system-specific factors have been found to influence stone sizing. The degree of size overestimation seems to be correlated with greater stone depth and gain.[26] At increasing depths beyond the focus, US rays diverge, decreasing spatial resolution. Placing the focus at the stone therefore minimizes beam spread and maximizes stone resolution. In vitro, high gain settings increased measured stone size by 18%.[26] High gain can saturate the US image, decrease stone contrast and detectability, and make the identification of stone edges more difficult. The greatest size overestimation is seen with spatial compounding, because the averaging of multiple images generates a smoother overall image but also blurs the stone and shadow

borders. In vitro, harmonic imaging has been found to minimize stone size overestimation.[27]

The posterior acoustic shadow has also been suggested as an adjunct to improve the accuracy of stone sizing (**Fig. 2**). In stone phantoms, measuring shadow width decreased average

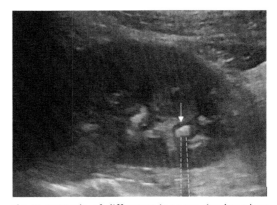

Fig. 2. Example of difference in stone size based on measurement of the echogenic stone signal and the posterior acoustic shadow width. Dashed guide-lines indicate the borders of the stone shadow. This stone (*arrow*) measured 5 mm on computed tomography, 9.7 mm on ultrasound examination, and 6.8 ± 3 mm by shadow measurement among 26 novice reviewers. (*From* Dai JC, Dunmire B, Liu Z, et al. Measurement of Posterior Acoustic Shadow is a Learnable Skill for Inexperienced Users to Improve Accuracy of Stone Sizing." J Endourol. 2018;32(11):1033–38; with permission.)

overestimation error to 0.5 mm, regardless of imaging depth or modality. Shadow size was significantly more accurate than measured stone size on US images and reduced misclassification of stone size in clinically relevant size categories (>5 mm vs ≤5 mm) from 50% to 15%. Using this technique, 78% of stones had a less than 1 mm size error. Notably, 53% of stones less than 5 mm did not demonstrate a shadow, suggesting that the absence of a shadow may indicate a small stone.[27]

Studies in human subjects support these findings. On a research US system, 55% of imaged stones demonstrated a shadow width within 1 mm of corresponding CT size. Average shadow size overestimation was 1.1 mm for stones 10 mm or smaller.[28] Evaluation of clinical US images from a commercial system demonstrated that shadow measurements resulted in less than 1 mm sizing error for 42% of stones, with respect to CT.[29] Additionally, up to 83% of nonshadowing stones measured less than 5 mm on CT, further suggesting that nonvisualization of a shadow on US imaging indicates a smaller stone.[29] Even among pediatric patients, shadow sizes were significantly smaller than reported US stone sizes (mean difference, 2.9 mm; P<.001) and resulted in downsizing of 68% of stones by at least 1 size category (P<.001).[30] The availability of such information prospectively may potentially influence provider decisions regarding patient management.

Because the shadow sizing technique requires no additional hardware or software modification, it was thought to be easily adoptable into clinical practice. A single-institution study examined the uptake of this technique among clinicians. Providers familiar but inexperienced with the training technique demonstrated that shadow measurements on clinical US images were no more accurate than reported US sizes (with respect to CT scans) at initial adoption. However, after a brief

training module, there was significant improvement in overestimation bias and more stones with 1 mm concordance between shadow and CT size. No improvements were seen with repeated practice alone.[31] Techniques reviewed in the training module included careful identification of the shadow, evaluation for confounding artifacts, tracing the entire shadow path using guidelines to project the shadow back to the stone, and measuring the shadow perpendicular to the direction of the US beam.[31]

Future Directions in Stone Imaging

The development of stone-specific algorithms to optimize stone imaging is an area of active research. One such research system, coined S-mode, maximizes stone contrast and highlights the posterior acoustic shadow by avoiding speckle reduction and spatial compounding.[32] It uses a higher frequency transducer and higher scanning line density to improve resolution. Side-by-side imaging can be performed with grayscale and color flow Doppler modes (**Fig. 3**). A custom Doppler mode uses lower frequency to enhance the twinkling signal and suppress blood flow signal. In human subjects, sensitivity for stones was 84%, with 44% of stone sizes demonstrating 1 mm concordance with corresponding CT measurements.[28] Additional refinement of this system may further enhance stone detection capabilities on US imaging.[19]

Other investigators have explored advanced beamforming techniques, such as plane wave synthetic focusing, short-lag spatial coherence imaging, mid-lag spatial coherence imaging with incoherent compounding, and aperture domain model image reconstruction. When Tierney and colleagues[33] compared stone size and contrast on each mode to traditional B-mode imaging in vitro, stone sizing error was minimized with plane wave synthetic focusing (0.3 ± 2.9 mm vs

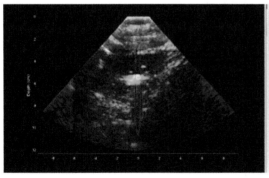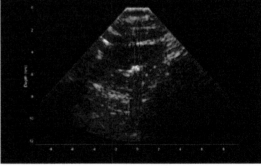

Fig. 3. Example of stone imaging output platform on a customized S-mode imager. Color flow Doppler mode is visualized on the left, with twinkling signal displayed in green. Simultaneous grayscale imaging is shown on the right for the same stone. The *red oval* represents a focal zone for ultrasonic propulsion therapy that can be delivered using the same probe, discussed elsewhere in this article.

1.2 ± 1.1 mm). Further work to compare and integrate these techniques into existing imaging platforms remains.

Three-dimensional (3D) US imaging is another area of emerging research, because it provides unique information about stone morphology. Three-dimensional US imaging with surface rendering of stones has been shown to be feasible and has been used in pregnant patients.[34] A transrectal 3D US approach has been proposed to evaluate the success of SWL for distal ureteral stones.[35,36] This technology may also offer radiation-free opportunities for improved percutaneous stone treatment planning and enhanced trainee and patient learning.[37–39] Reconstruction of the pelvicalyceal system from 3D US images has been shown to be feasible and anatomically comparable to casts of the collecting system.[40] This technique may ultimately help to optimize stone treatment outcomes.

MOVEMENT OF STONES WITH ULTRASOUND ENERGY

Noninvasive movement of kidney stones and stone fragments has generated significant interest over the past decade. Specifically, the conundrum of how to clear residual fragments after stone treatment has spurred much research. Inversion therapy, mechanical percussion, and diuresis have been shown to help, but are nonspecific and can be labor intensive.[41,42] The "Lithecbole," a novel mechanical percussion device, has also been shown to significantly improve stone-free rates and expedite passage of stone fragments following SWL,[43,44] as well as symptomatic distal ureteral stones.[45]

Recent application of US technology to this space has led to novel methods of noninvasive stone manipulation. The movement of kidney stones using US energy has been termed "ultrasonic propulsion." This innovative technology is currently in clinical trials under an investigational device exemption from the Food and Drug Administration.

Ultrasonic Propulsion: Development and Evolution

Ultrasonic propulsion was first described in 2010 by Shah and colleagues[46] at the University of Washington. This technology is based on the acoustic radiation force resulting from the transfer of acoustic wave momentum to a visualized stone. In the initial prototype, an annular array of elements was incorporated into a handheld probe, yielding a focused acoustic beam. Combined with a coaxial imaging probe, this could target stones visualized on US for real-time pushing.[46]

Since the initial feasibility study, several refinements have been made to improve device efficacy. The evolution of this technology and treatment details are summarized in **Table 1**. After the original research prototype in 2010, a second-generation probe was developed in 2013, which integrated imaging and treatment capabilities into a single commercial US probe. This system used lower peak pressures and a shorter 1-s burst of push pulses.[47] The device was modified again in 2014 to improve stone targeting by integrating a touchscreen to both visualize stone targets and activate push pulses. Push burst duration was also decreased to limit the amount of ineffective, off-target energy delivered to the treatment focus after the stone moves out of the focal field.[48,49]

The first human clinical study was performed in 2016. Ultrasonic propulsion was applied to 13 awake subjects in the clinic and 2 anesthetized subjects at the time of endoscopic stone treatment. Of the awake subjects, 6 had residual fragments after lithotripsy less than 5 mm, 3 had less than 5 mm de novo stones, and 4 had 5 mm or greater de novo stones. Stone compositions included calcium oxalate monohydrate (COM), calcium oxalate dihydrate, apatite, and brushite. Stone motion was achieved at 50 and 90 V power settings. Four of 6 patients passed postlithotripsy fragments. Notably, there was symptomatic pain relief in 1 subject with a 10-mm ureteropelvic junction stone. Ultrasonic propulsion provided additional diagnostic information in 4 patients by dispersing a collection of small fragments thought to be a larger stone on pretreatment imaging.

Safety

Multiple safety studies of ultrasonic propulsion in porcine models have demonstrated no histologic evidence of injury to the kidney.[47,48,50] Preclinical animal studies demonstrated that even at maximal treatment settings of 90 V, no histologic injury was induced with transcutaneous or direct organ treatment. Survival studies in pigs demonstrated no adverse events or deaths at moderate or high dose treatment settings, with normal hematologic and urinary parameters at time of necropsy after 1 week.[48]

Although treatment-level settings have not been shown to cause tissue injury, power settings in excess of typical treatment parameters can still induce tissue injury. Thermal coagulation injury was caused in 6 of 7 porcine kidneys treated at excessive exposures (1900 W/cm^2), with a maximal injury size of 1 cm. In contrast, treatment-level exposure was only 325 W/cm^2.[50] Connors and colleagues[51] further demonstrated that at high power settings (240 W), no renal injury occurred with

Table 1
Evolution of ultrasonic propulsion technology and effectiveness over time, from initial feasibility studies to the first human clinical study

Publication, Year	Probe	Treatment Parameters	Study Type	Experimental Setup	Outcomes
Shah et al,[46] 2010	*Therapy:* 6-cm annular probe, 8 elements, 2 MHz, 4.5–8.5 cm focal depth *Imaging:* Philips 5000 HDI imaging system, P4-2 transducer	Five to 40 W; 2–5 s pulse duration; 50% duty cycle	In vitro	Glass beads (2.5–4 mm) and human COM, COD, or CaP stones (3–8 mm) implanted in kidney phantom	Stones or beads repositioned from lower pole to renal pelvis.
Shah et al,[50] 2012	*Therapy:* 6 cm annular probe, 8 elements, 2 MHz, 4.5–8.5 cm focal depth *Imaging:* Philips 5000 HDI imaging system, P4-2 transducer	Average treatment exposure of 325 W/cm^2; 1–4 s pulse duration; 50% duty cycle	Animal model	Glass/metal beads (3–5 mm) and human cystine, COM, or CaP stones (1–8 mm) implanted endoscopically or percutaneously into lower or interpolar calyces of 6 anesthetized pigs	Stones or beads repositioned from mid or lower pole calyces to renal pelvis and UPJ in all 6 pigs within 10 min.
Harper et al,[47] 2013	Integrated imaging and therapy probe: HDI ATL C5-2 or Philips P4-2; Verasonics imaging system	Push burst duration of 0–1 s (250 pulses of 0.1 ms duration per 1 s burst); 3% duty cycle	Animal model	There were 26 COM stones or beads (2–8 mm) endoscopically implanted in 12 kidneys (interpolar or lower pole calyces) of 8 anesthetized pigs	Seventeen stones (65%) successfully relocated from calyx to renal pelvis, UPJ, or ureter; 2 moved out of calyx but did not reach renal pelvis; 7 stones moved within calyx. Average displacement time 14.2 ± 7.9 min using a mean of 23 ± 16 push bursts. Average displacement 5.6 ± 2.7 linear cm.

Harper et al,[48] 2014	HDI ATL C5-2 probe; Verasonics imaging system; integrated touchscreen monitor	Fifty or 90 V settings; 50 millisecond push burst duration; 73% duty cycle	Animal model	1. Six COM stones (2–5 mm) endoscopically implanted into right lower pole calyces of 5 anesthetized pigs 2. De novo stones in 3 pigs in a diet-induced hyperoxaluria model; 2 < 3 mm stones identified in 6 renal units	1. Six stones (100%) successfully repositioned from lower pole to UPJ or proximal ureter. Average displacement time 14 ± 8 min using a mean of 13 ± 6 bursts. 2. Two stones (100%) repositioned to collecting system. Average displacement time 20 ± 13 min using a mean 10 ± 8 push bursts.
Harper et al,[53] 2016	HDI ATL C5-2 probe, Verasonics imaging system	Fifty or 90 V settings; 50 millisecond push duration; 73% duty cycle; maximum of 40 pushes	Human subjects	1. Six patients with <5 mm residual fragments following lithotripsy 2. Three patients with <5 mm de novo stones 3. Four patients with ≥5 mm de novo stones 4. Two patients with ≥5 mm de novo stones undergoing ureteroscopy	1. Four of 6 patients passed stone fragments; 47% moved <3 mm and 18% moved ≥3 mm. Mean of 39 push bursts. 2. No stones passed; 25% moved <3 mm. Mean of 39 push bursts. 3. 19% moved <3 mm. Mean of 23 push bursts. 4. 30% moved <3 mm, 12% moved ≥3 mm. Mean of 28 push bursts.

Abbreviations: CaP, calcium phosphate; COD, calcium oxalate dihydrate; COM, calcium oxalate monohydrate; UPJ, ureteropelvic junction.

transcutaneous treatment, but direct treatment of the kidney resulted in hemorrhagic injury similar to that of SWL; thermal coagulation injury occurred at lower power treatments. The resulting area of injury was still less than one-third that caused by SWL (0.46% vs 1.56% of the total renal volume).

Further work to determine more precise tissue injury thresholds was conducted by Wang and colleagues,[52] who demonstrated that a spatial peak intensity of 16,620 W/cm^2 was needed to cause significant kidney injury with direct treatment. In comparison, the maximum spatial peak intensity generated during transcutaneous treatment in animal models was nearly 7 times lower. As this work transitioned to human trials, the spatial peak intensity remained more than 330 times lower than this injury threshold.[49,53]

In the first human clinical study, none of the 13 awake subjects reported any sensation with a 50 V push burst. All reported warming of the skin at the transducer interface at 90 V, and 2 subjects reported a brief internal sensation that was not considered painful. There were no unanticipated or serious adverse events.[53]

Clinical Use

Ultrasonic propulsion has many potential clinical applications. These include facilitating passage of postlithotripsy fragments, repositioning stones preoperatively or intraoperatively, dislodging obstructing stones, and providing endpoint detection for SWL or other transcutaneous lithotripsy modalities. Combined with treatments such as diuresis, inversion therapy, or mechanical percussion, this technology may optimize residual stone passage after stone treatment, particularly for lower pole stones.[42]

Ultrasonic propulsion is envisioned as part of a clinic-based, noninvasive approach to kidney stone management. However, provider education might be necessary to facilitate its adoption among urologists. Hsi and colleagues[54] developed and piloted a training curriculum on the fundamentals of renal US and ultrasonic propulsion among 10 board-certified urologists. After completing the curriculum, all participants successfully moved lower pole stones within a phantom model, and 90% successfully repositioned stones into the renal pelvis with a mean of 15.7 pushes and a mean time of 4.5 minutes.

Optimization and Future Work

To better optimize clearance of stone fragments, further modifications to the ultrasonic propulsion system have been made since the first human trial. A custom probe with an integrated imaging transducer and water-circulating coupling head was developed, with less probe heating (**Fig. 4**). This incorporated a longer focal beam and burst duration (3 seconds vs 50 milliseconds). At 4.5 and 9.5 cm depths, 1 to 2 mm fragments, 3 to 4 mm fragments, and a 4 × 7-mm stone were successfully expelled out of a phantom calyx.[55] In a 7-day porcine survival study, there were no adverse clinical, laboratory, or histologic findings with treatments. Successful movement of larger 8 to 12 mm stones of varying compositions (COM, ammonium acid urate, calcium phosphate, and struvite) out of a phantom calyx model was achieved in 95% of cases.[56]

Recent clinical studies using the custom probe were performed during ureteroscopic stone treatment. Ultrasonic propulsion treatment was applied

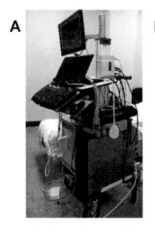 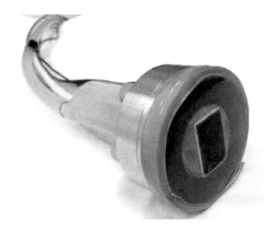

Fig. 4. The current ultrasonic propulsion system (*A*) and custom therapy probe (*B*). The annular therapy probe is visible in silver and the coaxial imaging probe is seen in red. A water-circulating coupling head minimizes overheating of the device.

simultaneously with direct endoscopic visualization of stone movement (**Fig. 5**). Stone targets ranged in size from dust to 7 mm. A blinded review of endoscopic videos demonstrated target movement greater than 3 mm in 14 of 15 kidneys. Ultrasonic propulsion obviated the need for stone basketing in 2 cases by repositioning stones to a more favorable intrarenal location. There were no serious or unanticipated adverse events.[57] A randomized, clinic-based trial using ultrasonic propulsion to facilitate clearance of residual fragments and an emergency department-based trial of ultrasonic propulsion to move obstructing ureteral stones are ongoing at the University of Washington.

Acoustic tractor beam technology is yet another emerging area of research in US-based stone movement. This technology may enable directed capture and navigation of a stone through the calyceal system.[58] In recent years, tractor beam technology has been shown to have the capability to move targets greater than 1 cm in size.[59] Integration with current ultrasonic propulsion technology may allow for more directed, noninvasive stone movements. However, its potential application in this space remains to be explored.

ULTRASONIC STONE FRAGMENTATION: BURST WAVE LITHOTRIPSY

SWL has greatly evolved since the development of the Dornier HM1 in 1980. A better understanding of the role of stone density, skin-to-stone distance, coupling, shockwave delivery rate, and power ramping have influenced treatment delivery.[60,61] Further technological developments such as wider focal zones and tandem or dual head lithotripters have also been suggested to improve treatment success. However, with continued advances in ureteroscopic technology, the role of SWL has been questioned.[62] Burst wave lithotripsy (BWL) is an emerging, US-based approach to extracorporeal lithotripsy that holds promise as a novel option for noninvasive stone treatment.

Proof of Concept

Current SWL machines typically use single-cycle pulses at a slow rate (≤ 2 Hz) and high peak pressures (30–100 MPa). In contrast, BWL uses short bursts of focused, sinusoidal US pulses. These are hypothesized to minimize the accumulation of cavitation bubbles that shield acoustic wave propagation to the stone, resulting in more effective stone comminution.[63] BWL is administered transcutaneously under US guidance using a hand-held probe at higher rates (<200 Hz) and lower peak pressures (<12 MPa) than SWL. Lower pressures are hypothesized to make BWL safer and more tolerable to awake patients.

Initial in vitro experiments by Maxwell and colleagues[63] demonstrated the potential of this technology. Using a 170, 285, or 800 KHz transducer, fragmentation of artificial Begostones occurred at peak pressures of greater than 2.3 MPa. At peak pressures of 6.5 MPa, stones of varying compositions were successfully comminuted to less than 4 mm fragments. Uric acid stones were treated most rapidly (0.17–1.40 minutes), followed by struvite (0.07–2.02 minutes), COM (8.0–18.1 minutes), and cystine stones (10.3–21.3 minutes). Finer fragments were generated by higher frequency treatment.

The efficacy of BWL has also been studied in animal models. Five COM stones 5 to 7 mm in size were surgically implanted into 3 pig kidneys and treated transcutaneously for 30 minutes with a 350 kHz transducer. Peak negative focal pressures were 6.5 to 7.0 MPa. Eighty-two percent of treated stone mass was fragmented to less than 2 mm. Three of 5 stones were entirely comminuted, and in all cases 58% or more of the stone was fragmented. **Fig. 6** shows an example of

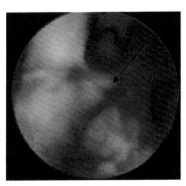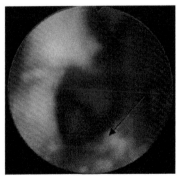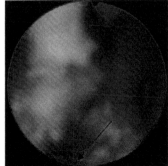

Fig. 5. Endoscopic visualization of a 5-mm stone being repositioned using ultrasonic propulsion (panels progress in time from left to right). *Arrows* indicate the direction of stone movement. The stone traveled about 1 cm in less than 1 second.

treatment effect. Gross examination of treated kidneys revealed only minor petechial injury to the urothelium where the stone was targeted, with no effects on the overlying skin or parenchyma.[64]

Safety

Tissue injury can occur with BWL, and this has been demonstrated on real-time US imaging. Using 170 kHz and 335 kHz transducers, May and colleagues[65] treated 10 porcine kidneys at exposures of 5.8 to 8.1 MPa. Cavitation during treatment was observed as echogenicity on US imaging. Treatment was deliberately continued to purposefully induce injury, which was seen in 10 of 21 treated sites. No injury greater than 0.1% of renal volume was seen with the 335 kHz transducer, but larger areas of injury less than 5.2% of renal volume were generated with the 170 kHz transducer. Histologic analysis demonstrated intraparenchymal hemorrhage, focal tubular injury and focal necrosis, similar to SWL-related injury.[66] Cavitation on US imaging predicted BWL-related renal injury with 100% sensitivity and specificity.[65] Thus, US imaging feedback may allow for the adjustment of treatment parameters in real time to avoid renal injury during BWL treatment.

Preliminary porcine studies provide further evidence for the safety of this technology under treatment conditions. Six pigs were treated at exposures of 7 MPa for 30 minutes. There were 4 untreated controls and histopathologic evaluation of kidneys was performed 1 week later. There were no chemistry abnormalities and no gross or histologic findings of injury.[67] These results have been submitted to the Food and Drug Administration for approval for an investigational clinical trial.

Future Directions

Recent in vitro studies have examined the combined efficacy of ultrasonic propulsion and BWL

for stone fragmentation. Dispersion of comminuted stone fragments from the target with ultrasonic propulsion was hypothesized to increase BWL efficiency. When both technologies were used together, fragmentation was increased for artificial crystalline calcite stones, Begostones, and human COM stones. The most pronounced effect was noted when push pulses were interweaved with BWL pulses.[68] This study suggests that the integration of these 2 technologies during a single treatment may optimize the usefulness of both.

Remaining challenges include optimizing targeting in vivo, determining treatment end points, and defining optimal treatment parameters. Moreover, the ideal stone and patient characteristics for this technology are unknown. Ultimately, treatment parameters may be potentially adjusted in real time and guided by advanced imaging feedback to tailor treatment sessions to the individual patient. Future studies assessing the efficacy and safety of this therapeutic technology in humans remain to be completed.

SUMMARY

US has significantly evolved as a diagnostic and therapeutic modality for kidney stones since over the past 60 years. Identification and optimization of sonographic features such as the twinkling signal and the posterior acoustic shadow may help improve stone detection and sizing. Novel beamforming techniques and 3D US are future areas for research. Novel therapeutic US technologies have also been developed. Ultrasonic propulsion has been shown to be safe and feasible in human subjects, and its clinical impact is beginning to be explored. BWL development is ongoing and progressing toward human trials. For both, there remain many unknowns regarding the optimal candidates, treatment parameters, and ultimate adoption of into clinical practice. As future research continues, such innovations in US technology may open up new avenues for stone management and treatment.

ACKNOWLEDGMENTS

The authors gratefully acknowledge funding support from the National Institutes of Health, National Institute of Diabetes and Digestive and Kidney Diseases (NIDDK), through grant P01 DK043881. This material is the result of work supported by resources from the Veterans Affairs Puget Sound Health Care System, Seattle, Washington. The authors thank their colleagues at the Center for Industrial and Medical Ultrasound, Department of Urology at the University of

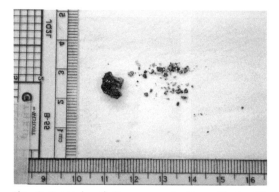

Fig. 6. Example of stone comminution effect with burst wave lithotripsy on a calcium oxalate monohydrate stone.

Washington, and within NIH Program Project DK043881 for their help in reviewing the article.

REFERENCES

1. Schlegel J, Diggdon P, Cuellar J. The use of ultrasound for localizing renal calculi. J Urol 1961;(86):367–9.

2. Fulgham PF, Assimos DG, Pearle MS, et al. Clinical effectiveness protocols for imaging in the management of ureteral calculous disease: AUA technology assessment. J Urol 2013;189(4):1203–13.

3. Fwu CW, Eggers PW, Kimmel PL, et al. Emergency department visits, use of imaging, and drugs for urolithiasis have increased in the United States. Kidney Int 2013. https://doi.org/10.1038/ki.2012.419.

4. Choosing Wisely. American College of Emergency Physicians. 2015. Available at: http://www.choosingwisely.org/wp-content/uploads/2015/02/ACEP-Choosing-Wisely-List.pdf. Accessed April 13, 2018.

5. Tzou DT, Usawachintachit M, Taguchi K, et al. Ultrasound use in urinary stones: adapting old technology for a modern-day disease. J Endourol 2017. https://doi.org/10.1089/end.2016.0584.

6. Fowler K a B, Locken JA, Duchesne JH, et al. US for detecting renal calculi with nonenhanced CT as a reference standard. Radiology 2002;222(1):109–13.

7. Ray AA, Ghiculete D, Pace KT, et al. Limitations to ultrasound in the detection and measurement of urinary tract calculi. Urology 2010;76(2):295–300.

8. Kanno T, Kubota M, Sakamoto H, et al. The efficacy of ultrasonography for the detection of renal stone. Urology 2014;84(2):285–8.

9. Sternberg KM, Eisner B, Larson T, et al. Ultrasonography significantly overestimates stone size when compared to low-dose, noncontrast computed tomography. Urology 2016;95:67–71.

10. Ganesan V, De S, Greene D, et al. Accuracy of ultrasonography for renal stone detection and size determination: is it good enough for management decisions? BJU Int 2017;119(3):464–9.

11. Rahmouni A, Bargoin R, Herment A, et al. Color Doppler twinkling artifact in hyperechoic regions. Radiology 1996. https://doi.org/10.1148/radiology.199.1.8633158.

12. Sorensen MD, Harper JD, Hsi RS, et al. B-mode ultrasound versus color doppler twinkling artifact in detecting kidney stones. J Endourol 2013;27(2):149–53.

13. Abdel-Gawad M, Kadasne RD, Elsobky E, et al. A prospective comparative study of color doppler ultrasound with twinkling and noncontrast computerized tomography for the evaluation of acute renal colic. J Urol 2016;196(3):757–62.

14. Masch WR, Cohan RH, Ellis JH, et al. Clinical effectiveness of prospectively reported sonographic twinkling artifact for the diagnosis of renal calculus in patients without known urolithiasis. Am J Roentgenol 2016. https://doi.org/10.2214/AJR.15.14998.

15. Lu W, Sapozhnikov OA, Bailey MR, et al. Evidence for trapped surface bubbles as the cause for the twinkling artifact in ultrasound imaging. Ultrasound Med Biol 2013;39(6):1026–38.

16. Simon JC, Sapozhnikov OA, Kreider W, et al. The role of trapped bubbles in kidney stone detection with the color Doppler ultrasound twinkling artifact. Phys Med Biol 2018;63(2):25011.

17. Shabana W, Bude RO, Rubin JM. Comparison between color Doppler twinkling artifact and acoustic shadowing for renal calculus detection: an in vitro study. Ultrasound Med Biol 2009;35(2):339–50.

18. Lee JY, Kim SH, Cho JY, et al. Color and power doppler twinkling artifacts from urinary stones: clinical observations and phantom studies. Am J Roentgenol 2001. https://doi.org/10.2214/ajr.176.6.1761441.

19. Cunitz BW, Harper JD, Sorensen MD, et al. Quantification of renal stone contrast with ultrasound in human subjects. J Endourol 2017. https://doi.org/10.1089/end.2017.0404.

20. Chelfouh N, Grenier N, Higueret D, et al. Characterization of urinary calculi: in vitro study of "twinkling artifact" revealed by color-flow sonography. Am J Roentgenol 1998. https://doi.org/10.2214/ajr.171.4.9762996.

21. Shang M, Sun X, Liu Q, et al. Quantitative evaluation of the effects of urinary stone composition and size on color doppler twinkling artifact: a phantom study. J Ultrasound Med 2017. https://doi.org/10.7863/ultra.16.01039.

22. Kielar AZ, Shabana W, Vakili M, et al. Prospective evaluation of Doppler sonography to detect the twinkling artifact versus unenhanced computed tomography for identifying urinary tract calculi. J Ultrasound Med 2012;31(10):1619–25.

23. Sharma G, Sharma A. Clinical implications and applications of the twinkling sign in ureteral calculus: a preliminary study. J Urol 2013. https://doi.org/10.1016/j.juro.2012.11.176.

24. Smith-Bindman R, Aubin C, Bailitz J, et al. Ultrasonography vs computed tomography for suspected nephrolithiasis. N Engl J Med 2014;371(12):1100–10.

25. Sternberg KM, Littenberg B. Trends in imaging use for the evaluation and follow-up of kidney stone disease: a single center experience. J Urol 2017; 198(2):383–8.

26. Dunmire B, Lee FC, Hsi RS, et al. Tools to improve the accuracy of kidney stone sizing with ultrasound. J Endourol 2015;29(2):147–52.

27. Dunmire B, Harper JD, Cunitz BW, et al. Use of the acoustic shadow width to determine kidney stone size with ultrasound. J Urol 2016;195(1):171–6.

28. May P, Haider Y, Dunmire B, et al. Stone-mode ultrasound for determining renal stone size. J Endo 2016; 30(9):958–62.

29. Dai JC, Dunmire B, Sternberg KM, et al. Retrospective comparison of measured stone size and posterior acoustic shadow width in clinical ultrasound images. World J Urol 2017. https://doi.org/10.1007/s00345-017-2156-8.

30. Dai JC, Dunmire B, Chen T, et al. Clinical outcomes in pediatric patients with ureteral stones are correlated with the posterior acoustic shadow measurement on ultrasound: a pilot study. Societies for Pediatric Urology, Pediatric Urology Fall Congress. Atlanta(GA), September 14, 2018.

31. Dai JC, Dunmire B, Liu Z, et al. Measurement of Posterior Acoustic Shadow is a Learnable Skill for Inexperienced Users to Improve Accuracy of Stone Sizing. J Endourol 2018;32(11):1033–8.

32. Cunitz B, Dunmire B, Paun M, et al. Improved detection of kidney stones using an optimized Doppler imaging sequence. IEEE Int Ultrason Symp 2014. https://doi.org/10.1109/ULTSYM.2014.0112.

33. Tierney JE, Schlunk SG, Jones R, et al. In vitro feasibility of next generation non-linear beamforming ultrasound methods to characterize and size kidney stones. Urolithiasis 2018. https://doi.org/10.1007/s00240-018-1036-z.

34. Shukunami KI, Nishijima K, Miyazaki M, et al. Visualization of renal stone using 3-D ultrasound with surface rendering in a pregnant woman [1]. Eur J Obstet Gynecol Reprod Biol 2006. https://doi.org/10.1016/j.ejogrb.2005.06.026.

35. Volkmer BG, Nesslauer T, Kuefer R, et al. Visualization of urinary stones by 3-D ultrasound with surface rendering. Ultrasound Med Biol 2002. https://doi.org/10.1016/S0301-5629(01)00493-8.

36. Volkmer BG, Nesslauer T, Kuefer R, et al. Evaluation of disintegration in prevesical ureteral calculi by 3-dimensional endo-ultrasound with surface rendering. J Urol 2002. https://doi.org/10.1016/S0022-5347(05)64656-3.

37. Li H, Chen Y, Liu C, et al. Construction of a three-dimensional model of renal stones: comprehensive planning for percutaneous nephrolithotomy and assistance in surgery. World J Urol 2013. https://doi.org/10.1007/s00345-012-0998-7.

38. Atalay HA, Ülker V, Alkan İ, et al. Impact of three-dimensional printed pelvicaliceal system models on residents' understanding of pelvicaliceal system anatomy before percutaneous nephrolithotripsy surgery: a pilot study. J Endourol 2016. https://doi.org/10.1089/end.2016.0307.

39. Atalay HA, Canat HL, Ülker V, et al. Impact of personalized three-dimensional (3D) printed pelvicalyceal system models on patient information in percutaneous nephrolithotripsy surgery: a pilot study. Int Braz J Urol 2017. https://doi.org/10.1590/S1677-5538.IBJU.2016.0441.

40. Ghani KR, Pilcher J, Patel U, et al. Three-dimensional ultrasound reconstruction of the pelvicaliceal system: an in-vitro study. World J Urol 2008. https://doi.org/10.1007/s00345-008-0276-x.

41. Pace KT, Tariq N, Dyer SJ, et al. Mechanical percussion, inversion and diuresis for residual lower pole fragments after shock wave lithotripsy: a prospective, single blind, randomized controlled trial. J Urol 2001. https://doi.org/10.1016/S0022-5347(05)65507-3.

42. Liu LR, Li QJ, Wei Q, et al. Percussion, diuresis, and inversion therapy for the passage of lower pole kidney stones following shock wave lithotripsy. Cochrane Database Syst Rev 2013. https://doi.org/10.1002/14651858.CD008569.pub2.

43. Long Q, Zhang J, Xu Z, et al. A prospective randomized controlled trial of the efficacy of external physical vibration lithecbole after extracorporeal shock wave lithotripsy for a lower pole renal stone less than 2 cm. J Urol 2016. https://doi.org/10.1016/j.juro.2015.10.174.

44. Wu W, Yang Z, Xu C, et al. External physical vibration lithecbole promotes the clearance of upper urinary stones after retrograde intrarenal surgery: a prospective, multicenter, randomized controlled trial. J Urol 2017. https://doi.org/10.1016/j.juro.2017.01.001.

45. Liu G, Cheng Y, Wu W, et al. Treatment of distal ureteral calculi using extracorporeal physical vibrational lithecbole combined with tamsulosin: a new option to speed up obstruction relief. J Endourol 2018. https://doi.org/10.1089/end.2017.0560.

46. Shah A, Owen NR, Lu W, et al. Novel ultrasound method to reposition kidney stones. Urol Res 2010; 38(6):491–5.

47. Harper JD, Sorensen MD, Cunitz BW, et al. Focused ultrasound to expel calculi from the kidney: safety and efficacy of a clinical prototype device. J Urol 2013;190(3):1090–5.

48. Harper JD, Dunmire B, Wang Y-N, et al. Preclinical safety and effectiveness studies of ultrasonic propulsion of kidney stones. Urology 2014;84(2):484–9.

49. Cunitz BW, Dunmire B, Bailey MR. Characterizing the acoustic output of an ultrasonic propulsion device for urinary stones. IEEE Trans Ultrason Ferroelectr Freq Control 2017. https://doi.org/10.1109/TUFFC.2017.2758647.

50. Shah A, Harper JD, Cunitz BW, et al. Focused ultrasound to expel calculi from the kidney. J Urol 2012; 187(2):739–43.

51. Connors BA, Evan AP, Blomgren PM, et al. Comparison of tissue injury from focused ultrasonic propulsion of kidney stones versus extracorporeal shock wave lithotripsy. J Urol 2014;191(1):235–41.

52. Wang YN, Simon JC, Cunitz BW, et al. Focused ultrasound to displace renal calculi: threshold for tissue injury. J Ther Ultrasound 2014;2(1). https://doi.org/10.1186/2050-5736-2-5.

53. Harper JD, Cunitz BW, Dunmire B, et al. First in human clinical trial of ultrasonic propulsion of kidney stones. J Urol 2016;195(4):956–64.

54. Hsi RS, Dunmire B, Cunitz BW, et al. Content and face validation of a curriculum for ultrasonic propulsion of calculi in a human renal model. J Endourol 2014;28(4):459–63.

55. Janssen KM, Brand TC, Cunitz BW, et al. Safety and effectiveness of a longer focal beam and burst duration in ultrasonic propulsion for repositioning urinary stones and fragments. J Endourol 2017;31(8):793–9.

56. Janssen KM, Brand TC, Bailey MR, et al. Effect of stone size and composition on ultrasonic propulsion ex vivo. Urology 2018;111:225–9.

57. Harper J, Dai JC, Chang H, et al. Quantitative assessment of effectiveness of ultrasonic propulsion of kidney stones. World Congress Endourology. Paris, September 20, 2018.

58. Ghanem MA, Maxwell AD', Krieder W, et al. Field characterization and compensation of vibrational non-uniformity for a 256-element focused ultrasound phased array. IEEE Trans Ultrason Ferroelectr Freq Control 2018. https://doi.org/10.1109/TUFFC.2018.2851188.

59. Démoré CEM, Dahl PM, Yang Z, et al. Acoustic tractor beam. Phys Rev Lett 2014. https://doi.org/10.1103/PhysRevLett.112.174302.

60. Lingéman JE, McAteer JA, Gnessin E, et al. Shock wave lithotripsy: advances in technology and technique. Nat Rev Urol 2009. https://doi.org/10.1038/nrurol.2009.216.

61. Bhojani N, Lingeman JE. Shockwave lithotripsy-new concepts and optimizing treatment parameters. Urol Clin North Am 2013. https://doi.org/10.1016/j.ucl.2012.09.001.

62. Vicentini F. In the era of flexible ureteroscopy is there still a place for Shock-wave lithotripsy? Int Braz J Urol 2015;41(2):203–6.

63. Maxwell AD, Cunitz BW, Kreider W, et al. Fragmentation of urinary calculi in vitro by burst wave lithotripsy. J Urol 2015;193(1):338–44.

64. Wang Y-N, Krieder W, Hunter C, et al. Burst Wave Lithotripsy: an in vivo demonstration of efficacy and acute safety using a porcine model. 176th Meeting of the Acoustical Society of America. Vancouver (BC), November 6 2018.

65. May PC, Kreider W, Maxwell AD, et al. Detection and evaluation of renal injury in burst wave lithotripsy using ultrasound and magnetic resonance imaging. J Endourol 2017. https://doi.org/10.1089/end.2017.0202.

66. Matlaga BR, McAteer JA, Connors BA, et al. Potential for cavitation-mediated tissue damage in shockwave lithotripsy. J Endourol 2008. https://doi.org/10.1089/end.2007.9852.

67. Sorensen MD, Wang Y-N, Kreider W, et al. Preclinical safety and effectiveness of burst wave lithotripsy. In: World Congress Endourology, 2018.

68. Zwaschka TA, Ahn JS, Cunitz BW, et al. Combined burst wave lithotripsy and ultrasonic propulsion for improved urinary stone fragmentation. J Endourol 2018. https://doi.org/10.1089/end.2017.0675.

Emerging Mobile Platforms to Aid in Stone Management

Alexander C. Small, MD, Samantha L. Thorogood, BA,
Ojas Shah, MD, Kelly A. Healy, MD*

KEYWORDS

- Nephrolithiasis • Mobile health • Mobile applications • Social media • Telemedicine

KEY POINTS

- Various mobile applications are available for patients with kidney stone to promote hydration, diet modification, medication compliance, and stone symptom tracking.
- New mobile-compatible devices including the Hidrate Spark smart water bottle, ureteral stent tracker, mobile-integrated endoscopy, and wireless ultrasound continue to evolve and may transform stone diagnosis and management in the near future.
- Social media and telemedicine are making information access easier than ever before and are bringing urologists and stone formers closer together.
- Before widespread implementation of mobile platforms, imaging performance properties of newer devices need to be validated against the gold standard, and widely variable accuracy of the information available online to patients remains a concern.

INTRODUCTION

Nephrolithiasis is an increasingly common condition worldwide and mobile technology is revolutionizing how patients with stones are diagnosed and managed. Over the past 20 years, the dramatic increase in prevalence to 8.8% (10.6% men, 7.1% women) has been attributed to numerous dietary and lifestyle factors.[1] Kidney stones also commonly recur in approximately 50% of patients within 5 to 10 years of their initial episode.[2,3] Stone passage or surgical treatment only "reset the clock." Therefore, nephrolithiasis is best considered a chronic condition and should be approached with prevention measures. Mobile technology is rapidly changing kidney stone management, including during acute symptomatic stone episodes and chronic long-term prevention.

INCREASING ADHERENCE TO STONE PREVENTION

The medical management of kidney stones uses 2 main approaches: dietary strategies (ie, increased fluid consumption and modified intake of certain foods and nutrients) and pharmacologic therapies. The "stone clinic effect" has shown that dietary and lifestyle changes prevent stone growth or new stone formation in up to 60% of patients.[4] Despite its demonstrated efficacy, compliance is typically poor and more than half of patients are noncompliant at 6 months after dietary

Disclosure Statement: Dr O. Shah is a lecturer for Boston Scientific, on the advisory board for both Applaud Medical and Boston Scientific, and a wife shareholder for New Jersey Stone Center. Dr K.A. Healy is a consultant for Boston Scientific. Drs A.C. Small and S.L. Thorogood have nothing to disclose.
Department of Urology, Columbia University Medical Center, New York Presbyterian Hospital, 161 Fort Washington Avenue, 11th Floor, New York, NY 10032, USA
* Corresponding author.
E-mail address: kah2241@cumc.columbia.edu

Urol Clin N Am 46 (2019) 287–301
https://doi.org/10.1016/j.ucl.2018.12.010
0094-0143/19/© 2018 Elsevier Inc. All rights reserved.

counseling.[5] Medication compliance is equally as problematic. Although compliance is a multidimensional process, institution and maintenance of behavioral changes is critical.

Creative patients and physicians have used various home-grown strategies to adapt to the demands of medical stone management. For example, some develop their own schedules or spreadsheet logs to track foods, fluid intake, medication regimens, and even volume of urine output. These patients often cross-reference nutrition information sites to quantify oxalate, calcium, sodium, and protein intake. Others use alarms, pillboxes, or other memory tricks to remember medications and hydration. Others even condition themselves to stay hydrated in the absence of the satiety signal (not feeling "full") by reflexively reaching for fluids. No matter the strategy, all can become burdensome. Numerous stone-focused mobile applications (or "apps") now aim to increase patient compliance by exploiting known behavioral science principles. Many apps draw upon the similar "active ingredients" for behavioral interventions. The Behavior Change Technique Taxonomy identifies 93 specific techniques and clusters them into 16 broad categories.[6] For example, categories include scheduled consequences, rewards and threats, repetition and substitution, feedback and monitoring, and social support. Behavioral science may hold the keys to success for health-related behavior change apps and therefore increase the efficacy of medical management of urolithiasis.

As of 2018, there are dozens of stone-specific mobile behavior change/tracking tools and many more with potential relevance to stone patients. The apps fall into 5 broad categories: (1) hydration, (2) diet modification, (3) stone-specific apps, (4) medication adherence, (5) symptom trackers.

Hydration

Studies have repeatedly demonstrated an inverse relationship between fluid intake and rates of stone formation.[7,8] Fluid intake serves as a proxy for urine volume, which dictates the extent to which lithogenic factors are saturated in the urinary tract. Because individual metabolic parameters and diet compositions vary greatly, the American Urologic Association (AUA) deemed it inappropriate to offer a universal recommendation on daily fluid intake. Instead, the AUA Guidelines advise all stone formers to drink enough fluids to maintain a urine output of approximately 2.5 L per day.[9] The European Association of Urology (EAU) Guidelines recommend intake of 2.5 to 3.0 L of fluid per day.[10] Ideally, customized recommendations would be made based on total volumes from 24-hour urine collections; however, this is not practical, possible, or necessary in all comers. For example, the first-time stone former may agree to basic metabolic workup but not warrant comprehensive testing if low risk. In addition, 24-hour urine volumes are often inaccurate as determined by the calculated urinary creatinine (Cr) per kilogram (Cr 24/kg). In fact, one study found that nearly 40% of patients either under- or over-collected their specimens due to several possible factors such as baseline urinary incontinence, language barriers, or poor health literacy.[11] Because tracking daily urine output is burdensome, many patients track their daily fluid intake instead. Studies indicate that providing specific instructions regarding the volume and frequency of water intake achieved more consistent behavior changes.[12]

Despite the evidence and guidelines, patient adherence to hydration recommendations is low. More than 50% of patients are noncompliant with the medical management of stones.[5,13] One study surveyed kidney stone formers and found 3 main categories of barriers to increasing water intake.[14] First, patients were unaware of the benefits of fluid intake and did not remember to drink. Without the reminder of pain from active stone passage, many patients did not act beyond their native thirst mechanism to drink. Second, patients reported disliking the taste of water, lack of thirst, and lack of fluid availability. Third, increasing fluid intake to achieve the target urine output of 2.5 L can worsen baseline lower urinary tract symptoms such as frequency or incontinence. Consequently, patients are often noncompliant due to the work/life disruptions of drinking more fluids.

Among the aforementioned barriers to hydration, the cognitive burden of "remembering to drink" is readily targeted with mobile technologies integrated into smartphones, which are nearly omnipresent worldwide. Numerous mobile apps are currently available as stand-alone water trackers (**Table 1**). Although these vary in popularity and price, most share several common features: manual entry of fluid consumption, notifications to prompt fluid intake, customized goal setting, graphic representation of drinking trends, and performance feedback. Some apps provide a searchable database of nonwater drinks to estimate "water equivalents," whereas others allow users to create and save custom drinks with user-defined estimates water composition.

Water tracking apps have demonstrated efficacy. A systematic review of 16 nonpharmacologic intervention studies aiming to increase water intake in adults with stones, renal

Table 1
Top hydration mobile apps (apple iOS)

App (Publisher)	Popularity	Cost	Content and Features
WaterMinder (Funn Media, LLC)	• #17 in Health & Fitness • 4.8 stars (5590 reviews)	$4.99	• Track water intake, set goals, motivational achievements
Daily Water Tracker Reminder (Grassapper LLC)	• #26 in medical apps • 4.8 stars (4940 ratings)	Free (in-app purchases)	• Log water intake • Custom goals and reminders
Plant Nanny (Fourdesire)	• #52 in Health & Fitness • 4.6 stars (8420 reviews)	Free (in-app purchases)	• Fun design • Custom goals and reminders
My Water Balance (Viktor Sharov)	• #68 in Health & Fitness • 4.4 stars (1290 reviews)	$4.99	• Water requirement calculator, reminders, graphs, motivational awards, tips
Drink Water Reminder (Phoenix Games LLP)	• #122 in Health & Fitness • 4.5 stars (16,300 ratings)	Free (Pro upgrade $1.99)	• Track water intake, unlimited reminders, syncs to Apple Watch

dysfunction, or urinary tract infections (UTIs) found that the most effective interventions shared 2 features: specific instructions and self-monitoring tools (eg, dipsticks to measure urine-specific gravity or measurement of urine volume).[12] In 13 of the studies, the interventions successfully increased water intake by at least 500 mL. There was some support for counseling, education, and the provision of drinking containers; however, these interventions were present in a more limited number of studies.

Diet Modification

Current AUA guidelines offer dietary recommendations based on specific stone types and results of 24-hour urine studies, and EAU guidelines advise a balanced diet with the goal of normalizing general risk factors. Although it is widely accepted that diet and lifestyle affect the risk of developing stones, the contribution of each dietary component to an individual's risk is unclear. Perhaps more importantly, systemic metabolic conditions related to diet, including obesity, hypertension, and diabetes, may affect stone risk in profound ways.[15,16] With dietary recommendations to prevent stones, patients must interpret often vague guidelines, contend with an infinite number of dietary options, and self-regulate eating behaviors. In practice, some providers instruct stone formers to limit intake of a long list of specific foods known to be high in oxalate, nondairy animal proteins, or other dietary risk factors, which can become quite confusing to many patients. In response to these

demands and to assist with aspects of human fallibility including recall bias, smartphone apps have become useful tools for facilitating dietary interventions.

The field of diet-related apps is much broader than that of fluid tracking (**Table 2**). Even in 2013, a study counted 6 apps specifically targeted toward kidney stone formers to assist with diet recording and uric acid or gout management.[17] These comprise a small fraction of the total number of 100+ diet-related apps on the market. Diet apps excel in the extent to which they have been validated as effective behavioral interventions in stone formers. One study developed an internet program that informed stone formers of recommended dietary modifications, logged daily food, and fluid intake and delivered immediate feedback on compliance to recommendations.[18] Using 24-hour urine collections in 5 patients, the investigators demonstrated that the interactive program significantly reduced oxalate excretion, and it was as effective as a physician-controlled stone-preventative metabolic diet.

The long-term efficacy of diet tracking apps in stone formers is unclear. However, in other chronic conditions such as diabetes and heart disease, studies show sustained effects. A meta-analysis of 9 studies demonstrated a sustained decrease in HbA1c among diabetic patients with both short-term (3–6 months) and longer-term (10–12 months) use of lifestyle modification/tracking apps.[19] A prospective randomized trial between traditional diet/exercise counseling versus the addition of a smartphone app

Table 2
Top healthy diet mobile apps (Apple iOS)

App (Publisher)	Popularity	Cost	Content and Features
MyFitnessPal (MyFitnessPal.com)	• #1 Health and Fitness • 4.7 stars (489,000 ratings)	Free (upgrade to premium for $9.99/mo)	Recipe importer, robust nutrient tracker, syncs with many devices and apps, social networking
Lose It! Calorie Counter (FitNow)	• #11 Health and Fitness • 4.7 stars (158,000 ratings)	Free (in-app purchases)	Weight loss program and food diary
MyPlate Calorie Counter (Livestrong.com)	• #28 Health and Fitness • 4.5 stars (7390 ratings)	Free (Gold membership $9.99)	Food tracker, meal plans, community support
Lifesum—Diet & Food Diary (Lifesum AB)	• #31 Health and Fitness • 4.6 stars (20,200 ratings)	Free (upgrade to premium $21.99 USD/3-mo)	Many diet plan options, syncs with many devices and apps
Noom Coach (Noom, Inc.)	• #34 Health and Fitness • 4.6 stars (14,300 ratings)	Free (pro upgrade $9.99)	Structured course based on behavior change research, coaching, social networking

compared measurements of adiposity at 3 and 12 months.[20] The study found a beneficial effect of the app intervention at 12 months in the female-only subgroup, with decreased waist circumference (−0.67 cm) and decreased body adiposity estimator score compared with controls.

For stone patients, diet and nutrition apps may prove particularly beneficial because stones form over the course of years and modification of risk factors can significantly mitigate recurrence risk.

Stone-Specific Apps

Stone-specific mobile apps have broad availability, diverse functions, and very heterogeneous quality.[17] A 2015 survey of stone-specific apps identified 42 distinct apps with emphasis on patient information (52%), health professional resources (21%), patient dietary recording tools (10%), herbal remedies (10%), and uric acid/gout management (5%). Half of the apps required payment for download (mean cost $6.04, range $1.03–$58.87). Two-thirds of the apps lacked clear input from health professionals, and 62% were identified to have significant inaccuracies. The most popular free app currently available is *Stone MD* (Nariman Gadzhiev, Russia), which provides an individualized risk assessment, water and food diary, urine pH log, and stent tracker. The app has a solid 4.5/5 rating on the Google Play store from just 65 reviewers.

With a large number of apps specifically available for tracking fluid intake, modifying diets, and increasing medication adherence, one might wonder if there is enough demand for a similar stone-specific app that integrates these features. In fact, evidence suggests that patients prefer disease-specific apps. In a study of patients with cystic fibrosis (CF), participants all expressed interest in apps to support CF self-management.[21] Requested features included having multiple rather than single functions, information specific to CF, and automation of disease management activities (ie, medication reminders and pharmacy refills). Integrated stone-specific apps have great potential to ease management of this chronic disease.

To what extent is specificity accountable for the limited adoption of behavior change apps among stone formers? And could increasing disease specificity of an app lead to a secondary increase in clinical workflow integration, thereby further promoting standardized adoption?

Medication Adherence

Medication adherence for chronic disease is estimated to be about 50% in developed countries and much lower in developing countries.[22] A similar rate of nonadherence was found among kidney stone patients.[23] Using medical and pharmacy claims data, 8950 stone patients were identified, and only 51% were found to be adherent to preventive pharmacologic therapy at 6 months after prescription. Importantly, patients who were adherent to therapy had 27% lower odds of an emergency department visit, 41% lower odds of hospital admission, and 23% lower odds of surgery for stone disease than nonadherent patients. Frequency of medication dosing is a major barrier for many stone patients. Potassium citrate, for example, requires dose titration up to 15 mEq four times a day for optimization. Medication adherence and reminder apps provide a possible intervention for stone formers with poor compliance.

Medication adherence apps include features such as flexible scheduling, medication tracking history, visual aids to create "virtual pillboxes," refill reminders, and interaction warnings (**Table 3**).[24] There were 681 medication adherence apps identified in a recent study, but a mere 12% of those involved health care providers in their development. Despite often limited health care provider involvement, emerging evidence supports the effectiveness of mobile apps in increasing medication adherence in transplant patients, those with heart disease, and the elderly.[25,26] The highest rated medication management app is *Medisafe* (MediSafe Inc., Boston, MA), which touts more than 4.5 million users and has partnered with health care providers and insurance companies to increase medication compliance (**Fig. 1**). As these data mature, use of apps could become the standard of care, especially among patients with complex medication regimens or polypharmacy.

Symptom Trackers

Many stone patients suffer from lower urinary tract symptoms, recurrent infections, and chronic pain. Numerous apps have been released that offer users mechanisms to track their symptoms. These are useful for both patients to decide when to seek medical attention and for physicians to aid in diagnosis and treatment efficacy. One such app, UTI Tracker (Yourology Tracker, LLC, Mc Lean, VA), was created by a urologist in order to help patients identify lifestyle patterns that may trigger symptomatic episodes and to supply this information to physicians in a format conducive to quick review and treatment planning. The app allows users to log-in with their Facebook credentials, opt into receiving preventative tip, and share data with providers via email or printer-formatted hard copy. A study of a similar UTI diary app showed that younger participants tended to favor the app while older participants preferred an online survey.[27] Age and technological savvy seems to be an important limitation of outpatient workflows that involve symptom tracking apps.

Although not specific to stone formers, pain is another symptom targeted by mobile apps. A 2015 study identified 279 smartphone apps pertaining to pain self-management; these offered coping skill support, patient education, self-monitoring, social support, and goal setting. Only 8.2% involved a health care professional in development and only one underwent scientific evaluation.[28] Another review found 10 apps on the Android platform specifically designed for postoperative pain management. Similarly, there was a low rate of health care professional involvement in the development of these apps and none underwent scientific evaluation. Overall, symptom tracker apps lack evidence-based content and have limited support functions at this time.[29]

Table 3
Top medication tracker mobile apps (Apple iOS)

App (Publisher)	Popularity	Cost	Content and Features
WebMD (WebMD)	• #136 Health & Fitness • 4.7 stars (29,962 ratings)	Free	Pill identifier, interaction checker, medication reminders, physician directory
Medisafe (MediSafe Inc.)	• #28 medical apps • 4.7 stars (13,200 ratings)	Free (in-app purchases)	Reminders, Health app integration, report sharing, refill reminders
Round Health (Circadian Design)	• #74 medical apps • 4.4 stars (1200 ratings)	Free (in-app purchases)	Reminder, Apple Watch integration, refill reminders
CareZone (CareZone)	• #40 medical apps • 4.6 stars (8100 ratings)	Free	Medication bottle scanning, reminders, track health vitals (blood pressure, glucose, etc.)
Pill Reminder (Sergio Licea)	• #144 medical apps • 3.7 stars (2930 ratings)	Free (in-app purchases)	Similar to other pill reminder apps

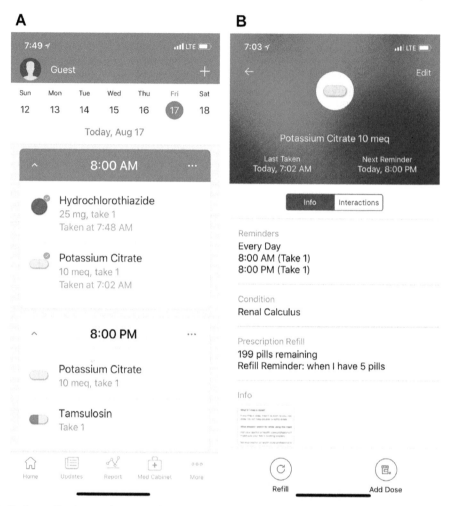

Fig. 1. Medisafe medication tracker app. The Medisafe medication tracker app allows users to set up reminders for daily pill schedules (*A*) and track detailed information about various medications (*B*). (*Courtesy of* MediSafe Inc.,copyright; with permission.)

MOBILE-COMPATIBLE HARDWARE
Smart Water Bottle

Despite the promise of mobile health behavior change apps, they are still far from being universally adopted by either clinicians or patients. An online poll conducted on the University of Chicago Kidney Stone blog received responses from 45 stone formers, 22 of whom (49%) said they prefer not to use an app to assist in managing their stone disease. Another 11 patients (25%) reported relying on "just a jug" to track their fluid intake.[30] In order to increase utilization of mobile platforms in this area, the current limitations of the technology must be addressed—chief among these limitations is the requirement to manually track and input fluid consumption data. The smart water bottle was developed to answer the demand for automated water tracking. A popular product is the

Hidrate Spark water bottle (Hidrate Inc., Minneapolis, MN) (**Fig. 2**). The water bottle was initially crowdfunded on the popular site Kickstarter and blew past its initial goal of $35,000 by raising $627,000 in presales to more than 8000 backers. Now for sale at $54.95, the Hidrate Spark bottle pairs via Bluetooth with an iOS- and Android-compatible smartphone app and uses a capacitive touch sensor embedded in the bottle to detect changes in water level and an accelerometer to detect movement. In a study composed of 9 non–stone-forming participants, fluid intake as measured by the Hidrate Spark was found to be accurate to within 3% of the "true" fluid intake as manually recorded in a research setting.[31] The companion app also calculates custom recommendations for daily water intake based on height, weight, age, and activity level, and it can also

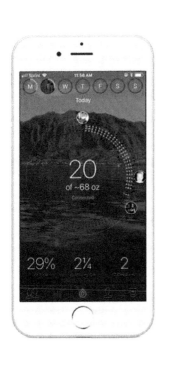

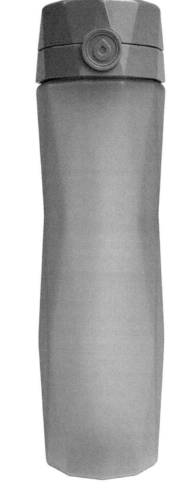

Fig. 2. Hidrate Spark smart water bottle and companion app. The Hidrate Spark bottle pairs via Bluetooth with an iOS- and Android-compatible smartphone app. It uses a capacitive touch sensor embedded in the bottle to detect changes in water level and an accelerometer to detect movement to log fluid consumption. The app provides pop-up reminders to drink and the bottle itself emits a glowing light when it detects static fluid levels over a prolonged period of time. (*Courtesy of* Hidrate Inc.,copyright; with permission.)

adjust the daily water goal based on local temperature, humidity, and elevation. The Hidrate Spark manages the need for reminders not only with pop-up smartphone notifications like its predecessor water tracking apps but also by emitting a glowing light from the bottle itself after it detects static fluid levels over a prolonged period.

Although the smart water bottle shows potential for the medical management of urolithiasis, the technology has yet to be validated in this population or studied for cost-effectiveness and scalability. There is currently a multiinstitutional randomized clinical trial underway titled "Investigation of Non-Invasive Hydration Monitoring with Smart Water Bottle to Increase Fluid Intake in Patients with Nephrolithiasis and Low Urine Volume"

(NCT02938884). Patients are being randomized to receive the Hidrate Spark water bottle or standard counseling alone, and the primary outcome is change from baseline in hydration adherence at 12 weeks, as determined by measurable increase in urine volume. Estimated enrollment is 150 patients, and it is scheduled to be completed by December 2018. In the future, this technology promises utility as a behavioral aide for recurrent stone formers and potential research tool research tool in clinical trials.

Stent Tracker

Indwelling ureteral stents are ubiquitous in endourology. Unfortunately, forgotten and retained stents occur in 4% to 13% of cases and can result in morbid complications, additional procedures, and increased treatment costs.[32,33] Furthermore, up to 16% of endourology lawsuits were for retained stents.[34] These high stakes have led to the development of several stent tracking systems. Early electronic registries capable of interfacing with patient electronic medical records (EMRs) and automating stent extraction reminders have shown promise, reducing incidence of overdue stents from 12.5% to 1.2%.[35,36]

The latest innovation in this space is the Ureteral Stent Tracker app (Visible Health Inc., Austin, TX, USA and Boston Scientific Corporation, Boston, MA, USA), which uses a Health Insurance Portability and Accountability Act (HIPAA)-compliant, cloud-based platform to bridge point-of-care stent placement and long-term tracking (**Figs. 3** and **4**). The proposed workflow starts when a clinician scans a stent's barcode after placement. A case record with planned extraction date is immediately generated and can be subsequently monitored via the app's visual dashboard. Patients can be filtered by overdue cases, incomplete cases, currently indwelling stents, and extracted stents. The Ureteral Stent Tracker system uses database encryption via Amazon Web Services and password protection of user accounts. A major limitation, however, is that the app can only automatically track Boston Scientific stents, and its use is limited to physicians who are preauthorized and registered by the company. Other stents can be manually

entered into the app once the user has registered to use the app. Other limitations include lack of automatic contact of patients flagged as overdue for stent removal, need for manual input of stent care plans and manual case status updates, and lack of a patient-facing portal. Despite these limitations, studies have demonstrated successful implementation of Ureteral Stent Tracker workflows. The first case series deployed the app to track 146 stent care plans in 115 patients over 2 years, and it helped to identify and call in 3 patients who did not return for scheduled extraction.[37] Another case series followed 194 patients over 6 months with the Ureteral Stent Tracker and reported identifying 9% of overdue stents and 0.5% of patients lost to follow-up.[32] Unfortunately, support for the Ureteral Stent Tracker has been discontinued, and it has been removed from the app stores. Because patient safety tools such as this one continue to mature and expand their scope to include other stent manufacturers, they will undoubtedly become valuable tools for endourologists.

Urinary Tract Infection Detection

UTI detection biosensors are another promising mobile technology. The gold standard for detecting and quantifying urinary pathogens remains the urine culture, but new microfluidic devices such as the micropad (or μPAD) may be able to improve speed, sensitivity, and specificity at the

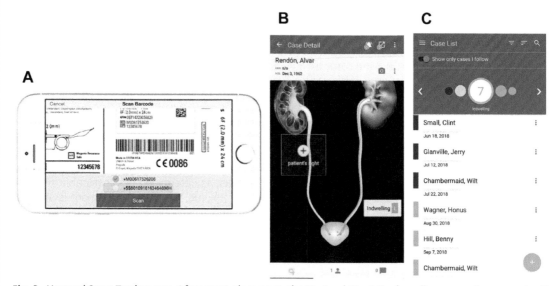

Fig. 3. Ureteral Stent Tracker app. After stent placement, the Ureteral Stent Tracker allows users to scan a stent's barcode (*A*) to immediately generate a case record with planned extraction date (*B*). The stent database can be subsequently monitored via the app's visual dashboard (*C*). Patients can be filtered by overdue cases, incomplete cases, currently indwelling stents, and extracted stents. (*Courtesy of* Stent Tracker is a registered trademark of Visible Health, Inc.; and Visible Health, Inc.,copyright, with permission.)

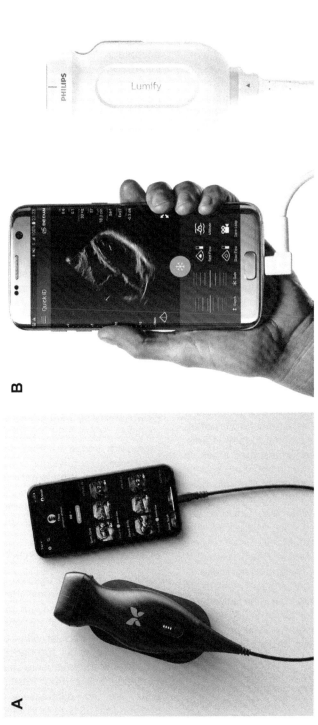

Fig. 4. Mobile-based ultrasound devices. The Butterfly IQ (*A*) and Philips Lumify (*B*) are 2 of the newest hand-held mobile ultrasound scanners capable of pairing with smartphones. (*Courtesy of* Butterfly Inc.,copyright; and Philips, with permission.)

point of care. The μPAD can provide rapid quantitative and qualitative results for UTI diagnosis—in one study anti-*Escherichia coli* antibodies were fixed to a microfluidic capillary platform, and human urine samples spiked with *E coli* were introduced into the platform. A smartphone camera was used to quantify the extent of immunoagglutination, and the assay was found to have a superior detection limit for bacteria compared with nitrite strips or rapid kits.[38] The ubiquity of smartphones paired with the favorable cost, speed, and operability of μPAD technology may enable point-of-care identification of UTIs.[39] μPADs have even been integrated with disposable undergarments to produce a wearable device, which could screen for UTI-associated biomarkers in real time.[40]

In addition to point-of-care diagnosis of UTIs, smartphones are now also becoming a platform for in-home urine testing. The iOS apps Cherto (Unicoms, Bulgaria) and Scanwell (Scanwell Health, Inc., Anaheim, CA, USA) use the iPhone's camera to automatically analyze proprietary urinalysis strips. Scanwell is approved by Food and Drug Administration (FDA) for urine testing and offers customers the ability to chat with a physician over the app interface and receive a prescription for antibiotics when necessary. There are currently no studies pertaining to either of these home diagnostic apps.

Smartphone Compatible Ultrasound

Briefly, mobile ultrasound scanners capable of pairing with smartphones have tremendous potential for diagnosing and managing kidney stones, especially in remote or resource-scarce areas. In the last few years, the FDA has approved several of these devices including Lumify (Android only; Philips, Amsterdam, The Netherlands), Butterfly iQ (Apple iOS only; Butterfly Inc., Guilford, CT, USA), Mobisante (Android only; Mobisante, Inc. Redmond, WA), and Clarius Mobile Health (Apple iOS and Android; Clarius Mobile Health, Burnaby, BC, Canada) (see **Fig. 4**). These devices make ultrasound a pocket-sized, bedside tool available to physicians at historically low cost—the Butterfly iQ is currently on preorder for about $2000 and the Philips Lumify can be leased for $199 per month. The apps for many of these devices are capable of pushing images to the cloud, further expanding the implications for telemedicine and education. Of note, these devices are currently considered prescription devices and are therefore only available to licensed health care practitioners.

Mobile Endoscopy

Mobile technology is already reshaping the world of endoscopy. The Endockscope (Endockscope, Orange, CA, USA) is a specialized lens and docking system that couples a flexible endoscope to a smartphone and a portable LED light source, thereby serving as a mobile endoscopic viewing system.[41] In a study, expert endoscopists found the overall image quality of the Endockscope acceptable for diagnostic purposes when used in cystoscopic and ureteroscopic image acquisition. Although this early study found the Endockscope system (paired with an iPhone 4S) to be inferior to images captured by the Storz HD camera in terms of image quality, image resolution, and color resolution, a subsequent test found comparable quality when the Endockscope was paired with a Galaxy S8, iPhone 7, and iPhone 6S.[42] The most problematic aspect of the Endockscope system seems to be the brightness of the LED light source—on evaluation of an iPhone 7 + LED light source and an iPhone 6S + LED light, 82% and 55% evaluators considered the platform appropriate for diagnostic purposes, compared with 100% who considered the Storz HD camera + xenon light source (standard for videocystoscopy) appropriate. As the quality of smartphone cameras continue to improve, this platform will improve as well. The Endockscope is now priced at $399 and touts a comparison with the average cost of an HD endoscopic system of approximately $45,000 (about $15,000 for the HD camera and $30,000 USD for the video system/receiver). Added benefits of smartphone compatibility for endoscopy include use of native camera application features (ie, one-touch recording, image capture, and sharing), global accessibility, lightweight portability, compatibility with cloud data storage networks, and live streaming capabilities onto secondary monitors. Other "digiscoping" universal adapters for smartphones are available as well for as little as $11.99.

EDUCATION AND SUPPORT

A review of mobile technologies in endourology would be remiss to omit the sweeping changes for patients and providers brought on by social media and "Web 2.0" developments. The Web is tremendously popular with 70% of all Americans using social media to connect with one another and 80% of Internet users searching for health information online (Pew Research Center). Urologists are no different—a Medscape survey showed that 56% to 81% of urologists use social media, depending on their age. In 2016, the AUA even published an Update Series on "The Role of Social Media in Urology" in an effort to help urologists understand how social media can play a role in augmenting medical practice and highlight potential pitfalls in its use related to professionalism and patient privacy.[43] The wave of disruption brought on by mobile technology has just begun, and there are already dozens of potential uses for patients and providers.

Provider Education

Providers have tapped into the power of mobile technology to optimize health care, especially through the personal education, dissemination of health information, advocacy, research, and streamlining patient-provider communication. Social media has created hundreds of "microcommunities" where specialists across every field of medicine can converge to discuss new research and challenging cases. Among urologists, Twitter has become the most popular platform. At conferences, use of a hashtag containing the abbreviation and year (ie, World Congress of Endourology 2018 becomes #WCE18) allows real-time discussion of presentations, interactions with moderators, and "remote" meeting access for those who want to follow along online. In a study of 8 international conferences in 2013, 12,363 tweets were sent, generating more than 14 million impressions. The most popular meeting was the #AUA13, with 573 participants.[44] By comparison, #AUA16 had 5 times the number of participants (2,877) writing 20,310 total tweets and generating more than 39 million impressions. The hashtag #StoneSmart was created by Boston Scientific and Urology Times to foster a virtual community for endourologists to explore the latest ideas and innovations in stone disease. Searching #StoneSmart on Twitter reveals dozens of interesting cases, technical videos, interviews, and discussions. When used appropriately, social media can provide significant education and engagement for health care providers.

Numerous other apps are designed specifically for provider education. The AUA has released its AUA Guidelines and AUA University apps to provide mobile resources for students, residents, and practicing urologists. Podcasts have also been produced by the AUA University and Journal of Endourology ("Endourology Sound Bites"), which cover topics such as new guidelines, research updates, and controversial management topics. Almost every major conference now also has an accompanying app to help attendees navigate sessions, review abstracts and presentations, and even interact with live audience questionnaires. Apps abound on the mobile devices of urologists everywhere and with good reason. They can serve to enrich providers' continuing medical education and expand their professional networks as nothing else ever before.

Patient Education

Patients with kidney stone commonly use social media communities as a resource for learning and support. On Twitter, a search for #KidneyStones revealed 10,333 tweets from 3426 users in 106 countries regarding stone prevention, symptoms, and treatment.[45] On Facebook, the largest page dedicated to stones is titled "Kidney Stones Suck - Support Group!!!" With close to 10,000 members and dozens of daily posts, patients turn to this page to share their personal experiences, treatment advice (including some interesting home remedies), and questions. Likewise, YouTube is a source of information for many patients. A study recently analyzed YouTube videos related to kidney stones for their content—despite hundreds of available videos, only 58% were deemed useful, 18% were misleading, and just 2% had content rated as "good."[46] The most popular current videos are "How do kidney stones form? How can we prevent them?" (2.5 million views) by a Florida private practice, VIP Urology, and "How to dissolve kidney stones naturally" (2.1 million views) by an Indian Ayurvedic home remedy enthusiast. Overall, these social media platforms may provide patients a good resource for seeking personal support. However, patients should be cautioned that most of the available resources online are inaccurate and often from unknown sources.[47] Alternative sites provide high-quality educational resources including the AUA Urology Care Foundation (http://www.urologyhealth.org/) and the noncommercial Website Kidney Stoners (http://www.kidneystoners.org/). Several industry-sponsored sites also provide patient-oriented information including the site for Urocit-K (Mission Pharmacal, San Antonio, TX, USA) and the site for Thiola (Retrophin, San Diego, CA, USA).

TELEMEDICINE AND MOBILE-INTEGRATED DEVICES

The AUA white paper on telemedicine broadly defines telemedicine and telehealth as the use of telecommunication tools such as the internet, video conferencing, and email to exchange information in the context of health care. Some examples include patient portals, mobile EMR apps, virtual patient visits, provider-to-provider eConsults, "telementoring," and "telesurgery." Mobile devices have greatly expanded the scope of telemedicine activities because they can aggregate multiple communication tools onto a single device. Given the workforce shortages in urology and maldistribution of urologists in urban and rural areas, telemedicine holds tremendous promise to expand access to specialty care.

Telemedicine services have been implemented successfully in urology on both small and large scales. The Department of Veterans Affairs (VA) has implemented video visits in urology in multiple states with excellent satisfaction reviews.[48] Patient savings were considerable when a telemedicine program was implemented at the Los Angeles VA Hospital—per visit savings amounted to an average of 277 travel miles, 290 minutes of travel time, $67 in travel expenses, and $126 in lost opportunity cost.[49]

Currently, telehealth has been tested along the full spectrum of urologic care from preoperative consultation to inpatient rounding to discharge.[50–52] The very idea of the mobile device is even being expanded. The VGo remote-controlled telemedicine robot (Vecna, Cambridge, MA, USA) seems to have versatile applications and has been deployed in skilled nursing facilities, Veterans Hospitals, and even pediatric hospitals. A pilot program at Boston Children's Hospital even supplied these robots to patients discharged from the hospital after urologic surgery in order to facilitate close, in-home monitoring and other institutions have routinely integrated telemedicine into the postoperative care of children.[52] The role of mobile platforms in telemedicine is sure to expand as the cost of technology responds to innovation and as regulatory bodies continue to react to industry demand and development.

Many urologists may be participating in patient care via telemedicine without fully realizing it. Exchange of information via text message is common practice within hospitals and practices—in 2015, it was estimated that 85% of physicians and 29% of nurses used their mobile phones to communicate clinical information at work.[53] Messaging apps such as WhatsApp and Apple iMessage provide free alternatives to standard SMS text messages and allow users to create group (multimember) chats composed of phone numbers registered anywhere in the world. WhatsApp was even specifically evaluated as a tool for use in tele-urology in the evaluation of hematuria—when compared with traditional in-person assessment, evaluation via photograph through WhatsApp had almost perfect agreement (kappa = 0.939) in grading hematuria severity.[54] Communication over text message can rapidly convey important information between providers and potentially reduce unnecessary medical visits and consultations.

True telesurgery may be the next frontier of telemedicine. This concept was born in the 1970s as a result of NASA's need for the delivery of nonearth-based health care as well as the Defense Advanced Research Projects Agency's hope for frontline battlefield intervention capabilities. Many of the developments in robotic surgery were born from these efforts. Urology has broadly experimented with telemanipulation. In endourology, telesurgery saw a burst of activity in the early 2000s with the development of PAKY (Percutaneous Access to the Kidney; Urobotics Laboratory, Johns Hopkins Medical Center, Baltimore, MD, USA). This device was a remotely controlled robot designed for fluoroscopic guided percutaneous needle insertion into the renal collecting system that was tested mostly in the laboratory.[55] Because robotic technology has matured and bandwidth for transmission of data has increased, these types of platforms may have renewed interest. At this time, robotic-assisted flexible ureteroscopy is only in its infancy, but telesurgery coupled with artificial intelligence may hold great promise in this field.[56]

LIMITATIONS AND FUTURE DIRECTIONS

There are important limitations to consider before many of these mobile platforms can be fully adopted for stone management. First and foremost, the quality of information within many of these platforms can be inaccurate or misleading—few mobile apps involved health care professionals during their development, some apps and Websites have clear commercial bias, and social media sites are riddled with false information and rumors that can limit the transfer of correct information.[17,47] Second, design and technical issues can hamper the usefulness of many technologies. Although some apps may embrace the building blocks of behavioral change theory, many are developed by engineers and not behavioral change experts. As such, most apps lack any objective evidence that they work, and those that have been studied use mostly small-scale cohort studies. Also, those that advertise cloud-based data sharing and EMR integration have run into HIPAA compliance problems and have limited native EMR integration. Third, the accessibility of new technology creates inherent limitations that may exclude certain populations such as those with lower socioeconomic status that cannot afford smart phones or mobile data service, non-English speakers, and the elderly or patients with less tech-savvy. Finally, although certainly convenient and exciting, many of the mobile-integrated hardware devices provide suboptimal imaging and should not be fully implemented until they have been validated compared with gold standards.

Even with these limitations, the future of mobile platforms in endourology is extremely promising. As technology continues to disrupt every aspect of our lives, software and hardware solutions will make diseases faster to detect and easier for patients and health care providers to manage. New platforms will have increased design input from health care professionals with more personalized recommendations for patients. These platforms will have the ability to synchronize across multiple devices and transmit data back to your doctor—for example, imagine a smart water bottle that reminds patients to drink through the TV or alarm clock, sends real-time data back to their physicians, and flags individuals with increasing stone risk. New classes of "smart" devices such as toilets or catheters could have the ability to detect changes in urine chemistry, presence of infection, or microhematuria. The implications for research are enormous as well. Apps could provide a secure, private, and easy mechanism for clinical trial enrollment and data collection. Apple has introduced the "ResearchKit" open source framework for app development to help medical researchers recruit patients and gather data. It is already being used for several large studies of diverse disease such as autism (Autism & Beyond app from Duke University and University of Capetown), epilepsy (EpiWatch app from Johns Hopkins University), and melanoma (Mole Mapper app from Oregon Health & Science University). Crowdsourcing has also become a hot topic and has allowed researchers to empower experts and nonexperts to analyze and validate data. In urology and surgery, crowdsourcing has been used to assess and give feedback on endoscopic and surgical skill.[57,58] Ultimately in the near future, these devices and applications could become linked to advanced artificial intelligence and machine learning algorithms to provide automated diagnosis, decision support, and integration with advanced forms of telemedicine.

SUMMARY

Emerging platforms to aid in stone management include software apps to increase adherence to stone prevention, mobile compatible hardware, online social media communities, and telemedicine. Apps and hardware specifically relevant to increasing hydration, diet modification, medication adherence, and rapid diagnosis (ie, mobile ultrasound and endoscopy) have the greatest potential reduce stone recurrence and speed treatment. Social media and online communities have also been rapidly adopted by patients and providers to promote education and support. There are important limitations to consider before widespread implementation of many of these mobile platforms, but the future holds great promise for patients, health care providers, and researchers.

REFERENCES

1. Scales CD, Smith AC, Hanley JM, et al, Urologic Diseases in America Project. Prevalence of kidney stones in the United States. Eur Urol 2012;62(1): 160–5.
2. Lotan Y, Pearle MS. Cost-effectiveness of primary prevention strategies for nephrolithiasis. J Urol 2011;186(2):550–5.
3. Strauss AL, Coe FL, Deutsch L, et al. Factors that predict relapse of calcium nephrolithiasis during treatment: a prospective study. Am J Med 1982; 72(1):17–24.
4. Hosking DH, Erickson SB, Van den Berg CJ, et al. The stone clinic effect in patients with idiopathic calcium urolithiasis. J Urol 1983;130(6):1115–8.
5. Khambati A, Matulewicz RS, Perry KT, et al. Factors associated with compliance to increased fluid intake and urine volume following dietary counseling in first-time kidney stone patients. J Endourol 2017; 31(6):605–10.
6. Michie S, Richardson M, Johnston M, et al. The behavior change technique taxonomy (v1) of 93 hierarchically clustered techniques: building an international consensus for the reporting of behavior change interventions. Ann Behav Med 2013;46(1): 81–95.
7. Curhan GC, Willett WC, Rimm EB, et al. A prospective study of dietary calcium and other nutrients and the risk of symptomatic kidney stones. N Engl J Med 1993;328(12):833–8.
8. Taylor EN, Curhan GC. Dietary calcium from dairy and nondairy sources, and risk of symptomatic kidney stones. J Urol 2013;190(4):1255–9.
9. Pearle MS, Goldfarb DS, Assimos DG, et al. Medical management of kidney stones: AUA guideline. J Urol 2014;192(2):316–24.
10. Türk C, Petřík A, Sarica K, et al. EAU guidelines on diagnosis and conservative management of urolithiasis. Eur Urol 2016;69(3):468–74.
11. Healy KA, Hubosky SG, Bagley DH. 24-hour urine collection in the metabolic evaluation of stone formers: is one study adequate? J Endourol 2013; 27(3):374–8.
12. Chua TXW, Prasad NS, Rangan GK, et al. A systematic review to determine the most effective interventions to increase water intake. Nephrology (Carlton) 2016;21(10):860–9.
13. Barcelo P, Wuhl O, Servitge E, et al. Randomized double-blind study of potassium citrate in idiopathic hypocitraturic calcium nephrolithiasis. J Urol 1993; 150(6):1761–4.

14. McCauley LR, Dyer AJ, Stern K, et al. Factors influencing fluid intake behavior among kidney stone formers. J Urol 2012;187(4):1282–6.

15. Taylor EN, Stampfer MJ, Curhan GC. Obesity, weight gain, and the risk of kidney stones. JAMA 2005; 293(4):455–62.

16. Borghi L, Meschi T, Guerra A, et al. Essential arterial hypertension and stone disease. Kidney Int 1999; 55(6):2397–406.

17. Stevens DJ, McKenzie K, Cui HW, et al. Smartphone apps for urolithiasis. Urolithiasis 2015;43(1):13–9.

18. Lange JN, Easter L, Amoroso R, et al. Internet program for facilitating dietary modifications limiting kidney stone risk. Can J Urol 2013;20(5):6922–6.

19. Lunde P, Nilsson BB, Bergland A, et al. The effectiveness of smartphone apps for lifestyle improvement in noncommunicable diseases: systematic review and meta-analyses. J Med Internet Res 2018;20(5):e162.

20. Gomez-Marcos MA, Patino-Alonso MC, Recio-Rodriguez JI, et al. Short- and long-term effectiveness of a smartphone application for improving measures of adiposity: a randomised clinical trial - EVIDENT II study. Eur J Cardiovasc Nurs 2018;17(6):552–62.

21. Hilliard ME, Hahn A, Ridge AK, et al. User preferences and design recommendations for an mHealth app to promote cystic fibrosis self-management. JMIR Mhealth Uhealth 2014;2(4):e44.

22. De Geest S, Sabaté E. Adherence to long-term therapies: evidence for action. Eur J Cardiovasc Nurs 2003;2:323.

23. Dauw CA, Yi Y, Bierlein MJ, et al. Medication nonadherence and effectiveness of preventive pharmacological therapy for kidney stones. J Urol 2016; 195(3):648–52.

24. Santo K, Richtering SS, Chalmers J, et al. Mobile phone apps to improve medication adherence: a systematic stepwise process to identify high-quality apps. JMIR Mhealth Uhealth 2016;4(4):e132.

25. Mira JJ, Navarro I, Botella F, et al. A Spanish pillbox app for elderly patients taking multiple medications: randomized controlled trial. J Med Internet Res 2014;16(4):e99.

26. Zanetti-Yabur A, Rizzo A, Hayde N, et al. Exploring the usage of a mobile phone application in transplanted patients to encourage medication compliance and education. Am J Surg 2017;214(4):743–7.

27. Duane S, Tandan M, Murphy AW, et al. Using mobile phones to collect patient data: lessons learned from the SIMPle study. JMIR Res Protoc 2017;6(4):e61.

28. Lalloo C, Jibb LA, Rivera J, et al. "There's a pain app for that": review of patient-targeted smartphone applications for pain management. Clin J Pain 2015; 31(6):557–63.

29. Lalloo C, Shah U, Birnie KA, et al. Commercially available smartphone apps to support postoperative pain self-management: scoping review. JMIR Mhealth Uhealth 2017;5(10):e162.

30. Worcester E, Coe F. Web apps and smart bottles. Chicago (IL): University of Chicago Kidney Stones; 2016. Available at: https://kidneystones.uchicago.edu/web-apps-and-smart-bottles/. Accessed July 30, 2018.

31. Borofsky MS, Dauw CA, York N, et al. Accuracy of daily fluid intake measurements using a "smart" water bottle. Urolithiasis 2018;46(4):343–8.

32. Molina WR, Pessoa R, Donalisio da Silva R, et al. A new patient safety smartphone application for prevention of "forgotten" ureteral stents: results from a clinical pilot study in 194 patients. Patient Saf Surg 2017;11(1):10.

33. Bultitude MF, Tiptaft RC, Glass JM, et al. Management of encrusted ureteral stents impacted in upper tract. Urology 2003;62(4):622–6.

34. Duty B, Okhunov Z, Okeke Z, et al. Medical malpractice in endourology: analysis of closed cases from the State of New York. J Urol 2012; 187(2):528–32.

35. Ather MH, Talati J, Biyabani R. Physician responsibility for removal of implants: the case for a computerized program for tracking overdue double-J stents. Tech Urol 2000;6(3):189–92.

36. Lynch MF, Ghani KR, Frost I, et al. Preventing the forgotten ureteral stent: implementation of a web-based stent registry with automatic recall application. Urology 2007;70(3):423–6.

37. Ziemba JB, Ludwig WW, Ruiz L, et al. Preventing the forgotten ureteral stent by using a mobile point-of-care application. J Endourol 2017;31(7):719–24.

38. Cho S, Park TS, Nahapetian TG, et al. Smartphone-based, sensitive μPAD detection of urinary tract infection and gonorrhea. Biosens Bioelectron 2015; 74:601–11.

39. Kamakoti V, Kinnamon D, Choi KH, et al. Fully electronic urine dipstick probe for combinatorial detection of inflammatory biomarkers. Future Sci OA 2018;4(5):FSO301.

40. Zhou J, Dong T. Design of a wearable device for real-time screening of urinary tract infection and kidney disease based on smartphone. Analyst 2018; 143(12):2812–8.

41. Sohn W, Shreim S, Yoon R, et al. Endockscope: using mobile technology to create global point of service endoscopy. J Endourol 2013;27(9): 1154–60.

42. Tse C, Patel RM, Yoon R, et al. The endockscope using next generation smartphones: "a global opportunity". J Endourol 2018;32(8). https://doi.org/10.1089/end.2018.0275.

43. Filson C, Davies B, Eggener SE. The role of social media in urology. AUA Update Ser 2016.

44. Wilkinson SE, Basto MY, Perovic G, et al. The social media revolution is changing the conference experience: analytics and trends from eight international meetings. BJU Int 2015;115(5):839–46.

45. Salem J, Borgmann H, Bultitude M, et al. Online discussion on #kidneystones: a longitudinal assessment of activity, users and content. PLoS One 2016;11(8): e0160863.

46. Sood A, Sarangi S, Pandey A, et al. YouTube as a source of information on kidney stone disease. Urology 2011;77(3):558–62.

47. Traver MA, Passman CM, LeRoy T, et al. Is the Internet a reliable source for dietary recommendations for stone formers? J Endourol 2009;23(4): 715–7.

48. Safir IJ, Gabale S, David SA, et al. Implementation of a tele-urology program for outpatient hematuria referrals: initial results and patient satisfaction. Urology 2016;97:33–9.

49. Chu S, Boxer R, Madison P, et al. Veterans affairs telemedicine: bringing urologic care to remote clinics. Urology 2015;86(2):255–60.

50. Viers BR, Lightner DJ, Rivera ME, et al. Efficiency, satisfaction, and costs for remote video visits following radical prostatectomy: a randomized controlled trial. Eur Urol 2015;68(4):729–35.

51. Park ES, Boedeker BH, Hemstreet JL, et al. The initiation of a preoperative and postoperative telemedicine urology clinic. Stud Health Technol Inform 2011;163:425–7.

52. Canon S, Shera A, Patel A, et al. A pilot study of telemedicine for post-operative urological care in children. J Telemed Telecare 2014;20(8): 427–30.

53. Mobasheri MH, King D, Johnston M, et al. The ownership and clinical use of smartphones by doctors and nurses in the UK: a multicentre survey study. BMJ Innov 2015;1(4):174–81.

54. Sener TE, Butticè S, Sahin B, et al. Whatsapp use in the evaluation of hematuria. Int J Med Inform 2018; 111:17–23.

55. Bauer J, Lee BR, Stoianovici D, et al. Remote percutaneous renal access using a new automated telesurgical robotic system. Telemed J E Health 2001; 7(4):341–6.

56. Saglam R, Muslumanoglu AY, Tokatlı Z, et al. A new robot for flexible ureteroscopy: development and early clinical results (IDEAL stage 1-2b). Eur Urol 2014;66(6):1092–100.

57. Kaler KS, Valley ZA, Bettir KC, et al. Crowdsourcing evaluation of ureteroscopic videos using the post-ureteroscopic lesion scale to assess ureteral injury. J Endourol 2018;32(4):275–81.

58. Lendvay TS, White L, Kowalewski T. Crowdsourcing to assess surgical skill. JAMA Surg 2015;150(11): 1086–7.

Assessing Cost-Effectiveness of New Technologies in Stone Management

David B. Bayne, MD, MPH*, Thomas L. Chi, MD

KEYWORDS

- Cost-effectiveness • Kidney stone surgery • Ureteroscopy • Percutaneous nephrolithotomy
- Shock wave lithotripsy • Disposables • Robotic surgery

KEY POINTS

- With economic pressures rising to provide value-based care, it is important to evaluate the cost-effectiveness of new technologies prior to their implementation.
- The literature demonstrates that at centers where costs of repair and maintenance for reusable ureteroscopes can be controlled, although they may decrease systems and personnel stress for scope care, disposable ureteroscopes may not represent a cost-effective technology.
- To thoroughly assess cost-effectiveness for new technologies in nephrolithiasis, labor costs of treatment, facility costs, and costs associated with clinical outcomes must be taken into account.

INTRODUCTION

Epidemiology and Economic Burden of Stone Disease

In the United States, rates of nephrolithiasis are on the rise. Between 1976 and 1994, prevalence of kidney stones increased in nearly all age groups, independent of race, with an overall rise from 3.8% to 5.2%.[1] It is estimated that from 2007 to 2010, kidney stone prevalence had increased to 8.4%.[2] This rising prevalence has been taxing to the health care system.

In 1993, the estimated annual cost of urolithiasis was $1.83 billion in the United States.[3] This cost was estimated to have increased to $2.07 billion in 2000[4] and is expected reach $4.1 billion in 2030 in part due to the impact of the rising prevalence of diabetes and obesity.[5]

This disease affects both adults and children, and, for pediatric patients alone, estimated hospital charges for kidney stones were as high as $375 million in 2009.[6]

Approximately 1.3 million people in the United States labor force between the ages of 18 years and 64 years receive treatment of nephrolithiasis each year.[7] When considering indirect costs, such as cost of labor, the economic cost of stone disease may be as high as $5.3 billion based on estimates from the year 2000.[7]

Urinary stones represent a costly and morbid disease, and new technologies are constantly being developed for their treatment. With economic pressures rising to provide value-based care, it is important to evaluate the cost-effectiveness of new technologies prior to their implementation. The aim of this review article is to provide an update on technologies that have been developed for kidney stone treatment and provide a framework by which the practicing urologist can assess their cost-effectiveness as it relates to their own

Disclosure Statement: The authors have nothing to disclose.
Urology, University of California San Francisco, San Francisco, CA, USA
* Corresponding author. Urology, University of California San Francisco, 400 Parnassus Avenue, 6th floor Urology Clinics A638, San Francisco, CA 94143.
E-mail address: david.bayne@ucsf.edu

Urol Clin N Am 46 (2019) 303–313
https://doi.org/10.1016/j.ucl.2018.12.011
0094-0143/19/© 2018 Elsevier Inc. All rights reserved.

practice environment. This article highlights areas where the literature provides guidance with regard to cost-effectiveness analysis as well as areas of need for further study.

Assessing Cost

Health care costs have been increasing at dramatic rates since 1970, and health care spending reached $2.7 trillion in 2011.[8] Current costs and future projections of cost increases have led many experts to rethink health care pricing and value.[9] Making accurate estimates on acceptable costs in health care requires assessing and incentivizing delivery of high-value care. Traditional reimbursement in health care is based on a fee-for-service model that tends to focus on intervention rather than outcomes or quality of care provided.[10] Alternative approaches, such as capitation and bundled payments, focus on reducing costs and provide incentive to reduce complications but do not completely align with the incentive to provide value.[10]

Time-driven activity-based costing (TDABC) has been proposed as a method to more accurately assess health care costs and expose opportunities for cost reduction without having a negative impact on outcomes.[11] TDABC focuses specifically on process mapping, where a patient's path through the health care system is recorded to assign costs to each step in the delivery of health care. In doing so, it better assigns dollar amounts to resource costs, such as health care provider labor, in addition to costs of equipment, space, and diagnostics. This better allows for the discovery of opportunities for health care process improvement and more efficient allocation of resources, which is particularly applicable to surgical processes.[12] There are examples of TDABC models in the urology literature exploring treatment of small renal masses,[13] prostate cancer,[14] benign prostatic hypertrophy,[15] and pediatric clinical practices,[16] but TDABC represents a new approach in cost assessments for the surgical treatment of nephrolithiasis.

Although there is a paucity of TDABC literature surrounding the treatment of kidney stones, its approach is valuable in that it encourages a focus on treatment value as defined by efficacy (ie stone-free status and limited morbidity) at a price that is cost-effective. Similarly, the approach of this review article is to present the literature through the lens of a more global assessment of health care delivery. Direct costs (eg, cost of equipment and operative time) and indirect costs (eg, cost of hospitalization, need for retreatment, costs of complications, and postoperative recovery) are both taken into account, where information is available.

TREATMENT MODALITIES

Multiple surgical modalities exist to treat kidney stones. Surgical management of urolithiasis has advanced dramatically alongside the advancement of modern medicine.[17] Treatment of stone disease has shifted from open surgery to minimally invasive and endoscopic approaches, both in the United States[18] and abroad.[19]

Shock Wave

Since its advent 4 decades ago, shock wave lithotripsy (SWL) has revolutionized treatment of kidney stones.[20,21] It provides patients with a noninvasive means to treat their kidney stones and as a result tends to be preferred by patients when successful.[22] SWL also has a shorter operative time with a lower complication rate relative to other stone treatment modalities[23,24] and requires a shorter hospital stay.[23,25] SWL has its treatment limitations, however, in that it has a higher retreatment rate and lower stone-free rate relative to other stone surgery modalities.[23] SWL has a poor success rate when treating dense stones,[26] anatomically abnormal kidneys, stones larger than 10 mm, and lower calyx stones.[27] Many new algorithms and guidelines exist to maximize effectiveness of SWL[28–30] and, when considering cost of SWL, in 2017, Chan and colleagues[31] calculated that a single treatment was calculated at £750 ($967.74) compared with £1261 ($1627.09) and £2658 ($3429.66), respectively, for retrograde ureteroscopic and antegrade percutaneous stone removal for the solitary 10-mm to 20-mm stone in a renal unity with simple anatomy. When SWL is likely to be effective with 1 treatment, it can be a cost-effective option.[31] Based on value, SWL may be cost-effective in instances where risk of complication from other treatment modalities is high and/or when likelihood of success with SWL is high. On the other hand, if risk of complication from SWL is high (patients on high-dose aspirin or antiplatelet therapy, for example[32]) or risk of stone clearance is low, SWL should be avoided in place of other treatment modalities. As a whole, SWL can be a cost-effective approach but its effectiveness is greatly dependent on appropriate patient selection.

Flexible Ureteroscopy

Retrograde intrarenal surgery using flexible ureteroscopy (URS) coupled with laser lithotripsy has been used to treat stones for many years.[33] Comparing shock wave versus URS, location of stone is relevant when determining which approach is more cost-effective. Cone and colleagues[34] found that when looking at treatment of ureteral stones, URS with laser lithotripsy was more cost-effective than shock wave. This was confirmed for distal ureteral stones by Wolf and colleagues.[22] Koo and colleagues,[35] on the other hand, showed that URS was less effective than shock wave when considering renal stones. A systemic review looking specifically and URS versus shock wave showed that overall URS is less costly than SWL per procedure with better stone-free rates.[36] This was confirmed in a recent meta-analysis, which also showed little difference in complication or retreatment rates.[37]

There exists substantial variability in costing from institution to institution,[38] however, and these institution-specific factors may greatly influence cost-effectiveness of flexible URS. Many investigators have expressed need to study treatment pathways in utilization of shock wave versus URS versus a combination of both in an attempt to standardize treatment.[39] This standardization in addition to more efficient approach to costing could lead to improvements in treatment efficiency and reduction in costs when looking at utilization of shock wave versus URS.

Traditional flexible URS employs reusable flexible scopes requiring eventual scope repairs and maintenance in addition to consideration of the costs of disposable adjunct equipment, such as laser fibers, baskets, wires, and exchange catheters.[40] Flexible ureteroscopes tend to deteriorate in visualization and deflection[40,41] as operative time and case count per scope increases.[42] This deterioration has been demonstrated in reusable flexible ureteroscopes from multiple manufacturers.[43] In addition to cost of repairs,[44] cost of sterilization and operating room time delay can factor into flexible URS costs.[45]

Disposable ureteroscopes

With the advent of disposable ureteroscopes, debates have ensued regarding cost-effectiveness of disposable scopes relative to reusable scopes. The concept of a disposable ureteroscope dates back as far back as 1996, when a disposable shaft rigid ureteroscope was first described in the literature,[46] but the modern era of disposable flexible ureteroscopes traces to Boylu and colleagues,[47] who published their in vitro experience with the SemiFlex Scope in 2009. Designed with convenience of use, concern for bacterial cross-contamination with suboptimal sterilization, and cost in mind, disposable flexible ureteroscopes have become more popularized since the introduction of the PolyScope (PolyDiagnost, Hallbergmoos,

Germany), LithoVue (Boston Scientific, Marlborough, Massachusetts, United States), and Uscope (Pusen, Zhuhai City, Guangdong China), first described in the literature in 2010, 2016, and 2018, respectively.[48–50] Clinical outcomes have been found equivalent between disposable and reusable scopes,[51] and costs have been studied most extensively for the LithoVue disposable ureteroscope. For LithoVue, cost has been demonstrated to range from $1300 to $3180 per procedure for disposable scopes.[51] The range in cost of disposable scopes are based on the manufacturer suggested retail price of $3180 and the estimated market price of $1300.[51] Martin and colleagues[52] use the market price of $1500 per disposable ureteroscope in their cost-benefit analysis, concluding that disposable ureteroscopes may be most cost-beneficial at centers with lower surgical volume but, with rising numbers of ureteroscopic cases per year, use of reusable ureteroscopes may be associated with cost savings per case. Isaacson and colleagues[45] used process mapping in a TDABC study to exploring labor and equipment costs for reusable ureteroscope processing. They determined that this added an additional cost of $139 per case for reusable scopes for a total cost of $965 per case for reusable flexible ureteroscopes at their institution, a high-volume stone treatment center. This was higher than the calculated per case costs of $436 to $708 in prior studies,[51,53] but utilization of process mapping accounted for additional costs compared with other costing studies. Isaacson and colleagues[45] also determined the opportunity to reduce reusable scope cost per case by improving efficiency in scope drying. Ultimately, when both purchase and maintenance costs were taken into account, cost of use for reusable flexible ureteroscopes was determined to range from $1212 to $1743 per procedure. The additional costs required to resterilize, maintain, and repair reusable scopes seems to greatly influence the cost-effectiveness of flexible URS when comparing reusable to disposable scopes,[54,55] because these costs do not exist with disposable scopes. Overall, the literature demonstrates that at centers where costs of repair and maintenance for reusable ureteroscopes can be controlled, although they may decrease systems and personnel stress for scope care, disposable ureteroscopes may not represent a cost-effective technology.

Laser fibers

Laser fiber costs must also factor into URS cost-effectiveness evaluation for stone treatment. When looking at cost-effectiveness of reusable versus disposable laser fibers, Kundsen and colleagues[56] show that reusable laser fibers were overall cost-effective compared with disposable fibers. They note that this is largely dependent on initial cost of the reusable fiber and that reusable fibers with a high initial cost, specifically the Lum 270 (Lumenis, Yokneam, Israel), were found cost-effective as a reusable fiber in their study. Disposable laser fibers have been demonstrated to reduce damage to ureteroscopes and, therefore, may provide cost savings overall during URS.[57]

Newer rounded-tip laser fibers have been shown to reduce working sheath trauma from laser fiber insertion.[58] Some investigators have found, however, these specialty designed laser fibers have a rapid degradation,[59] which limits their value outside of select situation, where likelihood of laser insertion trauma is high given their overall higher cost compared with flat-tipped laser fibers.

Although the Ho:YAG laser has become the laser of choice for lithotripsy due to its stone fragmentation efficiency and patient safety profile,[60] new technologies both in holmium and other laser types have been developed. Since the 2000s, Ho:YAG lithotripter manufacturers have introduced long-pulse lithotripsy, which limits laser tip fiber degradation and stone retropulsion.[61] It is believed that long-pulse lithotripsy also produces smaller residual fragments to make treatment more efficient.[60] Introduced in 2017, Moses technology (Lumenis, Yokneam, Israel) refers to a high power 120-W Ho:YAG lithotripter that aims to fragment stones more rapidly with faster treatment times compared with traditional lasers. When studied, however, some investigators have found that these differences were not found statistically significant.[60] In addition, the Moses technology is a more costly laser treatment platform.[62] Burst laser lithotripsy is a mode of Ho:YAG lithotripsy that has been shown to have more ablative efficiency than standard laser lithotripsy at the same energy settings[63]; however, this has not been demonstrated in vivo. Similarly, pulsed thulium laser has demonstrated potential for fragmentation[64] with reduced retropulsion in vitro,[65] but it has not been well studied in patients.

These new laser fiber platforms have promising potential in that they may reduce operative time and, therefore, operating room costs with more efficient stone fragmentation; however, they remain understudied as far as cost-effectiveness. There are not enough clinical data and, in many cases, no established price point to determine cost-effectiveness, and this area of new technology remains wide open for study.

Additional disposables

When considering stone removal, costs of additional disposables, such as ureteral access sheaths, wires, stents, and stone retrieval baskets, must be taken into account. Access sheathes range in price from $140 to $278, wires from $18 to $138, and stents from $12 to $18, and baskets can be priced as high as $611.[66] Over the course of 100 cases, Collins and colleagues[40] found that during URS, the costs of disposables was as high as £23,053 for disposables, not including the cost of laser fibers. Chasseigne and colleagues[67] were able to demonstrate a potential for annual cost savings of €100,000 ($113,682.20) for urologic, gynecologic, and general surgery procedures by eliminating the cost of wasted surgical supplies, and they propose price labeling of equipment and care provider education to reduce these costs. Although many investigators have indicated that the cost to the environment on waste generated from disposable devices must be taken into account, these costs are difficult to quantify. Given that cost of disposables varies greatly from institution to institution, the general viewpoint of the authors is that disposables should be used only when necessary, keeping in mind procedural efficiency and cost reduction.

Percutaneous Nephrolithotomy

Percutaneous nephrolithotomy (PCNL) has replaced open stone surgery for the removal of larger upper tract stones. It carries with it the advantage of improved stone clearance rates relative to shock wave and URS. PCNL has been shown associated with increased stone clearance rates compared with URS with proximal impacted stones, although hospitalization times are longer with PCNL.[68]

When considering the cost of PCNL, several aspects of the procedure must be taken into account. The utilization of interventional radiology to obtain renal access prior to surgery results in higher cost for PCNL.[69] The median cost of admission for PCNLs where access was obtained by a urologist was found to be $10,173 in comparison to a median cost of $11,287, when access was obtained by a radiologist. Urologist-obtained access was also associated with a shorter hospital stay and a lower rate of complications.[69] Tomaszewski and colleagues[70] also found that stone-free rate was higher in cases of urologists obtaining access relative to radiologists.

Access tract dilation methods also affect cost, with higher costs associated with Amplatz serial dilators relative to metal serial or metal single-step dilators,[71,72] without any difference in complication rates.[73,74] Single-step balloon dilators are associated with greater expense but shorter procedural length and reduced radiation exposure.[74]

In general for PCNL, urologists obtaining their own access using the most efficient set of disposables seems the most cost-effective approach to the procedure. New technologies and approaches, however, discussed later, should be factored into these assessments.

Ultrasound-guided percutaneous nephrolithotomy

Imaging modality used to gain access also has an impact on cost in PCNL, with Hudnall and colleagues[75] showing ultrasound a more cost-effective imaging modality. This cost comparison study showed that ultrasound guidance reduced operating room time from 98 minutes to 145 minutes for ultrasound and fluoroscopy, respectively. Ultrasound guidance also eliminated the need for a radiology technician. In total, use of ultrasound for guidance of PCNL may result in as much as a 30% savings compared with fluoroscopy,[75] without any associated increase in complication rates or worsening of clinical outcomes.[76] As an adjunct, retrograde ultrasound contrast injection has been demonstrated to facilitate ultrasound-guided PCNL[77] by providing the operative surgeon with a clearer collecting system target for renal access and dilation, although cost benefit analysis is still needed to determine cost-effectiveness of this novel use of contrast agents.

Tubeless approaches to percutaneous nephrolithotomy

Totally tubeless PCNL has been shown to reduce costs relative to traditional PCNL completed with a stent or nephrostomy tube.[78] Mean operating costs were found $2380 for totally tubeless PCNL in comparison to $2845 for traditional PCNL with a nephrostomy tube or stent. In the totally tubeless group, costs were additionally reduced for room and board, pharmacy, laboratory testing, radiology, stent removal, management of postoperative complications, and secondary treatment procedures.[78] Totally tubeless PCNL is generally performed, however, only in cases of no significant bleeding encountered and where the patient and was found stone-free with visual inspection at the end of the case.[78] Short of a totally tubeless approach, PCNL performed with a stent rather than a nephrostomy tube placed at the end of the procedure to provide renal drainage was found associated with reduced hospital stay and reduced analgesic requirement, providing evidence that this approach may be more cost-effective than PCNL performed with a nephrostomy tube. Again, patient selection is an important factor, given that generally tubeless

stented PCNL is performed in cases of minimal bleeding, no more than 1 access tract, and minimal residual stone burden.[79]

Mini–percutaneous nephrolithotomy

Over time, urologists have begun to perform PCNL through smaller access tracts. Standard PCNLs are performed through tracts 24F to 30F in diameter, whereas mini-PCNLs are performed through tracts 14F to 20F, ultra–mini-PCNLs are performed through tracts 11F to 13F, and micro-PCNLs are performed through tracts as small as 4.8F, with published cost of equipment priced at $8000, $8800, and $8679, respectively, for mini-PCNL, ultra–mini-PCNL, and micro-PCNL capital equipment.[80] Although smaller access tracts are associated with reduced complications, they also are associated with a slightly lower stone-free rate.[80,81] The balance of fewer complications against decreased stone-free rate may weigh into the cost evaluation. Compared with flexible URS, Schoenthaler and colleagues[82] show that for stones 10 mm to 20 mm, median cost for disposables and endoscopes for ultra–mini-PCNL was €656 ($745.76) compared with flexible URS cost of €1160 ($1318.71), with no difference in operating times, length of stay, and complications.[82]

Overall, PCNL is the most expensive of the procedures to treat stone disease when considering SWL, URS, or PCNL, but its cost-effectiveness is directly affected by clinical efficacy. PCNL should be used in cases of SWL and URS believed to have a low likelihood of success, such as for very large stones. Lower poles stones with unfavorable anatomy for shock wave or URS should also lead to consideration of PCNL. In cases of urologists having expertise in gaining access, cost-effectiveness favors urologist-obtained access over interventional radiologist–obtained access and ultrasound guidance over fluoroscopy.

Robotic-Assisted Laparoscopic Surgery for Stones

Open stone surgery has largely been replaced by endoscopic and other minimally invasive treatments of kidney stones. In a retrospective study comparing open stone renal surgery with percutaneous renal procedures, percutaneous procedures were found more cost-effective in that they reduced duration of anesthesia, hospitalization length, and transfusion requirement.[83] When comparing open stone surgery SWL, and PCNL, Charig and colleagues[84] found that procedural costs for SWL were more expensive than open surgery and PCNL. This same study, however, found that open surgery was more costly to the health system than nonopen treatment options, if taking into account cost of hospitalization and outpatient visits.[84]

In rare instances of congenital abnormalities and requirements of simultaneous reconstruction, the American Urological Association guidelines support the use of open surgery for kidney stones.[85] The open approaches in these rare circumstances, however, are being replaced with laparoscopic and robotic-assisted techniques that warrant discussion. These approaches may be more cost-effective in that they allow more than 1 procedure to be performed with 1 visit to the operating room.

Similar to open surgery, robotic-assisted laparoscopic surgery for kidney stone disease is not recommended for straightforward kidney stone surgery.[85] Procedures, such as robotic anatrophic nephrolithotomy, pyelolithotomy, and nephrolithotomy, have been shown both safe and effective.[86,87]

Although not much has been published regarding cost of robotic stone surgery, examples from the oncology literature provide parallels for cost analysis. Robotic surgery has been found to increase anesthesia time and operating room costs.[88] There is significant variation in robotic prostatectomy cost, for example, with mean hospital costs per procedure ranging from $2837 to $25,906. These costs tend to decrease as hospital robotic case volume increases.[89] When looking at the cost of robotic cystectomy compared with open cystectomy, robotic cystectomy costs approximately $2000 more per procedure, with the primary cost drivers operative time, length of stay, and case volume.[90] Nevertheless, robotic cystectomy may be more cost-effective when considering that the robotic approach results in fewer complications compared with the open approach.[91] Bijlani and colleagues[92] found that robotic prostatectomy relative to open prostatectomy may result in cost savings over time when considering decreased hospital stay, lower complication rate, and a faster return to work date, resulting in an estimated overall savings of $1202 for robotic relative to open prostatectomy. Buse and colleagues[93] also found similar cost savings for robotic partial nephrectomy relative to open partial nephrectomy in experienced centers due to reduction in complications and inpatient costs with robotic surgery. Mean inhospital costs for robotic partial nephrectomy were $14,824 compared with $15094 for open partial nephrectomy. Hughes and colleagues[94] found that when considering overall costs to the health care system at 360 days and 1080 days after surgery, robotic prostatectomy was significantly less costly relative to open prostatectomy due to reductions in inpatient admissions and

hospitalization days. They also demonstrated a reduction in cost for robotic partial nephrectomy relative to open partial nephrectomy, although these differences were not statistically significant. In addition to reductions in hospital stay, robotic prostatectomy also may reduce transfusion rates.[95]

Although robotic or laparoscopic assisted stone removal surgeries have not been evaluated from a cost-effectiveness standpoint, drawing from these examples, it is reasonable to perform robotic or laparoscopic surgery for kidney stones where the alternative treatment is open surgery in anticipation of cost reductions from limiting patient morbidity and recovery time.

DIAGNOSTIC IMAGING

Diagnostic imaging is crucial in the management and treatment of kidney stone disease but is not without cost to the health care system. Compared with the standard cost of a kidney, ureter, and bladder radiograph, CT scans cost approximately 10 times that amount, ultrasound costs 5 times that amount, and MRI costs up to 30 times that amount.[96] Ultrasound has come to be accepted as a reasonable first-line imaging to diagnose kidney stones, but preferred presurgical imaging for kidney stone diagnosis, according to the American Urological Association guidelines, is CT imaging.[85,96] In a comparison of diagnostic imaging for kidney stones in the emergency department (ED), Melnikow and colleagues[97] found that point-of-care ultrasound (POCUS) performed by an ED provider was priced at a mean of $98, radiology ultrasound was priced at a mean of $122, and CT scan was priced at a mean of $220; there was no statistically significant difference in overall 7-day inpatient and outpatient costs when comparing need for additional diagnostic studies through the course of the 7 days. Metzler and colleagues[98] found that although patients obtaining ultrasonography as initial imaging do not experience treatment delay, a majority end up getting CT scan eventually, and patients obtaining POCUS by an ED provider were as much as 2.6 times more likely to get a CT scan compared with patients getting a formal radiologist ultrasound at diagnosis, perhaps pointing to radiologic ultrasound as a more cost-effective initial imaging study relative to POCUS. Although expensive, there are some indications for MRI imaging in the diagnosis of kidney stones. Birsbane and colleagues[96] propose use of MRI in those cases of ultrasonography that is not diagnostic but when patients cannot be exposed to radiation, such as in pregnancy.

KIDNEY STONE PREVENTION

Although this article focuses mostly on the cost-effectiveness of new technologies in the treatment of urinary stones, the concept of new approaches from a nonsurgical vantage point warrants discussion, given the significant potential for impact. The opportunity to prevent kidney stone formation represents perhaps the most cost-effective means to treat nephrolithiasis from a population perspective, although it may be the most understudied. In a study looking at the cost-saving effects of the hypothetical intervention of 2 L of fluid intake daily on a population level, 100% compliance would reduce costs of kidney stone treatment by $273 million. A compliance of only 25% would prevent 2316 stone events and reduce costs by $68 million.[99] In addition to surgical treatments, preventative medical management when appropriate can be both cost-effective and efficient in preventing stone formation. A 1996 study by Parks and Coe[100] demonstrated potential cost savings of up to $3 million annually in 1092 patients, with medical prevention of stone events primarily through cost reductions from the prevention of hospitalizations and surgical procedures. To this end, medical prophylaxis may be particularly cost-effective with patients at risk for multiple stone episodes a year.[101]

The role of urease-producing bacteria in urinary tract infections in kidney stone formation is well established. There are instances, however, where patients present with kidney stones as a sequela of non–urease-producing bacteria. Tavichakorntrakool and colleagues[102] found non–urease-producing Escherichia coli in 69% of kidney stones taken from PCNL patients. Bauza and colleagues[103] hypothesize that there is opportunity for cost saving in the prevention of kidney stones, with a focus on preventing urinary tract infections in the general population. Consideration for developing better prevention strategies is an area of research that has lagged far behind development of new technologies in the field of urinary stone disease. From a global viewpoint, these preventative strategies may in the long term yield the greatest cost-effectiveness and warrant additional study and investment.

SUMMARY

Diagnosis, treatment, and follow-up are all influential in determining the overall cost to the health care system for kidney stones. To thoroughly assess cost-effectiveness for new technologies in nephrolithiasis, labor costs of treatment, facility costs, and costs associated with clinical outcomes must be taken into account. The most cost-effective strategy also changes between different institutions as well as between different sizes, locations, and types of stones. New innovations in the field of nephrolithiasis have been abundant, including disposable ureteroscopes, ultrasound-guided approaches to PCNL, and advanced laser lithotripters. Identifying cost-effective treatment strategies encourages practitioners to be thoughtful about providing value-based high-quality care and remains on important principle in the treatment of urinary stone disease.

REFERENCES

1. Stamatelou KK, Francis ME, Jones CA, et al. Time trends in reported prevalence of kidney stones in the United States: 1976-1994. Kidney Int 2003; 63(5):1817–23.
2. Scales CD Jr, Smith AC, Hanley JM, et al, Urologic Diseases in America Project. Prevalence of kidney stones in the United States. Eur Urol 2012;62(1): 160–5.
3. Clark JY, Thompson IM, Optenberg SA. Economic impact of urolithiasis in the United States. J Urol 1995;154(6):2020–4.
4. Wei JT, Calhoun E, Jacobsen SJ. Urologic diseases in America project: urolithiasis. J Urol 2005;173(4): 1256–61.
5. Antonelli JA, Maalouf NM, Pearle MS, et al. Use of the national health and nutrition examination survey to calculate the impact of obesity and diabetes on cost and prevalence of urolithiasis in 2030. Eur Urol 2014;66(4):724–9.
6. Wang HHS, Wiener JS, Lipkin ME, et al. Estimating the nationwide, hospital based economic impact of pediatric urolithiasis. J Urol 2015;193(5):1855–9.
7. Saigal CS, Joyce G, Timilsina AR. Direct and indirect costs of nephrolithiasis in an employed population: opportunity for disease management? Kidney Int 2005;68(4):1808–14.
8. Moses H, Matheson DHM, Dorsey ER, et al. The anatomy of health care in the United States. JAMA 2013;310(18):1947.
9. Porter ME. What is value in health care? N Engl J Med 2010;363(26):2477–81.
10. Porter ME, Kaplan RS. How to pay for health care. Harv Bus Rev 2016;94(7–8):88–98, 100, 134.
11. Kaplan RS, Porter ME. How to solve the cost crisis in health care. Harv Bus Rev 2011. https://doi.org/ 10.1037/e632682011-011.
12. Porter ME, Lee TL. The strategy that will fix health care - harvard business review. Harv Bus Rev 2013;(I):1–39.
13. Laviana AA, Tan HJ, Hu JC, et al. Retroperitoneal versus transperitoneal robotic-assisted laparoscopic partial nephrectomy: a matched-pair,

bicenter analysis with cost comparison using time-driven activity-based costing. Curr Opin Urol 2018; 28(2):108–14.

14. Ilg AM, Laviana AA, Kamrava M, et al. Time-driven activity-based costing of low-dose-rate and high-dose-rate brachytherapy for low-risk prostate cancer. Brachytherapy 2016;15(6):760–7.

15. Kaplan AL, Agarwal N, Setlur NP, et al. Measuring the cost of care in benign prostatic hyperplasia using time-driven activity-based costing (TDABC). Healthc (Amst) 2015;3(1):43–8.

16. Merguerian PA, Grady R, Waldhausen J, et al. Optimizing value utilizing Toyota Kata methodology in a multidisciplinary clinic. J Pediatr Urol 2015;11:228. e1-6.

17. Shah J, Whitfield HN. Urolithiasis through the ages. BJU Int 2002;89(8):801–10.

18. Ghani KR, Sammon JD, Karakiewicz PI, et al. Trends in surgery for upper urinary tract calculi in the USA using the Nationwide Inpatient Sample: 1999-2009. BJU Int 2013;112(2):224–30.

19. Marchini GS, Mello MF, Levy R, et al. Contemporary trends of inpatient surgical management of stone disease: national analysis in an economic growth scenario. J Endourol 2015;29(8):956–62.

20. Chaussy C, Schmiedt E, Jocham D, et al. First clinical experience with extracorporeally induced destruction of kidney stones by shock waves. J Urol 1981;127:417–20.

21. Madaan S, Joyce AD. Limitations of extracorporeal shock wave lithotripsy. Curr Opin Urol 2007;17(2): 109–13.

22. Wolf JS, Carroll PR, Stoller ML. Cost-effectiveness v patient preference in the choice of treatment for distal ureteral calculi: a literature-based decision analysis. J Endourol 1995;9(3):243–8.

23. Srisubat A, Potisat S, Lojanapiwat B, et al. Extracorporeal shock wave lithotripsy (ESWL) versus percutaneous nephrolithotomy (PCNL) or retrograde intrarenal surgery (RIRS) for kidney stones (Review). Cochrane Database Syst Rev 2014;11: 1–43.

24. Pearle MS, Lingeman JE, Leveillee R, et al. Prospective, randomized trial comparing shock wave lithotripsy and ureteroscopy for lower pole caliceal calculi 1 cm or less. J Urol 2005;173(6): 2005–9.

25. Albala DM, Assimos DG, Clayman RV, et al. Lower pole I: a prospective randomized trial of extracorporeal shock wave lithotripsy and percutaneous nephrostolithotomy for lower pole nephrolithiasis-initial results. J Urol 2001;166(6):2072–80.

26. Kim SC, Burns EK, Lingeman JE, et al. Cystine calculi: correlation of CT-visible structure, CT number, and stone morphology with fragmentation by shock wave lithotripsy. Urol Res 2007;35(6): 319–24.

27. Al-ansari A, As-sadiq K, Al-said S, et al. Prognostic factors of success of extracorporeal shock wave lithotripsy (ESWL) in the treatment of renal stones. Int Urol Nephrol 2006;24:63–7.

28. Tran TY, McGillen K, Cone EB, et al. Triple D score is a reportable predictor of shockwave lithotripsy stone-free rates. J Endourol 2015;29(2):226–30.

29. Park HS, Gong MK, Yoon CY, et al. Computed tomography-based novel prediction model for the outcome of shockwave lithotripsy in proximal ureteral stones. J Endourol 2016;30(7):810–6.

30. El-Nahas AR, El-Assmy AM, Awad BA, et al. Extracorporeal shockwave lithotripsy for renal stones in pediatric patients: a multivariate analysis model for estimating the stone-free probability. Int J Urol 2013;20(12):1205–10.

31. Chan LH, Hons B, Good DW, et al. Primary SWL is an efficient and cost-effective treatment. J Endourol 2017;31(5):510–6.

32. Schnabel MJ, Gierth M, Bründl J, et al. Antiplatelet and anticoagulative medication during shockwave lithotripsy. J Endourol 2014;28(9):1034–9.

33. Beaghler M, Poon M, Ruckle H, et al. Complications employing the holmium:YAG laser. J Endourol 1998;12(6):533–5.

34. Cone EB, Pareek G, Ursiny M, et al. Cost-effectiveness comparison of ureteral calculi treated with ureteroscopic laser lithotripsy versus shockwave lithotripsy. World J Urol 2017;35(1):161–6.

35. Koo V, Young M, Thompson T, et al. Cost-effectiveness and efficiency of shockwave lithotripsy vs flexible ureteroscopic holmium:yttrium-aluminium-garnet laser lithotripsy in the treatment of lower pole renal calculi. BJU Int 2011;108(11):1913–6.

36. Matlaga BR, Jansen JP, Meckley LM, et al. Economic outcomes of treatment for ureteral and renal stones: a systematic literature review. J Urol 2012; 188(2):449–54.

37. Geraghty RM, Jones P, Herrmann TRW, et al. Ureteroscopy is more cost effective than shock wave lithotripsy for stone treatment: systematic review and meta-analysis. World J Urol 2018. https://doi.org/10.1007/s00345-018-2320-9.

38. San Juan J, Hou H, Ghani KR, et al. HHS public access. J Urol 2018;199(5):1277–82.

39. McClinton S, Cameron S, Starr K, et al. TISU: Extracorporeal shockwave lithotripsy, as first treatment option, compared with direct progression to ureteroscopic treatment, for ureteric stones: study protocol for a randomised controlled trial. Trials 2018;19(1):1–11.

40. Collins JW, Keeley FX Jr, Timoney A. Cost analysis of flexible ureterorenoscopy. BJU Int 2004;93(7): 1023–6.

41. Afane JS, Olweny EO, Bercowsky E, et al. Flexible ureteroscopes: a single center evaluation of the durability and function of the new endoscopes smaller than 9Fr. J Urol 2000;164(4):1164–8.

42. Monga M, Best S, Venkatesh R, et al. Durability of flexible ureteroscopes: a randomized, prospective study. J Urol 2006;176(1):137–41.

43. Knudsen B, Miyaoka R, Shah K, et al. Durability of the next-generation flexible fiberoptic ureteroscopes: a randomized prospective multi-institutional clinical trial. Urology 2010;75(3):534–8.

44. Kramolowsky E, McDowell Z, Moore B, et al. Cost analysis of flexible ureteroscope repairs: evaluation of 655 procedures in a community-based practice. J Endourol 2016;30(3):254–6.

45. Isaacson D, Ahmad T, Metzler I, et al. Defining the costs of reusable flexible ureteroscope reprocessing using time-driven activity-based costing. J Endourol 2017;31(10):1026–31.

46. D'Amico F, Belis J. Treatment of ureteral calculi with an 8.3-Fr. disposable shaft rigid ureteroscope. Tech Urol 1996;2(3):126–9.

47. Boylu U, Oommen M, Thomas R, et al. In vitro comparison of a disposable flexible ureteroscope and conventional flexible ureteroscopes. J Urol 2009; 182(5):2347–51.

48. Bader MJ, Gratzke C, Walther S, et al. The polyscope: a modular design, semidisposable flexible ureterorenoscope system. J Endourol 2010;24(7): 1061–6.

49. Leveillee RJ, Kelly EF. Impressive performance: new disposable digital ureteroscope allows for extreme lower pole access and use of 365 μm holmium laser fiber. J Endourol Case Rep 2016;2(1): 114–6.

50. Salvadó JA, Olivares R, Cabello JM, et al. Retrograde intrarenal surgery using the single – use flexible ureteroscope Uscope 3022 (PUSEN TM): evaluation of clinical results. Cent European J Urol 2018;202–7. https://doi.org/10.5173/ceju. 2018.1653.

51. Mager R, Kurosch M, Höfner T, et al. Clinical outcomes and costs of reusable and single-use flexible ureterorenoscopes: a prospective cohort study. Urolithiasis 2018;46(6):587–93.

52. Martin CJ, McAdams SB, Abdul-Muhsin H, et al. The economic implications of a reusable flexible digital ureteroscope: a cost-benefit analysis. J Urol 2017;197(3):730–5.

53. Tosoian JJ, Ludwig W, Sopko N, et al. The effect of repair costs on the profitability of a ureteroscopy program. J Endourol 2015;29(4):406–9.

54. Hennessey DB, Fojecki G, Papa N, et al. Single use disposable digital flexible ureteroscopes: an ex-vivo assessment and cost analysis. BJU Int 2018; 121:55–61.

55. Taguchi K, Usawachintachit M, Tzou DT, et al. Micro-costing analysis demonstrates comparable costs for lithovue compared to reusable flexible fiberoptic ureteroscopes. J Endourol 2018. https:// doi.org/10.1089/end.2017.0523.

56. Knudsen B, Pedro R, Hinck B, et al. Durability of reusable holmium:YAG laser fibers: a multicenter study. J Urol 2011;185(1):160–3.

57. Chapman RA, Somani BK, Robertson A, et al. Decreasing cost of flexible ureterorenoscopy: single-use laser fiber cost analysis. Urology 2014; 83(5):1003–5.

58. Shin RH, Lautz JM, Cabrera FJ, et al. Evaluation of novel ball-tip holmium laser fiber: impact on ureteroscope performance and fragmentation efficiency. J Endourol 2016;30(2):189–94.

59. Kronenberg P, Traxer O. Lithotripsy performance of specially designed laser fiber tips. J Urol 2016; 195(5):1606–12.

60. Kronenberg P, Somani B. Advances in lasers for the treatment of stones — a systematic review. Current urology reports 2018;19(6):45.

61. Bell JR, Penniston KL, Nakada SY. In vitro comparison of holmium lasers: evidence for shorter fragmentation time and decreased retropulsion using a modern variable-pulse laser. Urology 2017;107: 37–42.

62. Kastin A, Goldin O, Kravtsov A, et al. Initial Clinical experience with a modulated holmium laser pulse — moses technology : does it enhance laser lithotripsy efficacy ? Rambam Maimonides Med J 2017;8(4):1–5.

63. Kronenberg P, Traxer O. Mp22-13 burst laser lithotripsy – a novel lithotripsy mode. J Urol 2016; 195(4):e258.

64. Fried NM. Thulium fiber laser lithotripsy: an in vitro analysis of stone fragmentation using a modulated 110-watt Thulium fiber laser at 1.94 ??m. Lasers Surg Med 2005;37(1):53–8.

65. Kamal W, Kallidonis P, Koukiou G, et al. Stone retropulsion with Ho: YAG and Tm: YAG lasers: a clinical practice-oriented experimental study. J Endourol 2016;30(11):1145–9.

66. Gurbuz C, Atiş G, Arikan O, et al. The cost analysis of flexible ureteroscopic lithotripsy in 302 cases. Urolithiasis 2014;42(2):155–8.

67. Chasseigne V, Leguelinel-Blache G, Nguyen TL, et al. Assessing the costs of disposable and reusable supplies wasted during surgeries. Int J Surg 2018;53:18–23.

68. Bozkurt IH, Yonguc T, Arslan B, et al. Minimally invasive surgical treatment for large impacted upper ureteral stones: Ureteroscopic lithotripsy or percutaneous nephrolithotomy? Can Urol Assoc J 2015;9(3–4):122.

69. Speed JM, Wang Y, Leow JJ, et al. The effect of physician specialty obtaining access for percutaneous nephrolithotomy on perioperative costs and outcomes. J Endourol 2017;31(11):1152–6.

70. Tomaszewski JJ, Ortiz TD, Gayed BA, et al. Renal access by urologist or radiologist during percutaneous nephrolithotomy. J Endourol 2010;24(11): 1733–7.

71. Arslan B, Fatih M, Ozkan A, et al. A comparison of Amplatz dilators and metal dilators for tract dilatation in mini - percutaneous nephrolithotomy. Int Urol Nephrol 2017;49(4):581–5.

72. Ozok HU, Sagnak L, Senturk AB, et al. A comparison of metal telescopic dilators and amplatz dilators for nephrostomy tract dilation in percutaneous nephrolithotomy. J Endourol 2012; 26(6):630–4.

73. Falahatkar S, Neiroomand H, Akbarpour M, et al. One-shot versus metal telescopic dilation technique for tract creation in percutaneous nephrolithotomy: comparison of safety and efficacy. J Endourol 2009;23(4):615–8.

74. Li Y, Yang L, Xu P, et al. One-shot versus gradual dilation technique for tract creation in percutaneous nephrolithotomy: a systematic review and meta-analysis. Urol Res 2013;41(5):443–8.

75. Hudnall M, Usawachintachit M, Metzler I, et al. Ultrasound guidance reduces percutaneous nephrolithotomy cost compared to fluoroscopy. Urology 2017;103:52–8.

76. Usawachintachit M, Masic S, Allen IE, et al. Adopting ultrasound guidance for prone percutaneous nephrolithotomy: evaluating the learning curve for the experienced surgeon. J Endourol 2016;30(8): 856–63.

77. Usawachintachit M, Tzou DT, Mongan J, et al. Feasibility of retrograde ureteral contrast injection to guide ultrasonographic percutaneous renal access in the nondilated collecting system. J Endourol 2017;31(2):129–34.

78. Choi SW, Kim KS, Kim JH, et al. Totally tubeless versus standard percutaneous nephrolithotomy for renal stones: analysis of clinical outcomes and cost. J Endourol 2014;28(12):1487–94.

79. Garofalo M, Pultrone CV, Schiavina R, et al. Tubeless procedure reduces hospitalization and pain after percutaneous nephrolithotomy: results of a multivariable analysis. Urol Res 2013;41(4):347–53.

80. Wright A, Rukin N, Smith D, et al. "Mini, ultra, micro" - Nomenclature and cost of these new minimally invasive percutaneous nephrolithotomy (PCNL) techniques. Ther Adv Urol 2016;8(2):142–6.

81. Mishra S, Sharma R, Garg C, et al. Prospective comparative study of miniperc and standard PNL for treatment of 1 to 2 cm size renal stone. BJU international 2011;108(6):896–900.

82. Schoenthaler M, Wilhelm K, Hein S, et al. Ultra-mini PCNL versus flexible ureteroscopy: a matched analysis of treatment costs (endoscopes and disposables) in patients with renal stones 10–20 mm. World J Urol 2015;33(10):1601–5.

83. Brown MW, Carson CC, Dunnick NRWJ. Comparison of the costs and morbidity of percutaneous and open flank procedures. J Urol 1986;135(6): 1150–2.

84. Charig CR, Webb DR, Payne SR, et al. Comparison of treatment of renal calculi by open surgery, percutaneous nephrolithotomy, and extracorporeal shockwave lithotripsy. Br Med J (Clin Res Ed) 1986; 292(6524):879–82.

85. Assimos D, Krambeck A, Miller N. American Urological Association (AUA) Guideline: Surgical Management of Stones. J Urol 2016;196(4):1161–9.

86. Madi R, Hemal A. Robotic pyelolithotomy, extended pyelolithotomy, nephrolithotomy, and anatrophic nephrolithotomy. J Endourol 2018;32: 73–81.

87. Swearingen R, Sood A, Madi R, et al. Zero-fragment nephrolithotomy: a multi-center evaluation of robotic pyelolithotomy and nephrolithotomy for treating renal stones. Eur Urol 2017;72(6): 1014–21.

88. Sugihara T, Yasunaga H, Horiguchi H, et al. Robot-assisted versus other types of radical prostatectomy: Population-based safety and cost comparison in Japan, 2012-2013. Cancer Sci 2014; 105(11):1421–6.

89. Cole AP, Leow JJ, Chang SL, et al. Surgeon and hospital level variation in the costs of robot-assisted radical prostatectomy. J Urol 2016; 196(4):1090–5.

90. Bansal SS, Dogra T, Smith PW, et al. Cost analysis of open radical cystectomy versus robot-assisted radical cystectomy. BJU Int 2018; 121(3):437–44.

91. Michels C, Wijburg CJ, Leijte E, et al. A cost-effectiveness modeling study of robot-assisted (RARC) versus open radical cystectomy (ORC) for bladder cancer to inform future research. Eur Urol Focus 2018. [Epub ahead of print].

92. Bijlani A, Hebert AE, Davitian M, et al. A multidimensional analysis of prostate surgery costs in the united states: robotic-assisted versus retropubic radical prostatectomy. Value Health 2016;19(4):391–403.

93. Buse S, Hach CE, Klumpen P, et al. Cost-effectiveness analysis of robot-assisted vs. open partial nephrectomy. Int J Med Robot 2018;1–6. https://doi.org/10.1002/rcs.1920.

94. Hughes D, Camp C, O'Hara J, et al. Health resource use after robot-assisted surgery vs open and conventional laparoscopic techniques in oncology: analysis of English secondary care data for radical prostatectomy and partial nephrectomy. BJU Int 2016;117(6):940–7.

95. Basto M, Sathianathen N, Te Marvelde L, et al. Patterns-of-care and health economic analysis of robot-assisted radical prostatectomy in the Australian public health system. BJU Int 2016;117(6): 930–9.

96. Brisbane W, Bailey MR, Sorensen MD. HHS public access. Nat Rev Urol 2016;13(11):654–62.

97. Melnikow J, Xing G, Cox G, et al. Cost analysis of the STONE randomized trial can health care costs be reduced one test at a time? Med Care 2016; 54(4):337–42.

98. Metzler IS, Smith-Bindman R, Moghadassi M, et al. Emergency department imaging modality effect on surgical management of nephrolithiasis: a multi-center, randomized clinical trial. J Urol 2017; 197(3):710–4.

99. Lotan Y, Jimenez IB, Lenoir-Wijnkoop I, et al. Primary prevention of nephrolithiasis is cost-effective for a national healthcare system. BJU Int 2012; 190(3):902.

100. Parks JH, Coe FL. The financial effects of kidney stone prevention. Kidney Int 1996;50(5):1706–12.

101. Chandhoke PS. When is medical prophylaxis cost-effective for recurrent calcium stones? J Urol 2002; 168(3):937–40.

102. Tavichakorntrakool R, Prasongwattana V, Sungkeeree S, et al. Extensive characterizations of bacteria isolated from catheterized urine and stone matrices in patients with nephrolithiasis. Nephrol Dial Transplant 2012;27(11):4125–30.

103. Bauza JL, Pieras EC, Grases F, et al. Urinary tract infection's etiopathogenic role in nephrolithiasis formation. Med Hypotheses 2018;118:34–5.

Moving?

Make sure your subscription moves with you!

To notify us of your new address, find your **Clinics Account Number** (located on your mailing label above your name), and contact customer service at:

Email: journalscustomerservice-usa@elsevier.com

800-654-2452 (subscribers in the U.S. & Canada)
314-447-8871 (subscribers outside of the U.S. & Canada)

Fax number: 314-447-8029

Elsevier Health Sciences Division
Subscription Customer Service
3251 Riverport Lane
Maryland Heights, MO 63043

Printed and bound by CPI Group (UK) Ltd, Croydon, CR0 4YY

03/10/2024

01040371-0017